Applied Pathophysiology for Nurses and Healthcare Students at a Glance

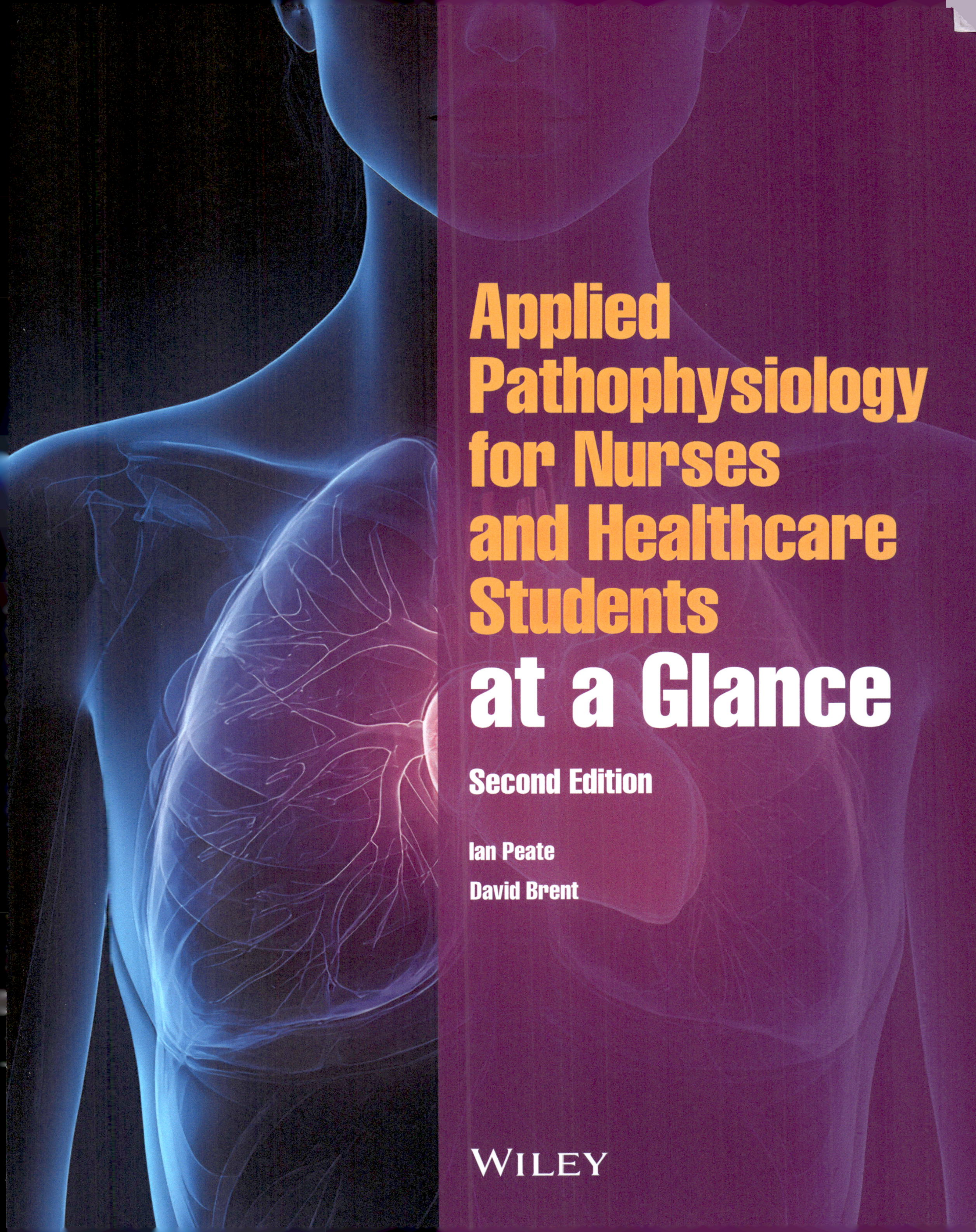

Applied Pathophysiology for Nurses and Healthcare Students

at a Glance

Second Edition

Ian Peate

David Brent

WILEY

This edition first published 2026

Edition History

First Edition (2015) by John Wiley & Sons Ltd

The right of Ian Peate and David Brent to be identified as the authors of this work has been asserted in accordance with law.

Registered Offices

John Wiley & Sons, Inc., 111 River Street, Hoboken, NJ 07030, USA

John Wiley & Sons Ltd, New Era House, 8 Oldlands Way, Bognor Regis, West Sussex, PO22 9NQ, UK

For details of our global editorial offices, customer services, and more information about Wiley products visit us at www.wiley.com.

The manufacturer's authorized representative according to the EU General Product Safety Regulation is Wiley-VCH GmbH, Boschstr. 12, 69469 Weinheim, Germany, e-mail: Product_Safety@wiley.com.

Wiley also publishes its books in a variety of electronic formats and by print-on-demand. Some content that appears in standard print versions of this book may not be available in other formats.

Limit of Liability/Disclaimer of Warranty

Library of Congress Cataloging-in-Publication Data has been applied for:

Paperback ISBN: 9781394421022
ePDF ISBN: 9781394421046
ePUB ISBN: 9781394421039

Cover Design: Wiley
Cover Image: © Naim/stock.adobe.com

Set in 9.5/11.5pt Minion by Lumina Datamatics Ltd., Chennai, India
Printed and bound by CPI Group (UK) Ltd, Croydon, CR0 4YY
C9781394421022_290526

Contents

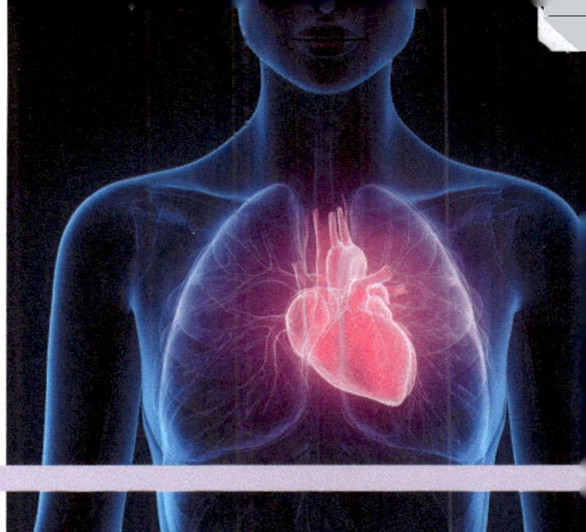

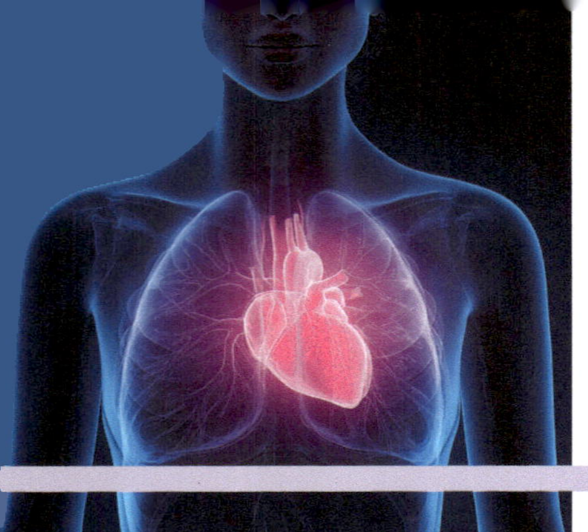

Preface

We are delighted to have been invited to prepare a second edition of the much-liked *Applied Pathophysiology for Nurses and Healthcare Students at a Glance*. Every chapter has been carefully reviewed and updated to reflect contemporary health and care practice, ensuring the content remains relevant and practical for today's learners and practitioners.

This new edition of *Applied Pathophysiology for Nurses and Healthcare Students at a Glance* continues to offer a concise and accessible overview of a wide range of health-related conditions. It retains the familiar *At a Glance* format that so many readers value for its clarity, structure and visual appeal. Full-colour illustrations are used throughout to enhance understanding and help readers link theory to real-world practice.

Our aim in writing *Applied Pathophysiology for Nurses and Healthcare Students at a Glance* has always been to make the some-times complex subject of pathophysiology both understandable and engaging and, above all, clearly connected to practice. The human body is extraordinary in its ability to adapt to disease through a range of physiological and psychological responses. This book explores those responses, outlining how disease processes disrupt normal body function and what this means for the person experiencing them.

Pathophysiology is the study of how normal mechanical, physi-cal and biochemical functions are altered by disease. The term itself combines the Greek 'pathos' (disease) and 'physiology' (the study of normal bodily functions). It examines both cellular and organ-level changes and how these changes influence the body's overall function. When the body's usual processes are disrupted by infection, injury or other conditions, a pathophysiological process occurs. However, it is important to remember that 'normal' health varies between individuals, and this variation should always be recognised in healthcare practice.

To deliver safe and effective care, health and care professionals must have the knowledge and skills to meet people's needs across hospital, community and social care settings. This is particularly vital in responding to the needs of an ageing population and those living with long-term conditions.

Applied Pathophysiology for Nurses and Healthcare Students at a Glance is written for all health and care students who encounter individuals with physical health challenges such as cancer, diabetes mellitus and many other conditions. While the focus is primarily on the adult person, the principles explored throughout the book apply broadly across care contexts.

Our goal is to help students and practitioners bridge the gap between theory and practice to understand not only what happens within the body during disease, but also why it matters for the peo-ple we care for. By linking normal body function to the changes that occur during illness, readers can develop the insight needed to deliver safe, effective and compassionate care.

Using *Applied Pathophysiology for Nurses and Healthcare Students at a Glance* will give readers a clear and practical under-standing of applied pathophysiology, supporting them to translate knowledge into confident, evidence-based practice.

Ian Peate
London, UK

David Brent
Bangor, UK

Acknowledgements

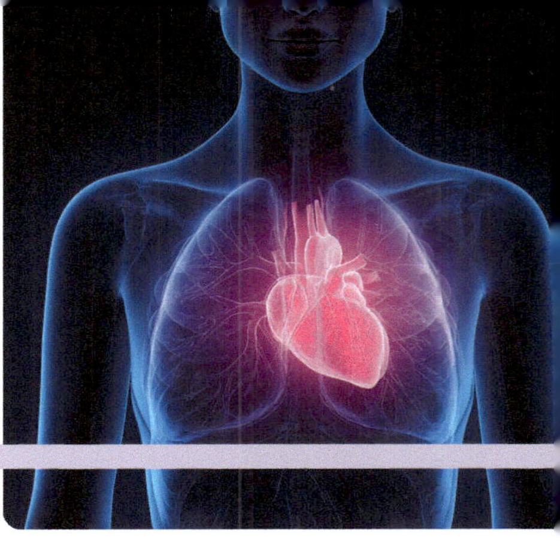

Ian would like to thank his partner Jussi Lahtinen for his continued support.
David thanks his partner Charlotte Ward for her ongoing encouragement.

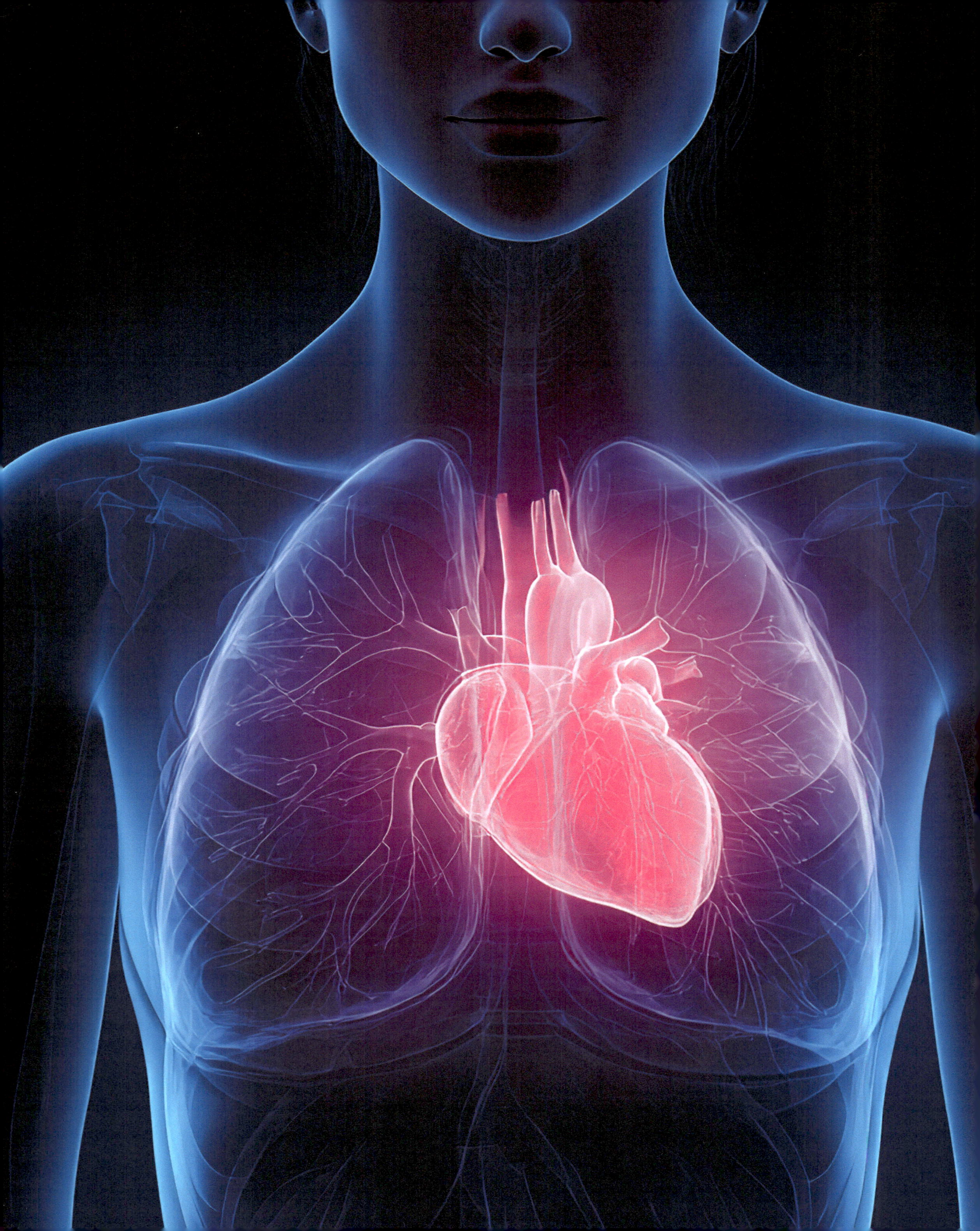

Pathophysiology

Chapters

1 Key principles of pathophysiology

Figure 1.1 Mendelian trait.

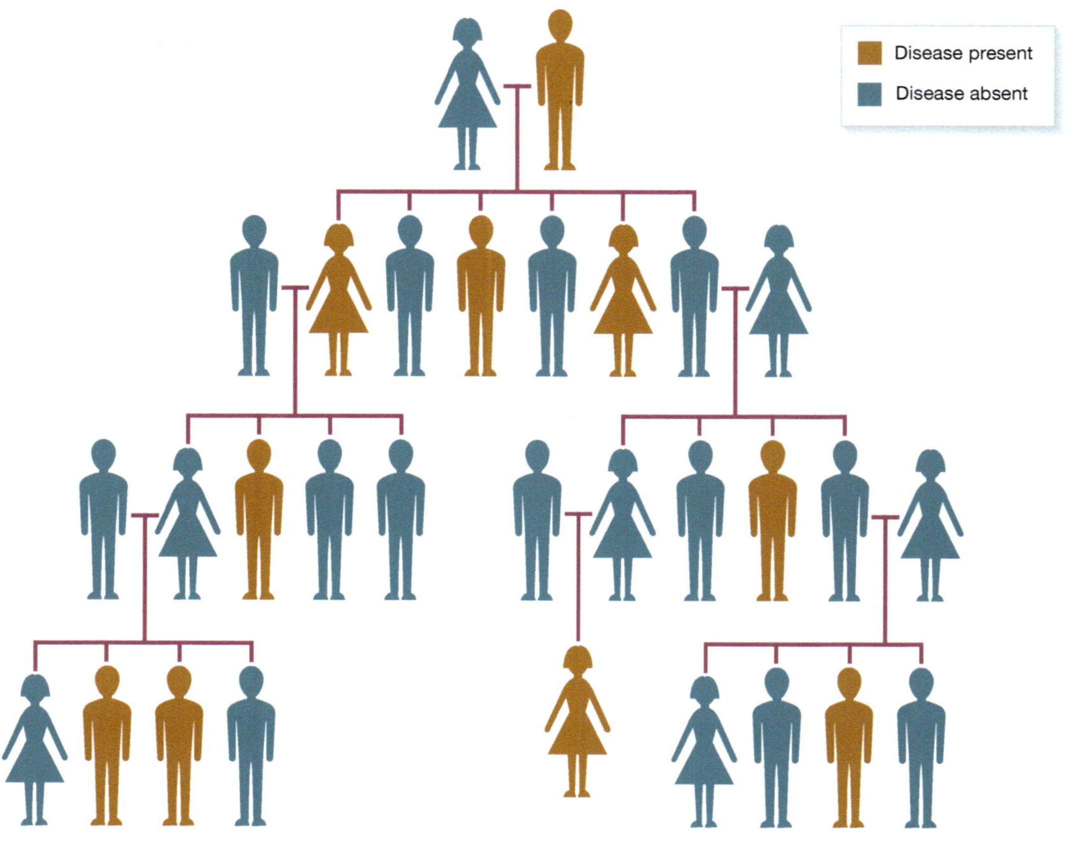

Figure 1.2 Fetal alcohol syndrome.

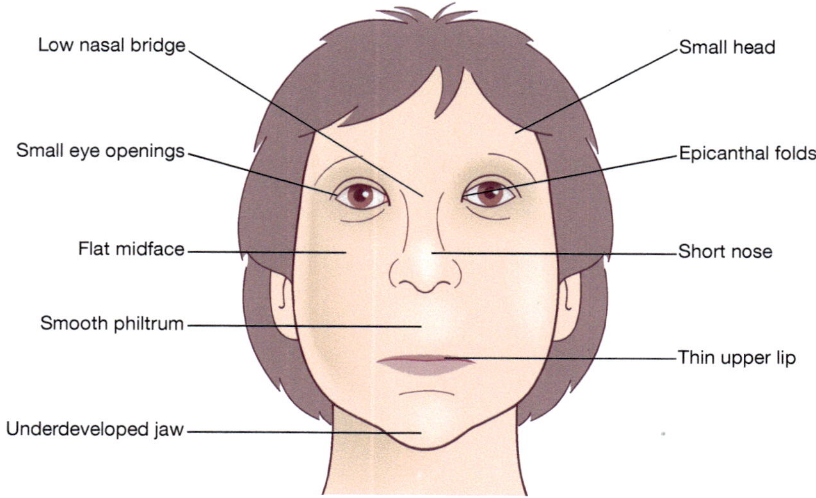

Pathophysiology versus pathology

Both of these terms indicate the study of disease. 'Pathology' is a broader term that deals with all aspects of a disease. This approach to disease is valuable for a physician or a pathologist who is interested in the macro- and microscopic characteristics of tissues and organs. On the other hand, in pathophysiology, the focus is on the abnormal function of diseased organs, with application to diagnostic procedures that lead to patient care. Healthcare professionals with face-to-face contact with patients are usually more concerned with pathophysiology when caring for patients.

Disease and aetiology

The study of the cause of disease is called aetiology, a fundamental concept in healthcare. Understanding aetiology enables healthcare professionals to identify why diseases occur, which factors contribute to their development and how these causes can be prevented or managed. Aetiology encompasses a wide range of influences, including biological factors (such as bacteria, viruses and genetic mutations), environmental factors (such as exposure to toxins or radiation) and lifestyle factors (such as diet, physical activity and smoking). By exploring the origins and mechanisms of disease, healthcare practitioners can make informed decisions about diagnosis, treatment and public health interventions.

The word 'aetiology' comes from the Greek *aitia*, cause + *logos*, discourse. Diseases are described as genetic, congenital or acquired.

Genetic

In diseases with a genetic origin, an individual may inherit a defective gene leading to the development of the condition. These faulty genes are often transmitted from parents to their children. Genetic abnormalities can vary widely, from a small mutation in a single gene to the loss or gain of an entire chromosome or set of chromosomes.

Some genetic conditions are known as Mendelian disorders (Figure 1.1), resulting from mutations in the DNA sequence of a single gene. These disorders include Huntington's disease and cystic fibrosis. Many genetic diseases, however, are multifactorial, meaning they arise from mutations in multiple genes combined with environmental influences. Common examples include heart disease, cancer and diabetes.

Congenital

In congenital disease, the genetic information is intact; however, problems with the intrauterine environment may result in congenital disorder. For example, cystic fibrosis is a genetic disorder, whereas fetal alcohol syndrome results from the mother's alcohol intake during pregnancy. This results in congenital abnormalities in a genetically normal child (Figure 1.2).

Acquired

In this type of disease, the person develops the condition after birth as a result of direct or indirect contact with another person or the environment. Examples include tuberculosis, emphysema, chickenpox or acquired heart diseases.

Signs and symptoms

A symptom is generally subjective, while a sign is objective. Any objective evidence of a disease, such as blood in the stool or a skin rash, is a sign – it can be recognised by the doctor, nurse, family members and the patient. However, stomach ache, lower-back pain and fatigue, for example, can only be detected or sensed by the patient – others only know about it if the patient tells them. Pain, for example, can either be acute or chronic. An example of acute pain is abdominal pain, which is sudden and may last only a few hours or longer.

Common chronic pain complaints include headache, low back pain, cancer pain, arthritis pain, neurogenic pain (pain resulting from damage to the peripheral nerves or to the central nervous system itself) and psychogenic pain (pain not due to past disease or injury or any visible sign of damage inside or outside the nervous system).

Pathogenesis

When assessing a patient's signs and symptoms, this can often identify the pattern and progression of a disease, which is known as its pathogenesis. Pathogenesis describes how a disease develops and causes tissue damage, leading to the observable clinical effects. As the disease progresses, it produces characteristic signs and symptoms that can change throughout its course, providing important clues for diagnosis and management.

Another key aspect of pathogenesis is the timeframe of disease development. Some diseases are acute, whereas others are chronic and develop more gradually, persisting over an extended period, often months or years. Understanding whether a condition is acute or chronic helps in planning appropriate investigations, treatment and follow-up care.

Investigations and diagnosis

To make a diagnosis, it may be necessary to carry out investigations to confirm the diagnosis. Some investigations may be invasive, while others are not. These may include blood tests, CT scans, chest X-rays, endoscopy and many more.

Diagnosis is the identification of a condition, disease, disorder or problem by systematic analysis of the background or history, examination of the signs or symptoms, evaluation of the research or test results and investigation of the assumed or probable causes. It is from the diagnosis that care or treatment is prescribed.

Treatment

Once a diagnosis is confirmed, treatment can proceed (e.g. medical or surgical). The aim of the treatment of a disease is to achieve a cure or minimise the patient's signs and symptoms to a degree where the patient can function near normal.

Prognosis

Prognosis is a prediction of the chance of recovery or survival from a disease. Most prognoses given are based on statistics of how a disease acts in studies on the general population. Prognosis can vary depending on several factors, such as the stage of disease at diagnosis, the type of disease and even gender.

Many factors can influence the prognosis of a patient with cancer. Among the most important are the type and location of the cancer, the stage of the disease (the extent to which the cancer has spread in the body) and how quickly the cancer is likely to grow and spread. Other factors that affect prognosis include the biological and genetic properties of the cancer cells (biomarkers), and the patient's overall general health and the extent to which the cancer responds to treatment.

Clinical considerations

Linking the underlying disease mechanisms to a patient's signs and symptoms can identify the cause of illness, anticipate complications and select the most appropriate interventions. For instance, recognising that shortness of breath in heart failure results from fluid accumulation in the lungs helps guide treatment with diuretics and oxygen therapy. Similarly, understanding that pyrexia and inflammation are part of the body's immune response assists in distinguishing between infection and autoimmune disease. Applying pathophysiological principles in clinical practice enhances diagnostic accuracy, improves treatment outcomes and supports the delivery of safe, evidence-based and person-centred care.

2 Cell injury, adaptation and death

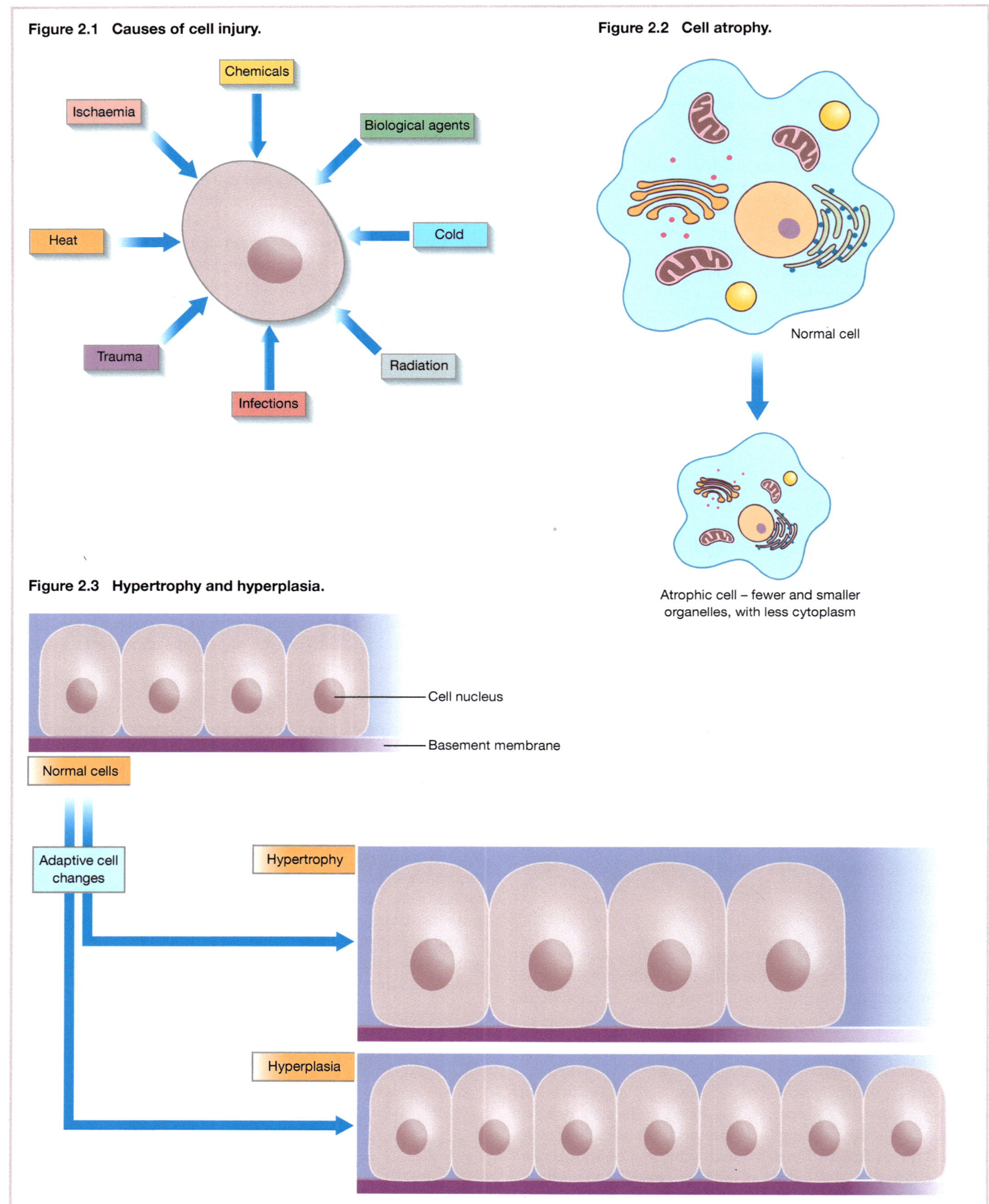

Figure 2.1 Causes of cell injury.

Figure 2.2 Cell atrophy.

Figure 2.3 Hypertrophy and hyperplasia.

Cell injury

The term 'cell injury' is used to specify a state in which the capacity for physiological adaptation has been exceeded by excessive stimuli, or when the cell is no longer able to adapt without experiencing some form of damage. Cell injury may be reversible or irreversible. Cell injury and cell death can result from exposure to toxic chemicals, infections and hypoxia (Figure 2.1).

Toxic chemicals

Chemical injury happens when toxic substances damage the cell's outer layer, the plasma membrane. Many different chemicals can harm cells and even cause them to die. Examples include:

- **Chemicals blocking oxygen use**, such as potassium cyanide, which stops cells from using oxygen properly.
- **Chemical carcinogens**, substances that can cause cancer. They produce reactive molecules that attach to important parts of the cell, such as proteins and DNA, and damage them.
- **Oxidising chemicals**, which create free radicals, unstable molecules that attack and destroy parts of the cell.
- **Chemicals that activate the immune system** in harmful ways, leading to cell damage.
- **Calcium ionophores**, which upset the normal balance of calcium inside cells and can trigger cell death.

Cell death is also an important part of how some chemicals can lead to cancer. Many cancer-causing chemicals, at high enough doses, first cause tissue damage and inflammation. When the body tries to repair this damage, abnormal cells may form, which can later develop into cancer.

Infections

Viruses can alter cells either by directly damaging them, causing injury or cell death, or by stimulating the cells to multiply uncontrollably, which may lead to tumour formation.

Bacteria are relatively complex, single-celled creatures with a rigid wall and a thin, rubbery membrane surrounding fluid inside the cell. They can reproduce on their own. Most bacteria are harmless, and some actually help by digesting food, destroying disease-causing microbes, fighting cancer cells and providing essential nutrients.

Hypoxia

Hypoxia is a deficiency of oxygen, causing cell injury by reducing aerobic oxidative respiration. Hypoxia is an extremely important and common cause of cell injury and cell death. Causes include reduced blood flow, inadequate oxygenation of the blood due to cardiorespiratory failure and decreased oxygen-carrying capacity of the blood, as in anaemia or carbon monoxide poisoning or after severe blood loss. Depending on the severity of the hypoxic state, cells may adapt, undergo injury or die.

Adaptation

Cells adapt to the environment to escape and protect themselves from injury. Cellular adaptations are common and a central part of many disease states. The most significant adaptive states include atrophy, hypertrophy, hyperplasia and metaplasia.

Atrophy

Atrophy is a decrease or shrinkage in cell size caused by loss of subcellular organelles and substances (Figure 2.2). Atrophy is most common in skeletal muscles, the heart, sex organs and the brain. However, physiological atrophy occurs in some glands. For example, the thymus gland undergoes physiological atrophy during childhood.

Hypertrophy

This is an increase in the size of the cells, thus enlarging the size of the organ (Figure 2.3). This can affect many types of cells, including those in the heart, kidneys and skeletal muscles.

Hyperplasia

Hyperplasia is increased cell production in a normal tissue or organ (Figure 2.3). Hyperplasia may be a sign of abnormal or precancerous changes (pathological hyperplasia). Hyperplasia may be harmless, an example of a normal hyperplastic response would be the growth and multiplication of milk-secreting glandular cells in the breast as a response to pregnancy, thus preparing for future breastfeeding.

Metaplasia and necrosis

Metaplasia

Metaplasia is when one type of mature cell is replaced by another type of mature cell. This is usually reversible. It can happen as part of normal development or in response to an abnormal stimulus. For example, in the lungs, the normal column-shaped, ciliated cells that line the bronchi can be replaced by flat, squamous cells.

Necrosis

When cells die from necrosis, they do not follow the controlled process of apoptosis. Instead, certain signals cause the cell membrane to break down, releasing the cell's contents into the surrounding tissue, triggering inflammation. Because nearby immune cells (phagocytes) cannot clear the dead cells properly, dead tissue and cell debris accumulate at or near the site of injury.

Cell death

Cell death eventually leads to necrosis of the cell. It occurs when there is not enough blood flowing to the tissue, whether from injury, radiation or chemicals. Necrosis is not reversible. One common type of necrosis is gangrene. There are many types of necrosis; it can affect many areas of the body, including bone, skin, organs and other tissues.

Apoptosis

'Apoptosis' is derived from the Greek words *apo*, meaning 'away from', and *ptosis*, meaning 'to fall'. The term 'falling away from' is derived from the fact that, during this type of prelethal change, cells shrink and undergo marked blebbing at the periphery. The blebs detach and float away. It is sometimes referred to as programmed cell death, and, indeed, the process of apoptosis follows a controlled, predictable routine. However, it is normal for many cells to die by apoptosis during the development of the nervous system, as this helps form the correct connections. Apoptosis also occurs in many other cell types after different kinds of toxic injury. It is particularly common in lymphocytes, where it is the main way that old or unnecessary lymphocyte clones are removed.

Fragments from apoptotic cells form the basophilic bodies that can be seen inside macrophages in lymph nodes. In other organs, apoptosis usually happens in individual cells, which are quickly removed by nearby tissue cells or macrophages. Because the process is controlled and the cell fragments are cleared efficiently, apoptosis usually does not cause inflammation. Before dying, apoptotic cells have a very dense cytoplasm, with mitochondria that are either normal or slightly condensed, and an endoplasmic reticulum that is normal or only slightly swollen.

Clinical considerations

Cell injury and death are central to many diseases. Necrosis causes tissue damage and inflammation (i.e. heart attacks, strokes and infections). Apoptosis is a normal process for tissue development and immune cell regulation. Cell adaptations such as metaplasia in smokers' lungs, may indicate chronic stress and can increase the risk of cancer.

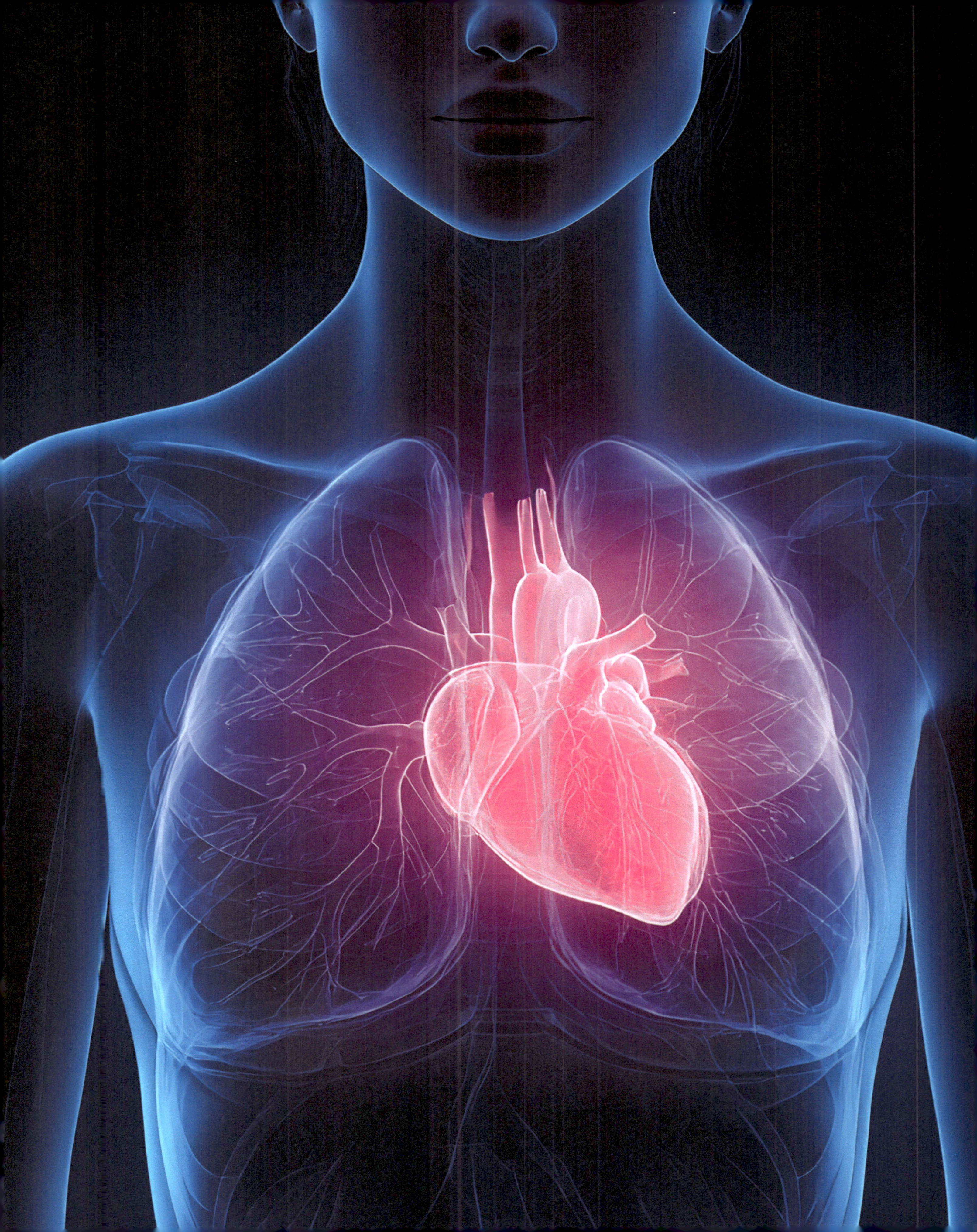

3 Inflammation, tissue repair and regeneration

Figure 3.1 Causes of inflammation.

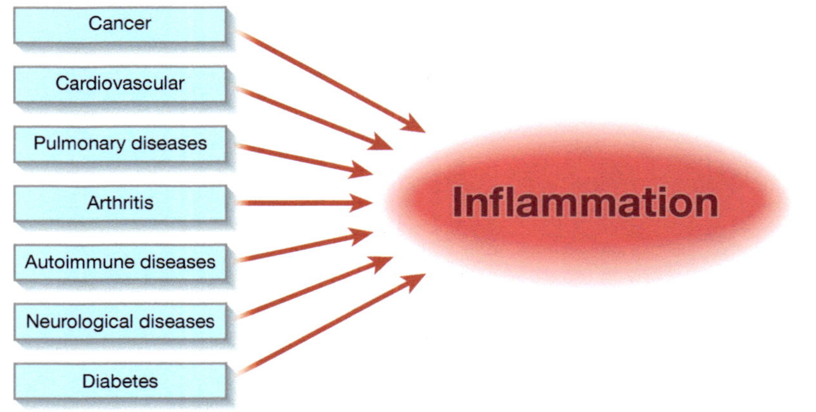

Figure 3.2 Tissue injury and the inflammatory process.

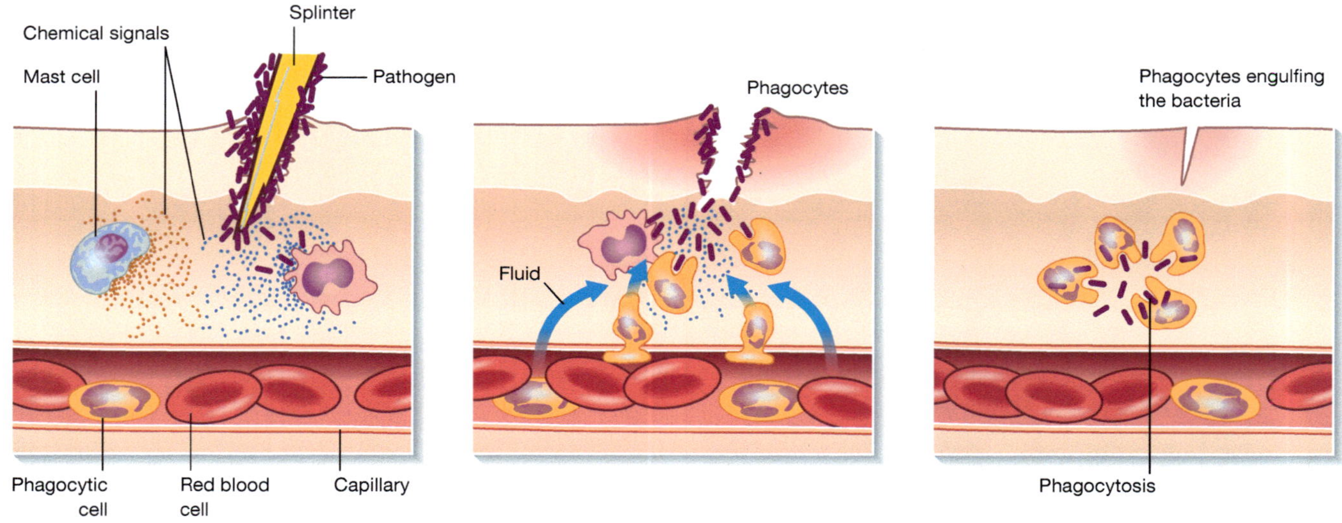

Figure 3.3 Phases of tissue repair.

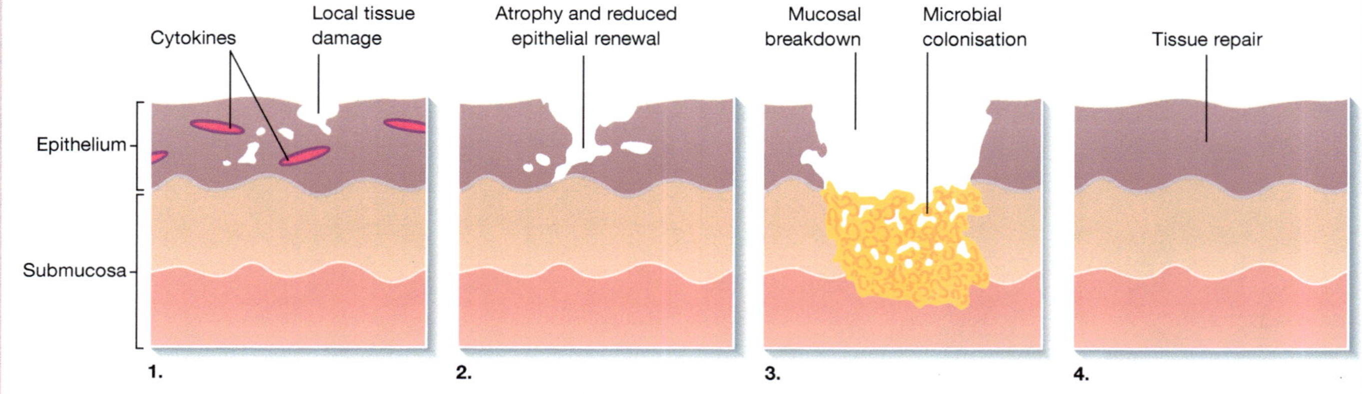

Inflammation

Inflammation is the body's attempt at self-protection; the aim is to remove harmful stimuli, including damaged cells, irritants or pathogens, and to begin the healing process. Inflammation can be clinically defined as the presence of swelling, redness and pain. Some diseases associated with inflammation include arthritis and neurological diseases (see Figure 3.1). The signs and symptoms of inflammation are caused by four processes: (1) mast cell degranulation, (2) activation of plasma proteins, (3) the immune response and (4) heat. All these processes occur simultaneously, producing what is known as the inflammatory response. First, mast cell degranulation is the release of granules containing serotonin and histamine from mast cells into tissues. These work with the other two processes to provide the complete inflammatory signs and symptoms.

The second process involves the activation of four plasma protein systems: complement (helps orchestrate the inflammatory response); clotting (stops bleeding, repairs damage); kinin (involved in vascular permeability); and immunoglobulins (destroys bacteria) working together to support the inflammatory process. This activates and assists inflammatory and immune processes and plays a major role in the destruction of bacteria. The third process is the movement of phagocytic cells to the area to phagocytose bacteria or any other non-self debris in the wound (Figure 3.2). The fourth process, heat, is a protective attempt by the organism to remove the injurious stimuli and initiate the healing process; without this, wounds would never heal.

Physical and mechanical barriers

These are part of the first-line defence against microorganisms. They include skin and epithelial cells of the viscera, genitourinary and respiratory tracts. Epithelial cells produce mucus to protect the lining of the tracts; some contain cilia to remove pathogens, and the temperature of the skin inhibits microorganisms from colonising.

Biochemical barriers

Epithelial surfaces also provide physical and biochemical barriers against infection. Some of these substances include sweat and saliva, which contain enzymes to destroy bacteria, and tears. Perspiration makes the skin slightly acidic, creating an environment that is less favourable for bacterial growth.

Acute and chronic inflammation

Acute inflammation begins rapidly (rapid onset) and quickly becomes severe. Signs and symptoms are only present for a few days; in some cases, this may persist for a few weeks. Some examples include acute bronchitis, appendicitis and sore throat.

Chronic inflammation means long-term inflammation, which may last for several months and even years. Some examples include chronic asthma, chronic peptic ulcer and chronic sinusitis.

Tissue repair

Wound healing is an intricate process in which the skin (or another organ tissue) repairs itself after injury. In normal skin, the epidermis (outermost layer) and dermis (inner or deeper layer) exist in a steady-state equilibrium, forming a protective barrier against the external environment. Once the protective barrier is broken, the normal (physiological) process of wound healing is immediately set in motion. The classic model of wound healing is divided into three or four sequential, yet overlapping, phases: (1) haemostasis (not considered a phase by some), (2) inflammatory, (3) proliferative and (4) remodelling. Upon injury to the skin, a set of complex biochemical events takes place in a closely orchestrated cascade to repair the damage. Within minutes post-injury, platelets (thrombocytes) aggregate at the injury site to form a fibrin clot. This clot acts to control active bleeding (haemostasis). The rate of wound healing can be affected by many factors, including hormone levels in the blood, such as oxytocin.

During the inflammatory phase, bacteria and debris are cleared by phagocytes, and signals are released that attract and stimulate the cells needed for the next, proliferative phase of healing.

The proliferative phase is characterised by angiogenesis, collagen deposition, granulation tissue formation, epithelialisation and wound contraction. In angiogenesis, new blood vessels are formed by vascular endothelial cells. In fibroplasia and granulation tissue formation, fibroblasts grow and form a new, provisional extracellular matrix by excreting collagen and fibronectin. Concurrently, re-epithelialisation of the epidermis occurs, in which epithelial cells proliferate and 'crawl' atop the wound bed, providing cover for the new tissue (Figure 3.3).

During wound contraction, myofibroblasts pull the edges of the wound together, using a mechanism that is similar to smooth muscle contraction. Once their job is nearly done, excess cells die through apoptosis. In the maturation and remodelling phase, collagen is reorganised along tension lines, and any remaining unnecessary cells are also removed by apoptosis.

Regeneration

In the regeneration phase, blood vessels are repaired, and new cells are formed in the damaged site, similar to the cells that were damaged and removed. Some cells, such as neurons and muscle cells (especially in the heart), are slow to recover. If the injury is minor, then it is possible to return the injured tissues to their original structure and function through regeneration. However, if the injury is severe, then regeneration is not possible and repair will not take place. Both regeneration and repair begin with phagocytosis, which includes fibrin from dissolved clots, microorganisms, erythrocytes and dead tissue.

Three phases occur in repairing the wound. These are the migratory, proliferative and maturation phases. In the migratory phase, the clot becomes a scab, and epithelial cells migrate beneath the scab to bridge the wound. During the proliferative phase, there is extensive growth of epithelial cells beneath the scab, deposition of collagen fibres by fibroblasts and continued growth of blood vessels. In the maturation phase, the scab drops off as the epidermis returns to normal thickness. In the dermis, the collagen fibres become more structured, fibroblasts decrease in number and blood vessels are restored to their normal function.

Clinical considerations

Inflammation helps fight infection and remove dead tissue, but excessive inflammation can worsen injury. Tissue repair, including scar formation, restores structural integrity after surgery, trauma or burns. Regeneration restores normal tissue where possible, and understanding these processes guides treatment decisions and wound management.

4 Cancer

Figure 4.1   Some of the organs affected by cancer.

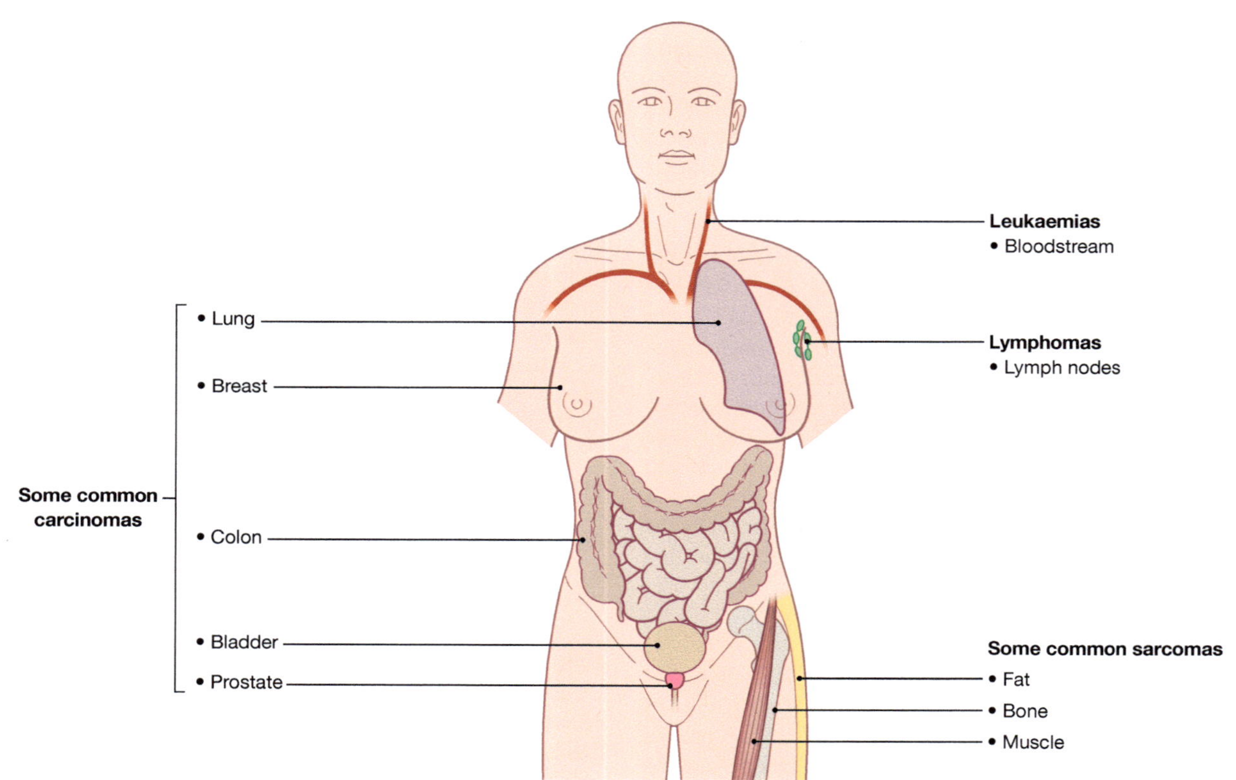

Figure 4.2   Staging of cancer.

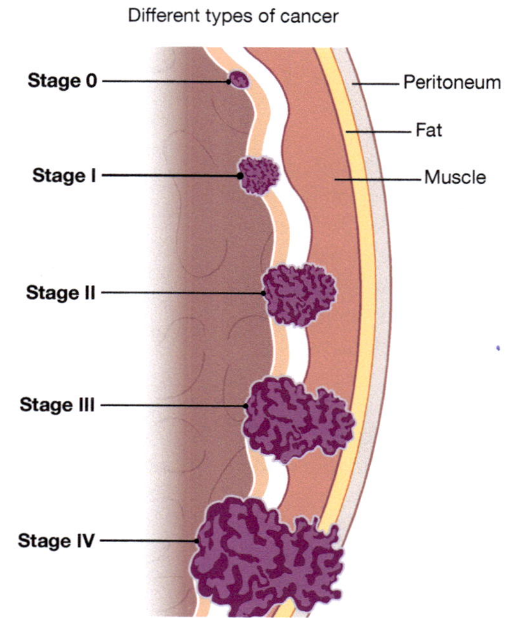

What is cancer?

Cancer is a disease that can affect the cells of the body. Because the body is made up of many different types of cells, there are many different types of cancer, each of them arising from a specific type of cell. What all cancers have in common is that the cells become abnormal, and they then multiply uncontrollably. If left untreated, a tumour can cause problems in a number of ways.

Cancer can develop from almost any type of cell, so multiple types of cancer can occur in the same organ. However, usually one type is much more common in a particular organ. For example, the bladder contains transitional cells, squamous cells and adenomatous cells. Although cancer can develop from any of these cells, it is far more common in transitional cells. Transitional cell carcinoma accounts for over nine out of ten cases of bladder cancer, while squamous cell carcinoma and adenocarcinoma are much less common (Figure 4.1).

How many types of cancer are there?

It is estimated that there are more than 200 different types of cancer, and they can develop in almost any organ of the body. The human body has over 60 organs, and each organ is made up of several different types of tissue, which in turn are composed of specific types of cells. For example, the skin contains multiple layers: the outer layer is made of epithelial cells, beneath which is connective tissue that may contain glandular cells, and deeper, still there are layers of muscle tissue. Each type of cell has a specific function, and cancer can arise from any of these cell types, depending on which cells become abnormal and begin to grow uncontrollably.

Causes of cancer

Causes of cancers can be classified into two groups: first, there are genotoxic carcinogens, which affect the DNA, causing mutations; and second, promoter substances, which may cause hormonal imbalance, altered immunity or long-term tissue damage, which can lead to the development of cancer.

Other risk factors include viruses, as they weaken the immune system; hormones, such as the ones found in contraceptive pills, which can lead to breast cancer; and chemical agents such as arsenic and radiation.

Genetic factors

A cell usually needs to acquire several genetic mutations before it becomes cancerous. Some people are born with one of these mutations, but this does not guarantee they will develop cancer. Having a mutation from birth increases the statistical likelihood of developing cancer over a lifetime, a situation doctors refer to as genetic predisposition.

The BRCA1 and BRCA2 genes provide well-known examples of genetic predisposition. Women who carry a faulty BRCA gene have a higher risk of developing breast cancer than women without these mutations. However, most cases of breast cancer are not caused by BRCA mutations. In fact, less than 3% of all breast cancers are linked to these genes. This shows that while inherited gene faults increase individual risk, the majority of breast cancer cases arise from other factors.

Age

Most types of cancer become more common as a person gets older. This is because the changes that make a cell become cancerous in the first place take a long time to develop. There has to be a number of changes to the genes within a cell before it turns into a cancer cell. These changes can happen by accident when the cell is dividing, or they can happen because the cell has been damaged by carcinogens, and the damage is then passed on to future cells when that cell divides. The longer a person lives, the more time there is for genetic mistakes to happen in the cells.

Viruses

Viruses can contribute to the development of certain cancers. However, this does not mean that these cancers are contagious like an infection. Instead, the virus can induce genetic changes within cells, increasing their likelihood of becoming cancerous.

Bacterial infection

Bacterial infections have not been thought of as cancer-causing agents in the past. However, studies have shown that people who have *Helicobacter pylori* (*H. pylori*) infection of their stomach develop inflammation of the stomach lining (gastritis), which increases the risk of stomach cancer. *H. pylori* infection can be treated with a combination of antibiotics.

Immune system

People with weakened or compromised immune systems are at an increased risk of developing certain types of cancer. This group includes individuals who have received organ transplants, as they take immunosuppressive medications to prevent organ rejection, and people living with HIV, whose immune systems are weakened by the virus. A reduced immune response makes it harder for the body to detect and destroy abnormal cells, allowing cancerous cells to grow more easily. Some cancers, such as Kaposi's sarcoma and certain types of lymphoma, are particularly associated with immune suppression.

Classification/Grading/Staging

Diagnosis of cancer involves three key steps: classification, grading, and staging. Classification refers to naming the tumour according to the type of cell it originated from. Grading describes the tumour's aggressiveness based on how the cells appear under the microscope. Staging reports how far the cancer has spread, including the size of the tumour and whether it has extended beyond its site of origin (see Figure 4.2).

- Stage 0: The cancer is in its original location (in situ) and has not spread.
- Stage I: The tumour is small (less than 2 cm), confined to its original site, with no spread.
- Stage II: The tumour is 2–5 cm in size, may involve nearby lymph nodes, but has not spread to distant sites.
- Stage III: The tumour is larger than 5 cm, or of any size but fixed to nearby structures such as the chest wall, muscle or skin, or has spread to lymph nodes above the collarbone.
- Stage IV: The tumour can be of any size, may involve lymph nodes, and has spread to distant organs or tissues.

Clinical considerations

Accurate cancer diagnosis, including tumour type, grade and stage, is essential for choosing appropriate treatment and estimating prognosis. Patients with risk factors such as genetic mutations, immune suppression or exposure to carcinogens require closer monitoring. Understanding these factors helps to plan therapy, follow-up and preventive strategies.

5 Genetics

Figure 5.1   A pictorial representation of a portion of the double helix.

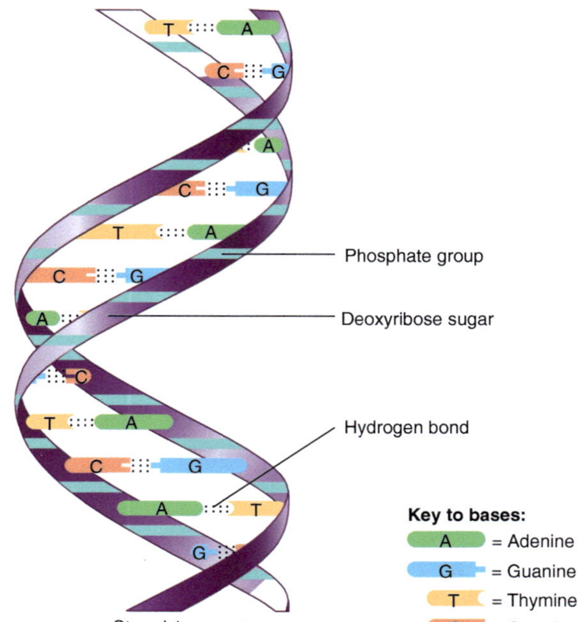

- DNA is made of two strands twisted in a spiral staircase-like structure called a double helix
- Each strand consists of nucleotides bound together
- Each nucleotide consists of a deoxyribose sugar bound to a phosphate group and one of Four nitrogenous bases [adenine (A), thymine (T), guanine (G), cytosine (C)]
- The nitrogenous bases pair together through hydrogen bonding to form the 'steps' of the double helix
- Adenine pairs with thymine and guanine pairs with cytosine

Source:
Tortora and Derrickson 2014/with permission of John Wiley & Sons

Figure 5.2   DNA from double helix to chromosome.

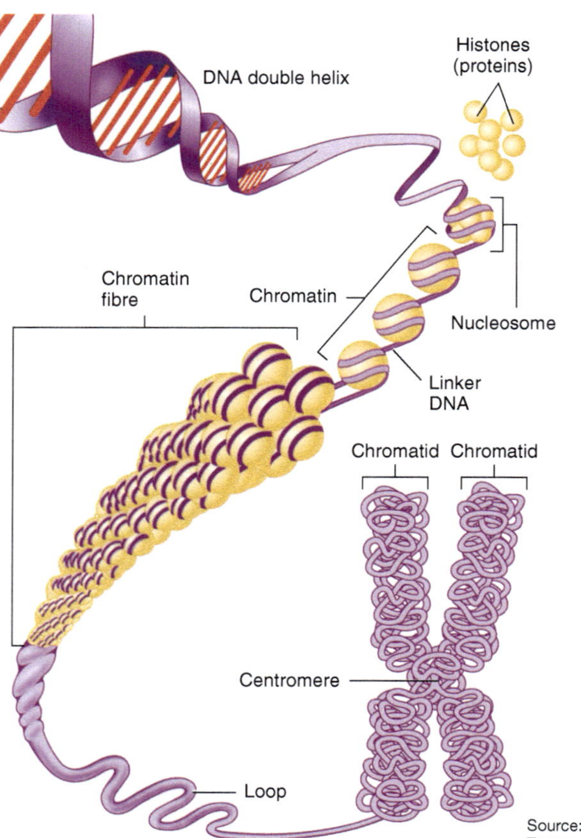

Source:
Tortora and Derrickson 2009/with permission of John Wiley & Sons

Figure 5.3   The separation of DNA for transcription. A small segment of DNA containing the gene to be transcribed opens up as the hydrogen bonds between complementary bases are temporarily broken. A strand of RNA is then formed, and when finished, it is released and the DNA bonds reform.

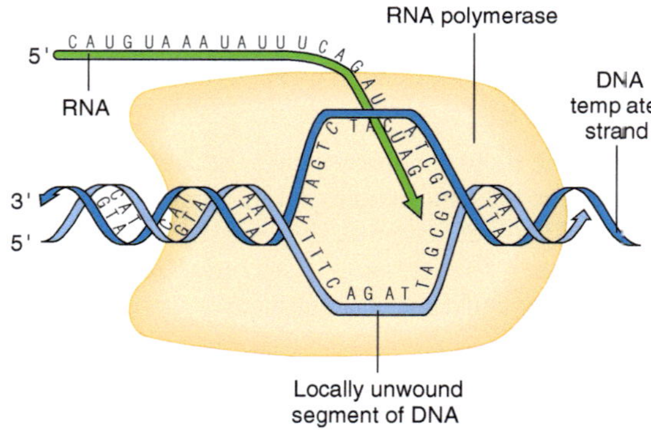

Source:
Snustad and Simmons 2012/with permission of John Wiley & Sons

Genetics is the study of heredity, the mechanisms by which traits are passed from one generation to the next. In healthcare, understanding genetics is fundamental for recognising disease risk, interpreting diagnostic tests and tailoring treatment. Pathophysiology is closely intertwined with genetics, as there are many diseases that arise from inherited or acquired genetic alterations. This chapter introduces the key concepts of genetics relevant to healthcare, focusing on deoxyribonucleic acid (DNA) structure, gene expression, inheritance patterns and the role of genetics in disease.

DNA, genes and chromosomes

At the core of genetics is DNA, which is the molecule that stores genetic information. DNA is composed of four nucleotides: adenine (A), thymine (T), cytosine (C) and guanine (G). These nucleotides pair specifically (A with T, C with G) to form the double-helix structure discovered by Watson and Crick in 1953 (see Figure 5.1).

Genes are segments of DNA that encode instructions for producing proteins; these are essential for cellular structure and function. The human genome contains approximately 20,000–25,000 genes. Genes are located on chromosomes; these are thread-like structures within the nucleus of each cell. Typically, humans have 46 chromosomes arranged in 23 pairs, including 22 pairs of autosomes and one pair of sex chromosomes (XX in females, XY in males) (see Figure 5.2).

Mutations, or changes in the DNA sequence, can alter gene function and this contributes to disease. These mutations may be inherited or acquired, affecting protein structure, function or regulation.

Gene expression: DNA to protein

The process by which genetic information is converted into functional proteins is known as gene expression. Gene expression occurs in two major steps: transcription and translation (see Figure 5.3).

1 Transcription – During transcription, the DNA sequence of a gene is copied into messenger RNA (mRNA). This process occurs in the nucleus and involves enzymes such as RNA polymerase.
2 Translation – The mRNA is transported to the ribosome in the cytoplasm; here it serves as a template for assembling amino acids into a specific protein. Transfer RNA (tRNA) molecules bring amino acids to the ribosome, matching the mRNA codons with their complementary anticodons.

Regulation of gene expression is complex; it ensures that proteins are produced at the right time, in the right cell and in the correct amount. Dysregulation of gene expression can occur and contribute to disease processes such as cancer, metabolic disorders and developmental abnormalities.

Patterns of inheritance

The way that genetic conditions are passed from parents to children is called inheritance. Some conditions are caused by a single faulty gene; others involve several genes and environmental factors.

In autosomal dominant conditions, only one copy of a faulty gene is needed for a person to be affected. This means if one parent has the condition, each child has a one-in-two chance of inheriting it (e.g. Marfan syndrome and Huntington's disease).

In autosomal recessive conditions, a person must inherit two faulty copies of a gene, one from each parent, to develop the disease. Parents who carry only one copy are usually healthy but can pass the gene on to their children (e.g. cystic fibrosis and sickle cell anaemia).

X-linked conditions involve genes on the X chromosome. Because males have only one X chromosome, they are more likely to be affected; females are usually carriers (e.g. haemophilia).

Some genes are passed on only from the mother through tiny structures in cells called mitochondria. This is known as mitochondrial inheritance and can affect how cells produce energy.

Not all conditions follow these clear patterns. Many common diseases, such as type 2 diabetes, heart disease and certain cancers, are influenced by several genes as well as lifestyle and environmental factors.

Genetic differences between people

Even though every human shares almost the same DNA, there are small differences that make each person unique. These differences are what give us our individual features, such as eye colour, hair type or height.

Some of these differences do not cause any problems, but others may change how our bodies work. Small changes in a gene might make one person more likely to develop high blood pressure or diabetes than another.

Genetic differences can affect how people respond to medicines. A drug that works well for one person might not work as well for someone else, or it might cause more side effects. In the future, genetic information may be used to help choose the safest and most effective medicine for each individual.

Genetics and disease

Genes play an important role in how and why some people develop certain illnesses. Sometimes a change in just one gene can cause disease, while in other cases, it's the result of many genes and lifestyle factors working together.

There are a few main ways that genes can lead to illness:

Single-gene conditions: these are illnesses caused by a change (or fault) in one gene. Cystic fibrosis: this condition affects the lungs and digestive system, causing thick, sticky mucus to build up. Sickle cell disease: this affects the red blood cells, making them an unusual shape. This can cause pain, tiredness and anaemia.

Chromosome conditions: sometimes, whole chromosomes are missing, extra or arranged differently. This can affect growth and development. Down syndrome: caused by an extra copy of chromosome 21. People with Down syndrome may have learning disabilities and certain physical features. Turner syndrome: occurs in girls who are missing part or all of one X chromosome. It can cause short height and problems with development during puberty.

Many conditions are multifactorial in origin. Rather than being caused by a single gene mutation, they result from the combined effects of multiple genes, often interacting with lifestyle and environmental factors. Examples include cardiovascular disease, type 2 diabetes and certain cancers. Things like diet, exercise, smoking and stress can also influence risk.

Genetic testing

Genetic testing has become an integral tool in modern medicine. Healthcare professionals must understand the indications, limitations and ethical considerations of genetic testing. Genetic counselling is essential to help patients understand the implications of test results, make informed decisions and manage potential psychological impacts.

Clinical considerations

As genetics continues to evolve, healthcare professionals will increasingly rely on genetic insights to provide personalised and precise care, making the study of genetics not just an academic exercise but a practical tool in improving patient outcomes.

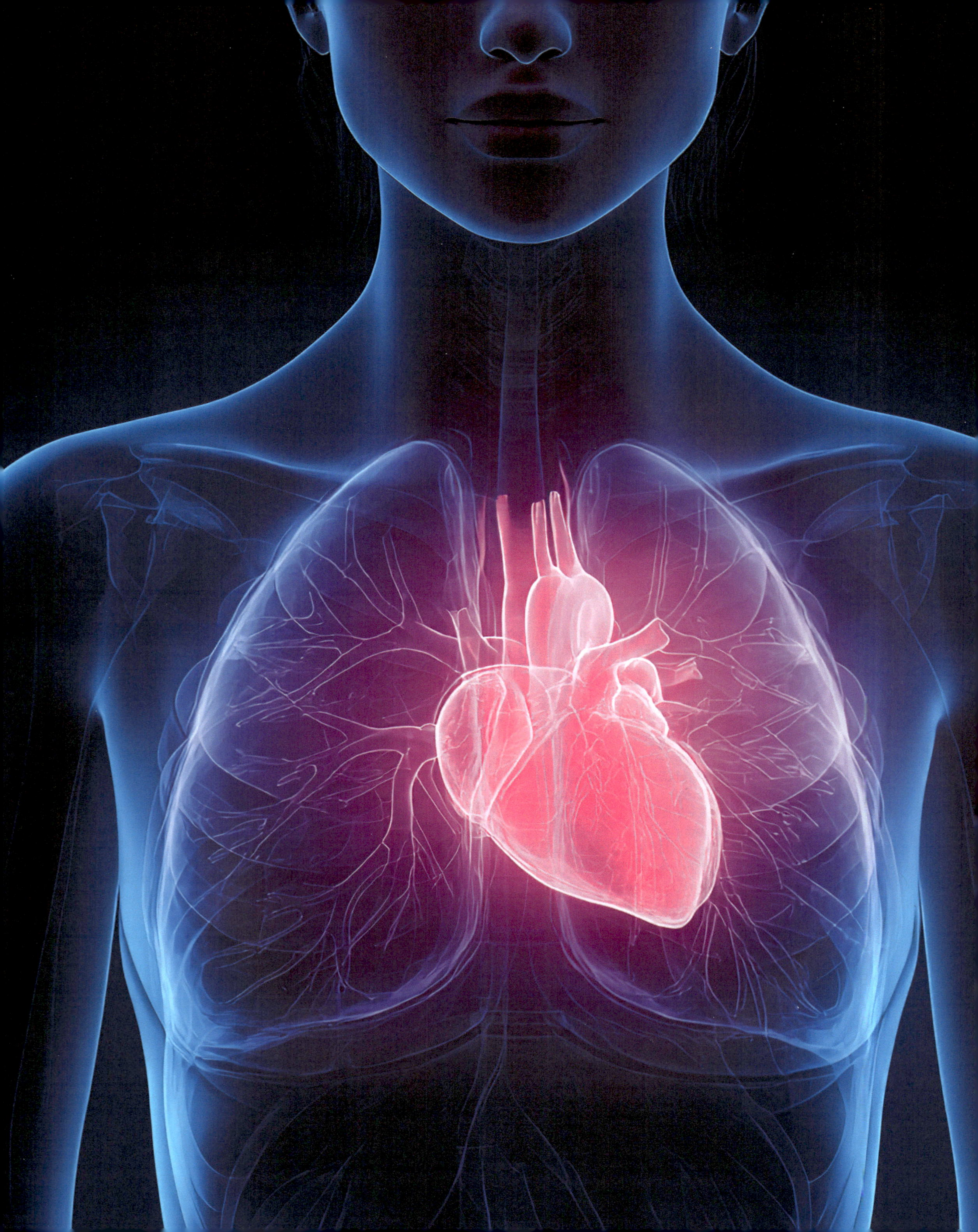

Shock

Chapters

6 Cardiogenic shock

Box 6.1   Detecting shock-related skin changes.

In patients with darker skin, detecting shock-related changes such as ashen, cyanotic, or mottled skin can be challenging because these visual signs are less apparent. Reliance on colour alone may delay recognition of poor perfusion. Clinicians should assess multiple indicators, including capillary refill, skin temperature, moisture, and mucous membrane colour, and interpret objective measures such as pulse oximetry and blood pressure cautiously, recognising that oximetry may underestimate hypoxaemia in darker skin. Awareness of these challenges is essential for the timely identification and management of shock in all patients.

Table 6.1   First-line investigations for suspected cardiogenic shock.

- Blood pressure
- ECG
- Urea, electrolytes and creatinine can assess renal function.
- Urine pregnancy test in women.
- Liver function tests.
- Full blood count to exclude anaemia.
- Cardiac enzymes, including troponins.
- Arterial blood gases.
- Brain natriuretic peptide (BNP)
- Chest X-ray
- CT pulmonary angiography (CTPA) or ventilation/perfusion lung scan (also known as V/Q scanning)
- Echocardiography

Table 6.2   Management options.

Medication	Medical procedures	Surgery
• Vasopressors (dopamine, epinephrine and norepinephrine). • Inotropes (dobutamine, dopamine and milrinone). • Aspirin. • Antiplatelet medicines. • Heparin.	• Angioplasty and stenting. This treatment can open clogged heart arteries. May be called percutaneous coronary intervention. • Intra-aortic balloon pump. Helps increase blood flow, also lowers strain on the heart. • Extracorporeal membrane oxygenation (ECMO). ECMO works like the lungs, removes carbon dioxide and adds oxygen to the blood.	• Coronary artery bypass grafting (CABG), open-heart surgery. • Surgery to repair an injury to the heart. Sometimes heart valve damage or a tear in a heart chamber can cause cardiogenic shock (valve replacement). • Ventricular assist device (VAD). Helps pump blood from the lower chambers of the heart to the rest of the body. • Heart transplant. May be needed if the heart is so damaged that no other treatments work.

Cardiogenic shock

Cardiogenic shock is a physiological state in which inadequate tissue perfusion results from low cardiac output due to cardiac dysfunction, usually systolic, despite adequate intravascular volume. It is a major and often fatal complication of acute and chronic cardiac disorders, most commonly occurring after acute myocardial infarction (MI), and remains a leading cause of death in post-MI patients. This is a life-threatening emergency and is treatable if it is diagnosed right away.

Pathophysiology

Cardiogenic shock occurs when the heart's pumping ability fails, resulting in reduced cardiac output and tissue hypoperfusion. It is typically defined by sustained hypotension (systolic blood pressure <90 mmHg for more than 30 minutes) accompanied by evidence of tissue hypoperfusion, such as cold extremities, oliguria, or both, regardless of adequate left ventricular filling pressure.

Acute deterioration of cardiac function can result from several conditions, including extensive left ventricular infarction, mechanical complications (e.g. ventricular septal defect and papillary muscle rupture) or right ventricular infarction. Other causes include acute myocardial ischaemia, myocarditis, sustained arrhythmias, severe valvular dysfunction and decompensation of end-stage cardiomyopathy.

In patients with cardiogenic shock following acute MI, progressive myocardial necrosis is often present, commonly involving multi-vessel coronary artery disease with limited coronary reserve. Decreased coronary perfusion pressure, along with increased myocardial oxygen demand, initiates a vicious cycle that further impairs cardiac function.

Cellular pathophysiology: Tissue hypoperfusion causes cellular hypoxia, leading to metabolic (or biochemical) consequences of tissue hypoxia and a cascade of cellular metabolic disturbances. Prolonged ischaemia can cause permanent damage to heart muscle cells. This includes swelling of mitochondria, build-up of damaged proteins, and breakdown of cell structures such as the nucleus and cell membrane, leading to cell death. Prolonged ischaemia can cause irreversible myocyte injury, including mitochondrial swelling, accumulation of denatured proteins, chromatin and lysosomal breakdown, and disruption of plasma membranes and nuclear envelopes.

Reversible heart muscle dysfunction can also contribute to cardiogenic shock. Areas of the heart that are still alive but temporarily weakened (known as stunned or hibernating myocardium) do not contract properly, even when blood flow has been restored. This reduces the amount of blood the heart pumps with each beat (stroke volume) and lowers overall cardiac output.

Haemodynamic consequences: When the heart's pumping ability (contractility) decreases, pressures in both the left and right ventricles rise, while the overall cardiac output falls. Because less oxygen-rich blood is delivered to tissues, the body extracts more oxygen from the blood, causing a drop in mixed venous oxygen saturation. Problems with oxygen exchange in the lungs (intrapulmonary shunting) and low blood oxygen levels (hypoxaemia) further reduce oxygen in the arteries. As the heart pumps less effectively, stroke volume and blood pressure fall, which worsens myocardial ischaemia and leads to poor tissue perfusion, lactic acidosis, and further decline in heart function.

Compensatory mechanisms: The body tries to maintain blood flow by activating the sympathetic nervous system, which increases heart rate and contractility, and by retaining fluid through the kidneys, which raises left ventricular filling (preload). However, these responses also increase the heart's oxygen demand, making ischaemia worse. Fluid backup in the lungs (pulmonary congestion) raises the resistance the heart must pump against (afterload), further reducing cardiac performance. If this vicious cycle continues, it can lead to progressive heart failure and multi-organ damage.

Diastolic dysfunction: When heart muscle ischaemia makes the ventricles stiffer (less compliant), the pressure inside the left ventricle rises even if the volume of blood remains the same. This can cause fluid to back up into the lungs (pulmonary congestion), leading to congestive heart failure and further reducing blood flow to the body.

Systemic consequences: Shock, irrespective of cause, is a syndrome initiated by acute systemic hypoperfusion, leading to tissue hypoxia and organ dysfunction. In cardiogenic shock, reduced coronary perfusion aggravates cardiac dysfunction, perpetuating global hypoperfusion. Renal hypoperfusion decreases glomerular filtration, resulting in oliguria and potential renal failure.

Signs and symptoms

These are hypotension, absence of hypovolaemia and clinical signs of poor tissue perfusion, including oliguria, cyanosis, cool extremities and confusion. Physical examination includes cool, ashen or cyanotic skin, and extremities are mottled (see Box 6.1). Peripheral pulses are rapid and faint and may be irregular if arrhythmias are present. Jugular venous distention and crackles in the lungs may be present; peripheral oedema can also be present. Heart sounds are distant, and third and fourth heart sounds may be present. Pulse pressure may be low, and patients are usually tachycardic. There is hypoperfusion, altered mental status and decreased urine output.

Investigations

First-line investigations can help to determine the underlying cause of cardiogenic shock. Table 6.1 outlines some of these investigations.

Management

Management is based on an individual assessment of each patient. Cardiogenic shock treatment focuses on repairing the damage to heart muscle and other organs caused by lack of oxygen. Emergency life support is a necessary treatment for most people who have cardiogenic shock.

Symptom relief may be needed (e.g. opiate analgesia). Treat any electrolyte abnormalities. Treat any cardiac arrhythmias (see Table 6.2).

> ### Clinical considerations
>
> Cardiogenic shock is a life-threatening condition where the heart cannot pump enough blood. Patient anxiety is common and can increase heart rate and blood pressure, making assessment more challenging. Clear, calm communication helps reassure patients and encourages cooperation with monitoring and treatment. Effective teamwork and situational awareness are essential to recognise changes in vital signs while managing patient distress. A calm bedside presence and simple explanations improve patient comfort and support timely, effective care.

7 Anaphylactic shock

Table 7.1 The most common causes of anaphylaxis.

Foods	Drugs	Venom
• Peanuts • Pulses • Tree nuts (e.g. Brazil nut, almond, hazelnut) • Fish and shellfish • Eggs • Milk • Sesame	Including: • Antibiotics • Opioids • Non-steroidal anti-inflammatory drugs (NSAIDs) • Intravenous (IV) contrast media • Muscle relaxants • Other anaesthetic drugs	For example: • Bee stings • Wasp stings

Figure 7.1 Signs and symptoms of anaphylactic shock.

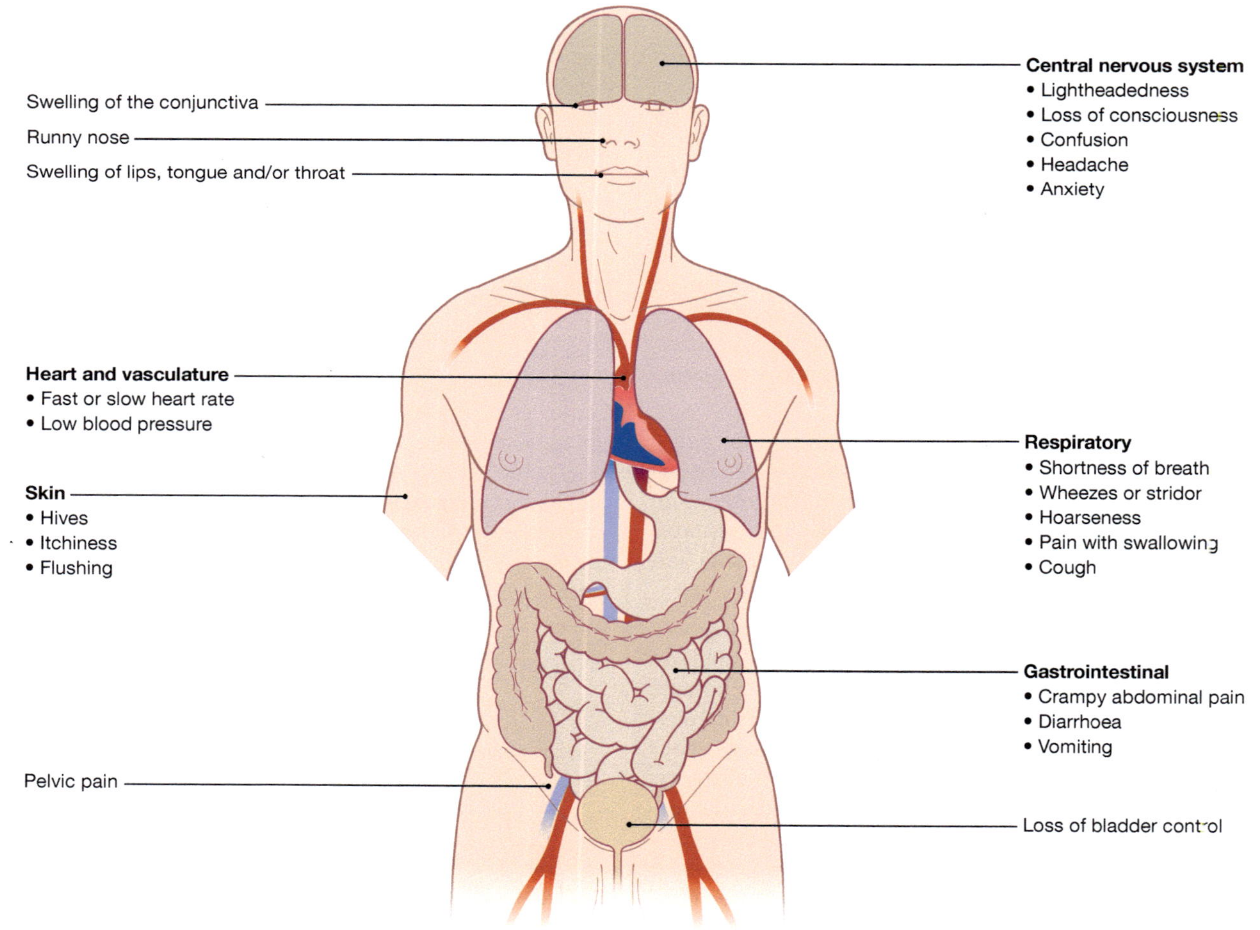

Anaphylaxis is a serious and potentially life-threatening allergic reaction. It can cause swelling (oedema), hives (urticaria), low blood pressure (hypotension) and widened blood vessels (vasodilation). In severe cases, it can lead to shock, which is life-threatening if not treated immediately.

Anaphylaxis happens when the immune system overreacts to a substance that is normally harmless, such as certain foods. The body may not react the first time it encounters the substance, but it can produce specific antibodies called immunoglobulin E (IgE). On later exposure, the allergen binds to these antibodies, triggering the release of large amounts of histamine, which causes those symptoms described.

Anaphylactic shock

Anaphylaxis can occur within seconds or minutes of exposure to an allergen, such as certain foods, including peanuts or shellfish. The immune system releases a flood of chemicals during anaphylaxis that can cause shock. Common triggers of anaphylaxis include certain foods, some medications, insect venom and latex (see Table 7.1). Anaphylaxis requires immediate emergency treatment; if the condition is not treated right away, unconsciousness or even death can occur.

Pathophysiology

The number of people experiencing severe, body-wide allergic reactions is increasing. However, because anaphylaxis is not always recognised, it may be under-reported.

An anaphylactic reaction occurs when an allergen interacts with specific IgE antibodies on cells called mast cells and basophils (a type I hypersensitivity reaction). This triggers a rapid release of histamine and other chemical mediators. These substances cause leaky blood vessels, swelling of mucous membranes, low blood pressure, and, in severe cases, shock or difficulty breathing (dyspnoea).

The severity and speed of anaphylactic reactions can vary. Some reactions can develop within minutes; others may occur in a biphasic pattern, where symptoms return after initial improvement. Rarely, reactions may be delayed by a few hours or last more than 24 hours, making diagnosis harder.

Anaphylactoid reactions are similar but do not involve IgE antibodies, though they still activate mast cells. In some cases, the cause is unknown (idiopathic). Table 7.1 lists the most common triggers of anaphylaxis.

Signs and symptoms

Often, but not always, there is a previous history of sensitivity to an allergen or a recent history of exposure to a new drug. Primarily, people frequently develop skin symptoms, including generalised itching (pruritus), urticaria and erythema, rhinitis, conjunctivitis and angiooedema. If the airway is affected, early signs may include itching of the roof of the mouth or ear canal, difficulty breathing (dyspnoea), stridor caused by swelling of the larynx, and wheezing or bronchospasm.

Other general symptoms can include tachycardia, palpitations, nausea, vomiting, abdominal pain, feeling faint and a sense of impending doom. Without prompt treatment, the person may collapse, and they may lose consciousness.

Signs of a severe or worsening allergic reaction include airway swelling, stridor, difficulty breathing, wheezing, hypotension, tachycardia and delayed capillary refill time. Bluish skin (cyanosis) is also a sign of severity; this may be harder to detect in those people with darker skin, so other indicators such as pale or grey lips, nail beds or mucous membranes, along with changes in breathing, consciousness and heart rate, should be carefully assessed. These are all warning signs of a potentially life-threatening reaction (see Figure 7.1).

Investigations

Anaphylaxis is diagnosed mainly by recognising its signs and symptoms. Those people who have had previous allergic reactions may be at higher risk of experiencing a severe reaction in the future. Skin tests can sometimes help in the identification of the substance that is causing the allergy, but these tests are not always safe if there is a risk of triggering an anaphylactic reaction.

A blood test measuring serum mast-cell tryptase can help to confirm the diagnosis when it is unclear. Tryptase (an enzyme, a type of protein) is released by mast cells during anaphylaxis. Levels are usually highest about 1 hour after a reaction has occurred, and they remain elevated for up to 6 hours. High tryptase levels indicate massive mast-cell activation, as seen in anaphylaxis or certain conditions such as mastocytosis (a condition in which the body produces too many mast cells or the mast cells behave abnormally). However, not all anaphylactic reactions cause tryptase to rise.

National guidelines exist for recognising and managing anaphylaxis. The basic principles of treatment are the same for all ages, though drug doses may vary between children and adults.

Because anaphylaxis can progress rapidly, diagnosis is clinical and urgent. A brief but focused history is taken to identify previous allergic reactions, exposure to new foods, medications, or insect stings, and any history of atopy (this is a genetic tendency to develop allergic conditions such as eczema, asthma, or hay fever and increases the risk of allergic reactions, including anaphylaxis). Treatment for anaphylaxis should be started immediately, even while assessment and monitoring continue.

Management

Rapid assessment

ABCDE assessment:

Airway: Look for obstruction, stridor, or swelling. Removal of allergens is appropriate (e.g. mouthwash for food fragments), but for bee stings, the stinger should be scraped off, not squeezed, to avoid injecting more venom.

Breathing: Observe for wheezing, dyspnoea and bronchospasm. Treat with oxygen and monitor respiratory effort.

Circulation: Check pulse, blood pressure, capillary refill and skin colour.

Disability: Check responsiveness and consciousness.

Exposure: Check skin for hives, flushing or swelling; maintain warmth.

Oxygen: High-flow oxygen (more than 10 L/min) via mask with reservoir is standard for severe reactions.

Positioning: Lie flat, unless breathing is difficult, then elevate the head slightly for comfort.

Epinephrine: IM injection given immediately. Auto-injectors are commonly used. IV adrenaline is reserved for severe refractory cases and managed by experienced staff.

IV fluids: Rapid fluid challenge may be needed for hypotension. Focus on giving rapid IV fluids for low BP.

Monitoring: Continuous pulse oximetry, ECG and BP are appropriate.

8 Hypovolaemic shock

Figure 8.1 Sequence of events in hypovolaemic shock.

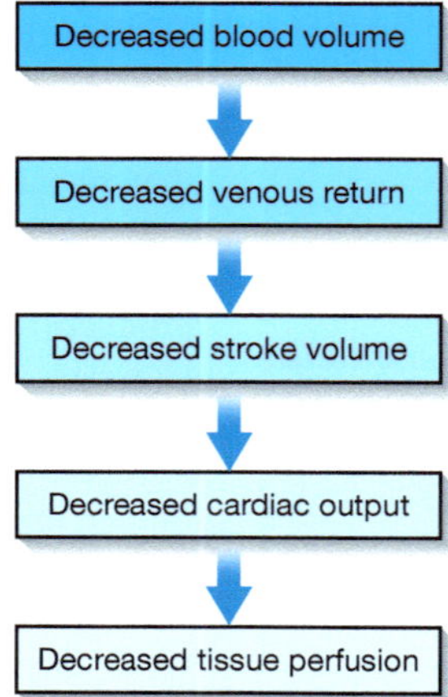

Figure 8.2 Stages of hypovolaemic shock.

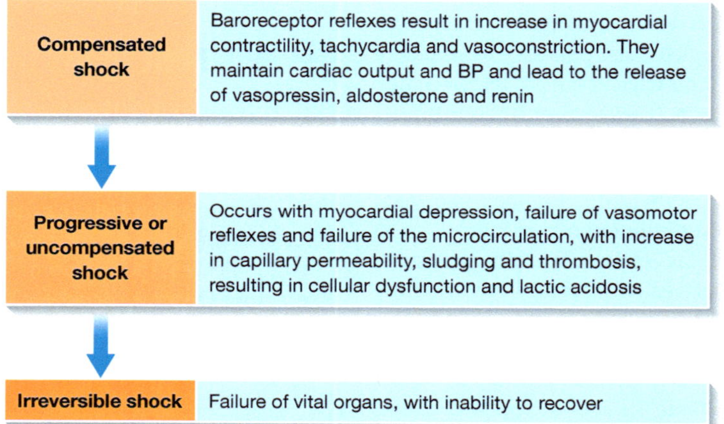

Table 8.1 Fundamentals of hypovolaemic shock management.

Category	Key measures	Notes/examples
General measures	Rapid ABCDE assessment; high-flow oxygen; positioning; fluid resuscitation; monitoring.	Fluids: crystalloids initially; blood products if haemorrhage. Monitor vital signs, urine output and perfusion.
Pharmacological	Vasopressors; analgesics and sedatives; correction of metabolic disturbances.	Vasopressors (e.g. norepinephrine) if hypotension persists; correct electrolytes, acidosis and coagulopathy.
Surgical/procedural	Control of bleeding; damage control surgery; repair of organs; interventional radiology if needed.	Examples: ligation of vessels, splenectomy, repair of ruptured ectopic pregnancy and drainage of fluids.

Hypovolaemic shock occurs when there is not enough circulating blood to maintain adequate perfusion of vital organs. Treatment aims to restore blood volume and organ perfusion to prevent irreversible damage, particularly to the brain and kidneys.

Hypovolaemic shock

Hypovolaemic shock is a medical or surgical condition; rapid fluid loss results in multiple organ failure as a result of inadequate circulating volume, causing inadequate perfusion. Hypovolaemic shock is very often due to rapid blood loss (sometimes referred to as haemorrhagic shock).

Two common causes of haemorrhagic shock are acute, external blood loss secondary to penetrating trauma and severe gastrointestinal bleeding. It can also be caused by a significant acute internal bleed into the thoracic and abdominal cavities. Hypovolaemic shock can result from significant fluid loss, other than blood loss (e.g. fluid loss due to severe gastroenteritis and extensive burns).

Pathophysiology

Hypovolaemic shock occurs; without rapid fluid or blood replacement and treatment of the underlying cause, circulation to the heart and other organs fails; this will eventually lead to multiple organ failure.

There are many causes of hypovolaemic shock. Blood loss may be visible or hidden (occult) and it can result from trauma, ruptured organs such as the spleen or liver, fractures (e.g. a femur may lose 0.5 L of blood and a pelvis about 1 L, depending on the person's age and size), gastrointestinal bleeding or ectopic pregnancy, where bleeding may not be obvious. Fluid loss also occurs in burns, severe diarrhoea or vomiting, when there is inadequate fluid intake, excessive sweating (diaphoresis) during strenuous activity or with the inappropriate use of diuretics. Other causes include reduced cardiac output from massive myocardial infarction, ruptured heart valves, massive pulmonary embolism, septic shock, acute pancreatitis or high spinal injury or anaesthesia, which can reduce vascular resistance and circulating volume.

The body can tolerate small blood losses (e.g. a healthy adult may lose around 0.5 L from their total circulation of around 5 L without major effects). Larger volumes or rapid loss, however, can cause progressively serious problems. The risk of complications rises with age and existing cardiovascular, respiratory or renal disease.

The body makes its response to acute hypovolaemia through several physiological systems. The haematological system will trigger clot formation and constriction of bleeding vessels. Platelets form an initial clot, while fibrin acts to stabilise it. The cardiovascular system increases heart rate and contractility, constricts peripheral vessels and prioritises blood flow to the brain, heart and kidneys at the expense of the skin, muscles and the gastrointestinal tract. The renal system releases renin that produces angiotensin II, which will cause vasoconstriction and stimulates aldosterone to help retain sodium and water. The neuroendocrine system releases antidiuretic hormone (ADH), which increases water and sodium reabsorption in the kidneys to restore circulating volume (see Figure 8.1).

Together, these mechanisms work to maintain vital organ perfusion, even when there is severe blood or fluid loss, by supporting blood pressure, conserving fluids and prioritising blood flow to the brain, heart and kidneys, thereby delaying the onset of irreversible organ damage.

Signs and symptoms

The person may feel cold, unwell, anxious, faint and short of breath. Dizziness or fainting can occur when standing or even sitting, as a result of postural hypotension. Symptoms may also reflect the underlying cause of the hypovolaemia, such as pain from a bleeding ulcer, a ruptured aneurysm, ectopic pregnancy, trauma or burns. Nausea and vomiting can result from reduced blood flow to the gut.

On examination, the patient may appear pale and sweaty, with rapid breathing (tachypnoea). Peripheral extremities may feel cold due to poor perfusion, and capillary refill time may be delayed. The heart rate is often fast and blood pressure may be low, sometimes only noticeable on standing (postural hypotension). Typically, tachycardia develops before hypotension, and hypotension occurs later, followed by confusion or even coma in severe cases.

Physiologically, hypovolaemic shock progresses through three stages (see Figure 8.2). In the compensated stage, the body attempts to maintain blood flow to vital organs by increasing heart rate and constricting blood vessels; blood pressure may remain normal, and the patient may feel concerned, dizzy or cold. In the decompensated stage, compensatory mechanisms will begin to fail, blood pressure drops and perfusion to non-essential organs is reduced; this leads to confusion, pallor, sweating and shortness of breath. In the irreversible stage, organ damage occurs despite treatment, the person's blood pressure remains very low, and the patient may become unconscious, making survival unlikely without immediate intervention.

Investigations

Investigations in hypovolaemic shock may include full blood count, urea and electrolytes, liver function tests, coagulation screen and arterial blood gas analysis. Ultrasound can help distinguish hypovolaemic from cardiogenic shock by assessing the filling of the vena cava. An echocardiogram may reveal heart pump failure. Central venous pressure monitoring can also be useful in those patients with evidence of shock to guide fluid management.

Management

Management of hypovolaemic shock focuses on rapid recognition, rapid restoration of circulating volume, supporting vital organs and addressing the underlying cause. General supportive measures, pharmacological interventions and surgical procedures all work together to improve perfusion and prevent irreversible multi-organ system failure. Table 8.1 outlines the fundamentals of management.

Clinical considerations

Infants and young children are at high risk due to small circulating blood volume and limited compensatory capacity, so even minor fluid or blood loss can rapidly precipitate shock; hypotension is a late and ominous sign. Older adults often have reduced cardiovascular reserve and comorbidities, which blunt compensatory responses. Clinical features may include tachycardia, delayed capillary refill, cool peripheries, altered mental status and hypotension. Both groups require urgent assessment, careful fluid resuscitation, haemodynamic monitoring and early intervention to prevent irreversible organ injury.

9 Septicaemia

Table 9.1 Sepsis.

Stage/term	Definition/description	Clinical features/implications
Septicaemia	Presence of bacteria in the blood causing systemic infection.	May produce fever, chills and malaise; can progress to organ dysfunction if untreated. Often considered a critical illness.
Sepsis	Life-threatening systemic response to infection.	Signs include fever, tachycardia, tachypnoea, hypotension and altered mental status. Can lead to organ dysfunction.
Septic Shock	Severe sepsis with circulatory and metabolic failure.	Persistent hypotension despite fluids, high lactate and multi-organ failure. Requires intensive care and carries high mortality.

Table 9.2 Six interventions for septic shock as outlined by the UK Sepsis Trust.

1. Administer high-flow oxygen if required: ensure that oxygen saturation levels are maintained above 94% to support adequate tissue oxygenation

2. Take blood cultures: collect blood cultures before administering antibiotics to identify the causative organism, which is crucial for effective treatment

3. Administer broad-spectrum antibiotics: start intravenous antibiotics within 1 hour of sepsis recognition to combat the infection effectively

4. Measure serum lactate levels: assess lactate levels to evaluate tissue perfusion and guide resuscitation efforts

5. Administer intravenous fluids: provide IV fluids to restore adequate circulating blood volume, which is essential for maintaining blood pressure and organ function

6. Monitor urine output (may require urinary catheter): keep track of urine output to ensure adequate renal perfusion and function

Box 9.1 Risk factors for developing sepsis.

- Those who are elderly and those who are very young
- Instrumentation or surgery
- Alcohol abuse
- People with diabetes mellitus
- Those with burns
- Immunosuppression
- Those who have undergone organ transplantation
- People who are undernourished
- Certain medications, such as high-dose steroids and chemotherapy

Sepsis remains a major clinical problem, causing significant morbidity and mortality and accounting for thousands of deaths each year. The terms used to describe septic shock and related conditions can vary, and while often similar, they have important differences.

Sepsis and septicaemia describe a range of clinical states in patients with bacteraemia, and in practice, these terms are sometimes used interchangeably. Bacteraemia refers to the presence of bacteria in the bloodstream. Small amounts of bacteria are often controlled by the immune system without causing systemic effects. When larger numbers of bacteria are present, they may trigger systemic symptoms or complications, such as pneumonia or abscess formation, which can occur with or without sepsis.

Septicaemia occurs when large numbers of bacteria are actively dividing in the blood, provoking a systemic inflammatory response that can lead to organ dysfunction. This is a critical and potentially fatal condition, which may be complicated by life-threatening events such as circulatory collapse. Septicaemia should never be considered merely an infection, as it represents a severe, systemic illness requiring urgent intervention.

Pathophysiology

Sepsis can be considered as a disease continuum (see Table 9.1). These stages form a disease continuum: septicaemia may trigger a systemic response (sepsis), which can worsen to septic shock, each stage representing progressively severe illness and higher risk of death. The pathophysiology associated with septic shock is not exactly understood; however, it involves a multifaceted interaction between the pathogen and the individual's immune system. The usual physiological reaction to a localised infection will include the initiation of host defence mechanisms, causing an increase of white blood cells, along with the release of inflammatory mediators, local vasodilation, increased leakage of fluid from blood vessels and the initiation of the various blood clotting pathways. Sepsis entails a variety of disorders, for example, abnormal coagulation, damage to the blood vessel lining, presence of tumour necrosis factor in excessive amounts and deficiency of steroid hormones.

There are a variety of causes of septic shock, and bacterial infection is most common; generally, this is responsive to antibiotic therapy. Sometimes the infection can overwhelm the person's defence mechanisms and progress rapidly to a serious illness called severe sepsis.

Pneumonia, perforated bowel, urinary tract infection and severe skin infections are the most frequent causes of severe sepsis. There is usually an abscess or a nidus (a focus) of infection associated with sepsis. Some risk factors for developing sepsis are outlined in Box 9.1.

Signs and symptoms

Sepsis is a life-threatening condition in which infection triggers a dysregulated host response, resulting in acute organ dysfunction. The term 'severe sepsis' is no longer used in current definitions, as organ dysfunction is now integral to the diagnosis of sepsis.

The person may have been seen by the practice nurse or GP and presented a few days earlier with a focus of infection. Antibiotics may have been prescribed for the condition. However, despite this, their condition may have declined quickly. Often the person presents with symptoms that are non-specific, such as tiredness, nausea and vomiting, abdominal pain and diarrhoea. The person may appear unwell, and there may be a spiking temperature that may or may not be accompanied by rigours. Tachycardia may be present, with a bounding pulse. There may be tachypnoea, along with cyanosis. The individual may have cold peripheries (they feel cold to touch), and they may also be sweating. Hypotension may be present. Drowsiness and impaired consciousness can occur; in the older person, this is common. Other features will relate to the infection itself; there may be a rash, the signs of a wound infection, and the person may be wheezing, or chest crackles can be heard in pneumonia. It is important to recognise that the features outlined here may not be present in older adults. Similarly, individuals who are immunocompromised may not exhibit these typical signs and symptoms.

Investigations

It is usual for a diagnosis to be made based on the clinical features the person presents with. A full blood count will be required, determining the presence of anaemia or other blood disorders; urinary tract infection needs to be ruled out. Renal function tests help to determine if there is dehydration or organ failure. Liver function tests can help to assess if there is liver damage. Blood cultures will be required. A chest X-ray, abdominal ultrasound and CT scan are needed. Oxygen saturation levels and an analysis of arterial blood gases are required. Invasive investigations may be required if the infection is covert, such as lumbar puncture or bronchoscopy.

Management

Those with septic shock are transferred to the intensive care unit, receiving ongoing support for organ dysfunction. Most patients require mechanical ventilation and treatment to support cardiac function. If renal impairment is present, renal replacement therapy may be needed, with haematological support for problems associated with abnormal blood clotting.

In preventing progression from infection and sepsis to death (the sepsis continuum), practitioners must have skills that can help identify key clinical indicators; timely and appropriate interventions are required in order to prevent complications and to avoid death.

The six interventions for septic shock outlined by the UK Sepsis Trust are detailed in Table 9.2. These six interventions must be carried out within an hour.

In an appropriate care environment, such as an intensive care unit, supportive care will include the need to resuscitate the person. Intravenous rehydration will be required; intravenous hydrocortisone may be administered, along with fludrocortisone. Monitoring the person's condition will be required, using NEWS2, central venous pressure and also hourly urinary output.

Broad-spectrum intravenous antibiotics are given in the first instance. Unusual organisms, including fungi, require specific treatment with specialist input from a microbiologist and virologist.

Surgery may be needed to debride wounds or drain an abscess.

Clinical considerations

Septicaemia is a life-threatening bloodstream infection that can rapidly progress to organ dysfunction. Its sudden onset and severity often evoke fear and anxiety. Early recognition, prompt antibiotics, supportive care and close monitoring are critical. Awareness of its seriousness ensures urgent, decisive clinical action to prevent progression to sepsis or septic shock.

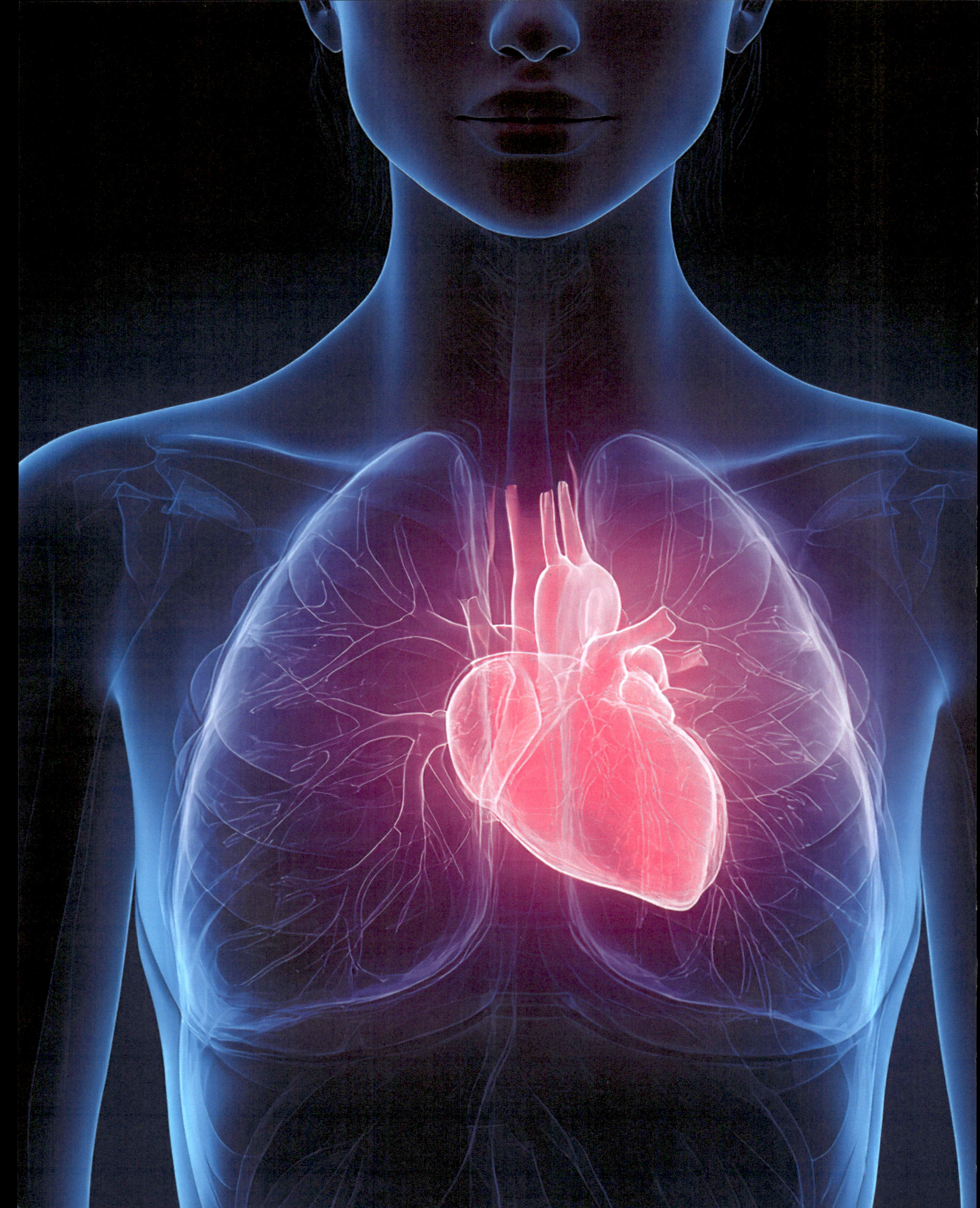

Immunity

Chapters

10 Human immunodeficiency virus

Figure 10.1   The structure of HIV.

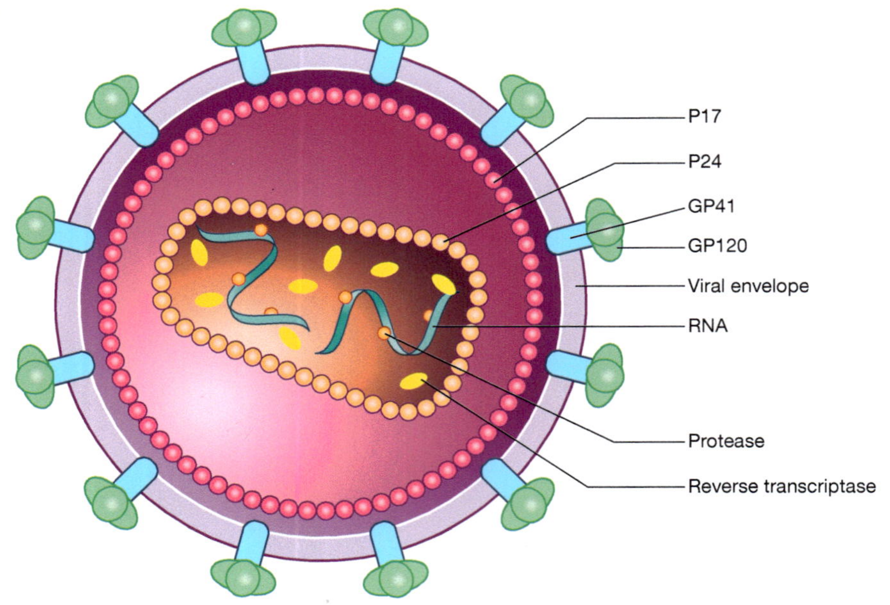

Figure 10.2   CD4 cell count and viral load (without treatment).

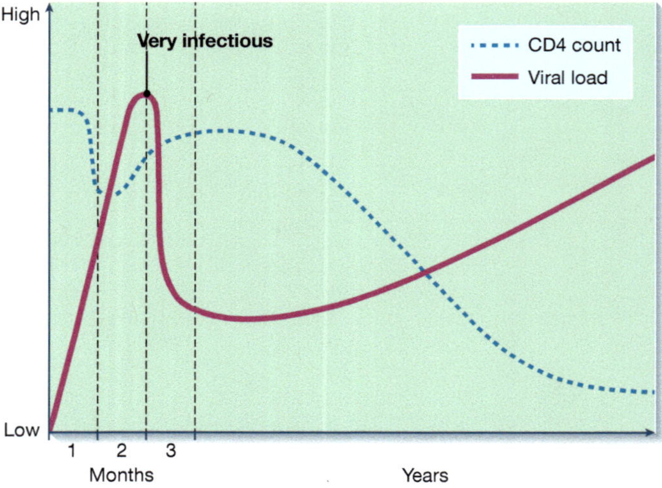

Table 10.1   HIV and AIDS.

Feature	HIV Infection	AIDS
Definition	Infection with Human immunodeficiency virus.	Advanced stage of HIV infection with severe immune system compromise.
Immune status	Gradual loss of CD4+ T cells, may remain asymptomatic for years.	CD4+ T-cell count <200 cells/µL or presence of opportunistic infections/cancers.
Symptoms	Often asymptomatic or mild flu-like symptoms.	Opportunistic infections, malignancies, HIV-related dementia, severe weight loss and fatigue.
Infectiousness	Person is infectious, even if asymptomatic.	Person remains infectious, generally with higher viral load.
Treatment goal	Early ART to preserve immune function.	ART to control viral replication, treat opportunistic infections, and manage complications.
Prognosis	Good with ART	Without treatment, life-threatening; prognosis improves significantly with ART.

Human immunodeficiency virus

Human immunodeficiency virus (HIV) is a retrovirus that was first identified in the early 1980s. Initially, it was called lymphadenopathy-associated virus (LAV) by French researchers and HTLV-III by US scientists. The virus was later universally renamed HIV, with HIV-1 being the most widespread type worldwide. HIV-2 was identified in 1985, mainly in West Africa, and is less virulent and less common outside that region.

HIV is blood-borne and transmitted via sexual contact, sharing of needles and mother-to-child transmission, which can occur during childbirth or breastfeeding. Understanding transmission routes is crucial for prevention and patient education.

It is important to distinguish HIV infection from acquired immunodeficiency syndrome (AIDS). A person can be infected with HIV yet remain asymptomatic for many years. Some untreated individuals have been known to live for over a decade without developing AIDS (see Table 10.1). AIDS is diagnosed when CD4+ T-cell counts fall below 200 cells/μL or when the person develops opportunistic infections (e.g. Pneumocystis jiroveci pneumonia, cytomegalovirus and toxoplasmosis), certain cancers, or HIV-associated dementia.

HIV progressively destroys CD4+ T lymphocytes, weakening the immune system and increasing susceptibility to infections and malignancies. Infection with HIV, even without symptoms, renders an individual infectious to others. Early diagnosis, monitoring of CD4+ counts and viral load, and initiation of antiretroviral therapy (ART) are essential for preserving immune function, reducing disease progression and preventing transmission.

HIV is a chronic, blood-borne virus with a long asymptomatic phase, but if left untreated, it can lead to severe immune compromise (AIDS). Awareness of its history, transmission and disease progression is fundamental for healthcare professionals in prevention, early recognition and management.

Pathophysiology

HIV gains entry to the cells by attaching to the CD4 receptor and a co-receptor via its envelope glycoproteins. It encodes the enzyme reverse transcriptase, permitting a DNA copy to be made from viral RNA. Once integrated into the cellular DNA, the provirus exists in the nucleus of infected cells, where it can remain dormant for lengthy periods of time. It can also become transcriptionally active using the machinery of the host cell to replicate. Viral RNA is then modified singly or in multiples, making numerous structural and regulatory and accessory proteins. Viral proteases further process proteins; mature viral particles are formed as budding of the virus occurs through the host cell membrane (see Figure 10.1).

There is a high level of viral replication in the blood within a few weeks of infection, and an associated decline in CD4 T-cells occurs. An immune response to HIV develops, curtailing viral replication, causing a decrease in viral load and a return of CD4 T-cell numbers close to normal levels. Immune control is said to be dependent on killer T cells and neutralising antibodies. It has been suggested that the host's initial response to HIV infection is critical and that this is genetically governed.

CD4 cells migrate to the lymphoid tissue, where the virus replicates and then infects new CD4+ cells. As the infection progresses, depletion or impaired function of CD4 cells predisposes to the development of immune dysfunction.

Signs and symptoms

There may be flu-like symptoms, a glandular fever-type illness, fever, malaise, myalgia, pharyngitis, headaches, diarrhoea, neuralgia or neuropathy, lymphadenopathy and/or a maculopapular rash. Rarely, meningoencephalitis occurs. Acute infection may be asymptomatic. HIV seroconversion illness includes oral candidiasis, recurrent shingles, leukopenia or central nervous system signs (e.g. seizures and dementia).

Investigations

HIV infection should be considered in any individual presenting with unexplained or recurrent infections, prolonged fever, weight loss or lymphadenopathy, especially when no other cause is identified. It is particularly important to consider HIV testing in people with known risk factors such as unprotected sexual contact, intravenous drug use or exposure to contaminated blood products.

The first test used to check for HIV infection is usually a fourth-generation HIV antigen/antibody test, which looks for both the p24 antigen and HIV antibodies. This test can usually detect infection within 2–4 weeks after exposure. If the result is positive, it must be confirmed using another test, such as an HIV-1/HIV-2 differentiation test or a Western blot. If HIV infection is strongly suspected but the antibody test is negative or unclear, a viral load test (HIV RNA test) can detect the virus's genetic material before antibodies have developed. Once HIV infection is confirmed, additional tests help guide treatment and monitor progress. The CD4+ T-cell count shows how well the immune system is functioning, while the HIV viral load measures the amount of virus in the blood. Resistance testing checks whether the virus has mutations that could affect how well medicines work. It is also important to test for other infections, such as hepatitis B and C, tuberculosis and sexually transmitted infections.

Early and accurate diagnosis is essential to begin ART as soon as possible and to reduce the risk of transmitting HIV to others.

Management

Early diagnosis and regular screening for HIV are vital; many people remain asymptomatic for years while the virus gradually weakens the immune system. Fourth-generation antigen/antibody tests are now the standard screening method.

Staging and monitoring of HIV infection are guided by both clinical features and laboratory results. The CD4+ count (normally 500–2,000 cells/μL) reflects immune function and risk of opportunistic infections. Over time, CD4+ levels decline if untreated, while a high viral load indicates rapid disease progression (see Figure 10.2). Regular monitoring of both markers is essential for guiding treatment and assessing response.

The cornerstone of modern HIV management is ART designed to suppress viral replication. The current approach is to start ART as soon as possible after diagnosis, regardless of CD4+ count, to improve long-term health and prevent transmission. Effective ART maintains viral suppression, restores immune function and allows near-normal life expectancy.

Prophylaxis against opportunistic infections may be required when CD4+ counts fall below specific thresholds. Ongoing management includes concordance support, management of comorbidities, mental health care and regular monitoring for treatment side effects.

> ### Clinical considerations
>
> As there is still no cure for HIV, prevention remains essential. Public health strategies focus on safer sex education, needle-exchange programmes, screening of blood products and the use of pre-exposure prophylaxis (PrEP) and post-exposure prophylaxis (PEP).

11 Non-hodgkin lymphoma

Figure 11.1 Lymph nodes and vessels.

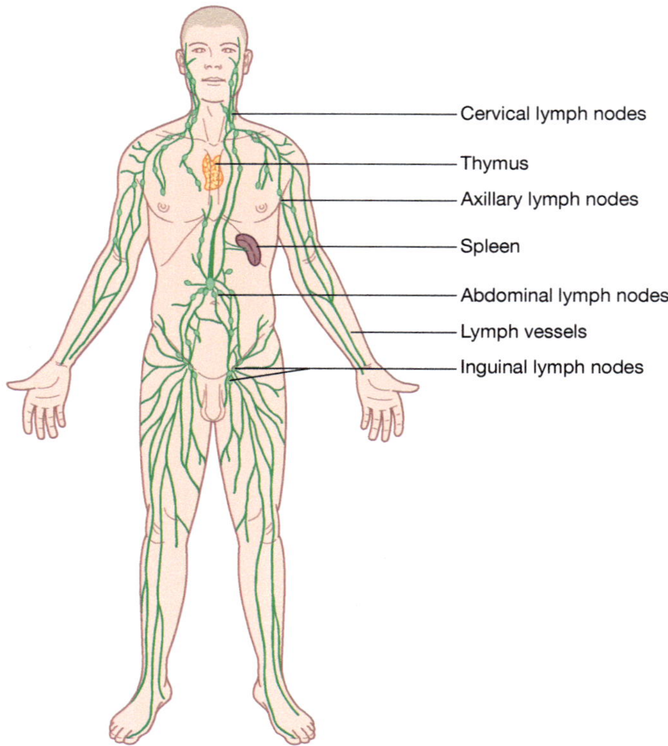

Figure 11.2 Structure of a lymph node.

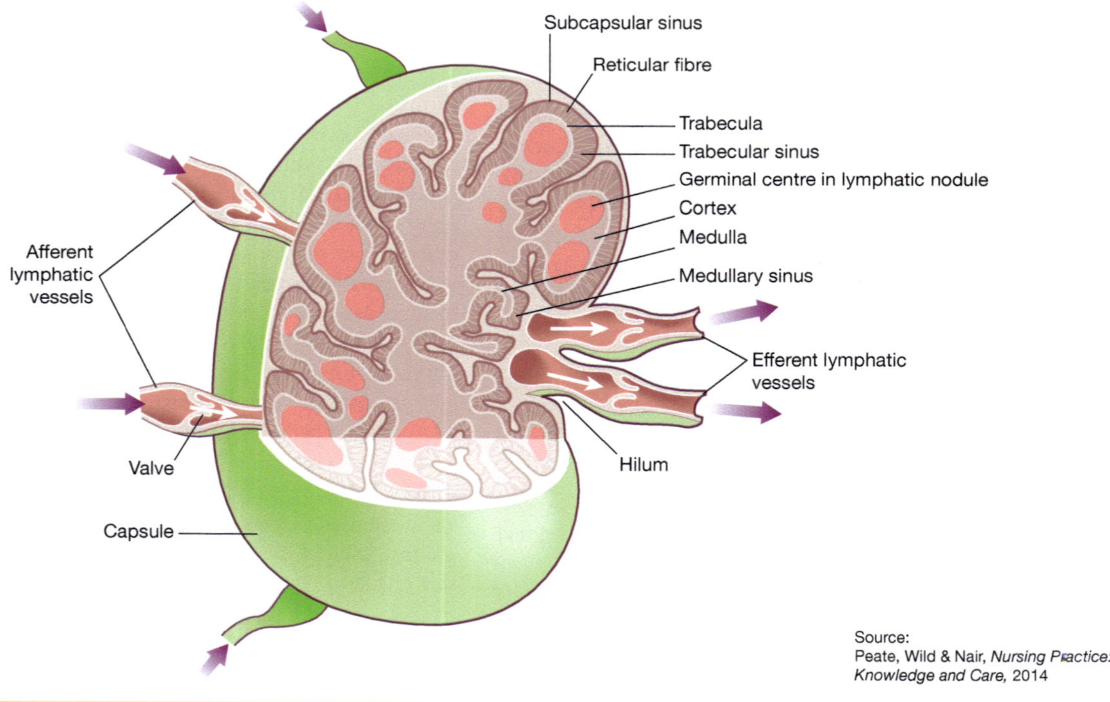

Source:
Peate, Wild & Nair, *Nursing Practice: Knowledge and Care*, 2014

Route of lymph flow through a lymph node:

Afferent lymphatic vessel ➡ Subcapsular sinus ➡ Trabecular sinus ➡ Medullary sinus ➡ Efferent lymphatic vessel

Non-hodgkin lymphoma

Non-Hodgkin lymphomas (NHLs) are the seventh most common cancer in the UK, with approximately 13,600 people diagnosed with it annually. There are several different types of NHL. Some of them will grow very slowly and treatment may not be required for months or years: other types have a tendency to grow quickly and treatment is required soon after a diagnosis is made. NHL is associated with ageing. As a person ages, there are increased chances of developing the condition. At diagnosis, the average age was around 65. Risk is higher in white people than in black and Asian people.

Pathophysiology

NHLs are a heterogeneous group of tumours that originate from lymphoid tissues, primarily of lymph nodes (a type of cancer of the lymphatic system) (see Figures 11.1 and 11.2). NHLs are lymphoproliferative malignancies (cancers of the lymph system) that vary widely in their behaviour, treatment response and prognosis. The outlook for each patient will depend on the histological type, stage at diagnosis and the treatment approach that is adopted. Unlike Hodgkin lymphoma, NHL more frequently spreads to extranodal sites, such as the gastrointestinal tract, skin or central nervous system.

NHL is commonly associated with a defective or weakened immune system. It occurs more often in those people who are receiving immunosuppressive therapy following organ transplantation, those with HIV infection, and also individuals with certain viral infections such as Epstein–Barr virus. Additional risk factors include a family history of lymphoma, male sex, white ethnicity, autoimmune diseases (e.g. rheumatoid arthritis) and previous exposure to radiotherapy.

The development of NHL may result from chromosomal translocations (these are genetic changes where parts of two different chromosomes swap places), viral or bacterial infections, environmental exposures, immunodeficiency and chronic inflammation. The key molecular feature of the disease is abnormal gene mutation during lymphocyte formation, maturation or activation. Mutations in a single lymphocyte can cause it to grow uncontrollably, producing many identical abnormal cells, a monoclonal population. The subtype of lymphoma, B-cell or T-cell, depends on which lymphocyte type was affected and at what stage of its development the mutation occurred, guiding diagnosis and treatment decisions.

B-cell lymphoma

The B cells develop and mature in the bone marrow before moving to lymph nodes and other lymphoid tissues to carry out immune functions. Mutations can occur at different stages of development: early precursor B-cell mutations may cause acute lymphoblastic leukaemia, while changes in immature, naïve or activated B cells can lead to various NHLs, including Burkitt lymphoma, diffuse large B-cell lymphoma and mantle cell lymphoma. Understanding the stage at which mutations occur helps explain the subtype of malignancy and guides clinical management.

T-cell lymphoma

The exact cause of most T-cell lymphomas remains unknown. However, mutations in genes that regulate T-cell growth, survival and signalling can cause cells to divide uncontrollably and in so doing form malignant populations. T cells originate in the bone marrow, but they mature in the thymus; it is in the thymus where they undergo selection and differentiation. Depending on the stage at which mutations occur, different subtypes of T-cell lymphoma can develop, each with unique behaviour, clinical features and treatment responses. Chronic immune stimulation and certain viral infections may also contribute to the development of T-cell malignancies.

Signs and symptoms

The clinical manifestations vary with such factors as the location of the lymphomatous process, speed of tumour growth and the function of the organ compromised or displaced by the malignancy. Clinical manifestations can include:

Low-grade lymphomas:

- Painless, slowly progressive and peripheral lymphadenopathy
- Primary extranodal involvement (lymphoma starts in an organ or tissue outside of the lymph nodes)
- Fatigue, weakness, fever, night sweats and weight loss
- Cytopenia (reduction in the number of one or more types of blood cells)
- Splenomegaly (enlarged spleen)
- Hepatomegaly (enlarged liver).

Intermediate- and high-grade lymphomas:

- Rapidly growing, bulky lymphadenopathy lymph nodes that enlarge quickly and become noticeably large or 'massive'
- Systemic symptoms and extranodal involvement
- Hepatomegaly
- Splenomegaly
- Testicular mass
- Skin lesions: associated with cutaneous T-cell lymphoma
- Burkitt's lymphoma: presents with a large abdominal mass and symptoms of bowel obstruction
- Pulmonary involvement and superior vena cava obstruction.

Investigations

- Full blood count
- Renal function tests and electrolytes
- Serology: may include HIV and hepatitis B/C
- Lactate dehydrogenase: elevated in aggressive lymphomas; prognostic marker
- Chest X-ray
- Lymph node excision core biopsy is for the diagnosis of follicular lymphoma; histology for assessment of the tumour grade
- Bone marrow aspiration and biopsy
- CT scan of neck, chest, abdomen and pelvis
- Bone scans
- Whole body positron emission tomography (PET) scan
- Scrotal ultrasound
- Lumbar puncture

Other investigations may be indicated, depending on the clinical presentation.

Management

Treatment depends on the type, grade, and stage of NHL and the patient's overall health. Watchful waiting may be appropriate for some people with slow-growing lymphomas. Chemotherapy is often given as single or combination therapy, sometimes with monoclonal antibodies such as rituximab to target malignant B cells. Radiotherapy is used for localised or bulky disease, while surgery is rarely needed. Supportive care is critical; those patients with severe neutropenia may require antibiotic prophylaxis. Therapy must be tailored to an individual's needs; there is often a need to balance effectiveness with side effects, and this will usually involve a multidisciplinary team including haematology, oncology and supportive care specialists.

Clinical considerations

Non-Hodgkin lymphoma presents variably, depending on tumour type, growth rate, and organ involvement. Key symptoms include rapidly enlarging lymph nodes, systemic 'B' symptoms (fever, night sweats and weight loss) and organ-specific signs. Investigations such as blood counts, lactate dehydrogenase, imaging, and biopsy guide staging, subtype classification and treatment planning. Aggressive lymphomas require urgent chemotherapy, while indolent forms may be monitored with watchful waiting. Patients are at high risk of infection due to immunosuppression, so supportive care – including prophylactic measures and vaccinations – is essential. A multidisciplinary approach, involving haematology, oncology, and supportive care teams, ensures optimal management and monitoring of complications.

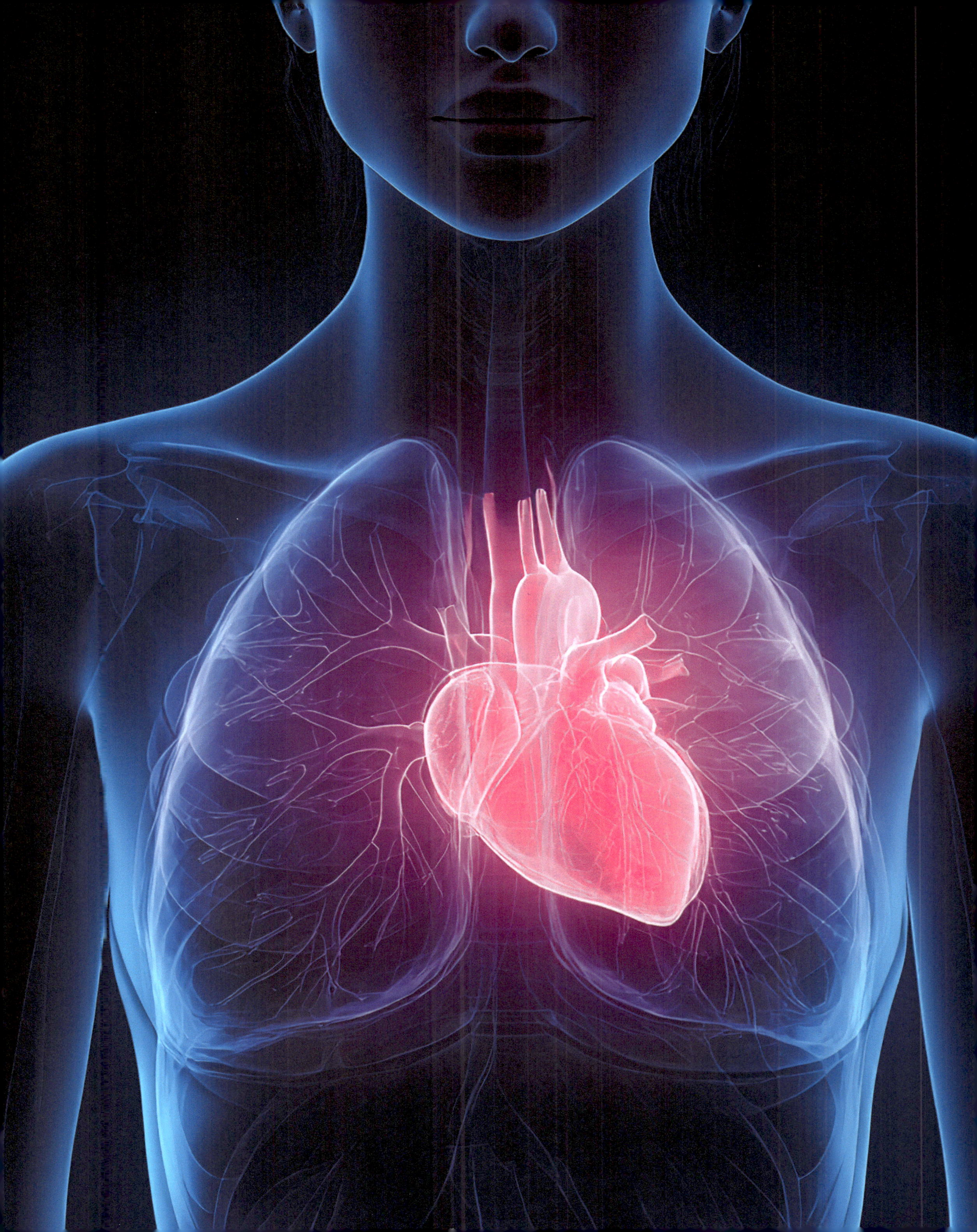

12 Infectious mononucleosis

Figure 12.1 Lymphadenopathy.

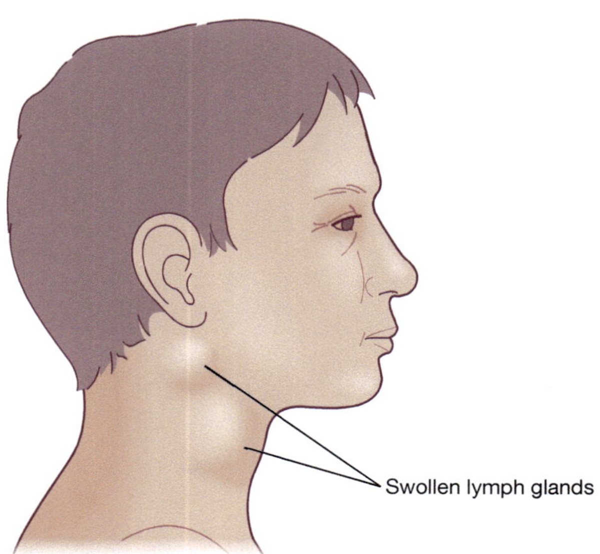

Figure 12.2 The main symptoms of infectious mononucleosis.

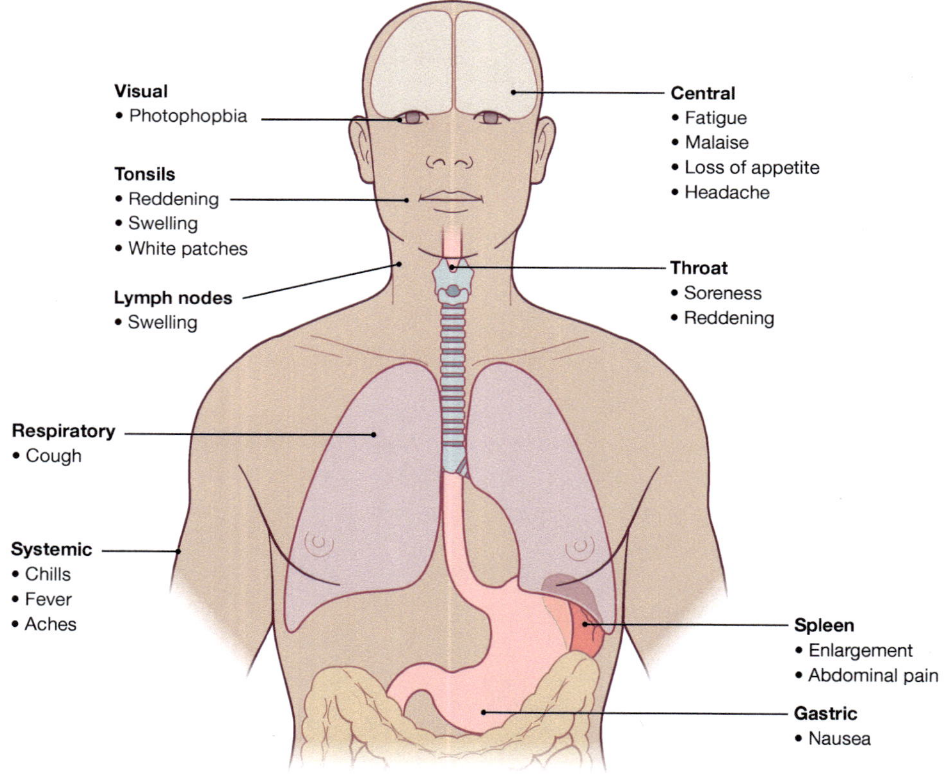

Infectious mononucleosis is also known as glandular fever.

Infectious mononucleosis

Infectious mononucleosis is a clinical syndrome that consists of fever, pharyngitis and adenopathy (enlargement or swelling of the lymph nodes). Most cases of glandular fever are caused by the Epstein–Barr virus (EBV), which is one of the most common viruses to affect humans. It is a member of the herpes virus family.

EBV is a viral infection that mainly affects adolescents and young adults. Most adults will show evidence of a past infection when their blood is tested. In most cases, EBV does not pose a serious health risk, but infection in early adulthood can cause glandular fever, which may be uncomfortable and can last several weeks. If a person develops an EBV infection during early adulthood, they can develop symptoms of glandular fever.

Pathophysiology

The EBV is transmitted primarily through saliva, earning it the nickname 'kissing disease'. Less commonly, EBV can spread through exposure to coughs or sneezes, sharing utensils, blood transfusions or organ transplantation. Genital transmission is rare.

EBV infects B lymphocytes in the oropharynx and can spread to the reticuloendothelial system, including the liver, spleen and peripheral lymph nodes. The body mounts two main immune responses. Humoral immunity, via antibodies against EBV proteins, forms the basis for diagnostic blood tests. Cellular immunity, mainly through CD8+ cytotoxic T cells and natural killer (NK) cells, is essential to control infected B cells and limit viral replication. A strong T-cell response usually leads to a mild or asymptomatic infection and lifelong viral suppression. In contrast, an ineffective T-cell response can allow uncontrolled B-cell proliferation, which in rare cases may contribute to malignancies such as B-cell lymphomas.

Clinical manifestations of infectious mononucleosis result from the immune response to the virus. Pyrexia occurs due to cytokine release. Pharyngitis develops from lymphoid tissue inflammation in the oropharynx, and lymphadenopathy results from reactive T-cell proliferation in lymph nodes (see Figure 12.1). Patients may also experience fatigue, malaise and splenomegaly. Blood tests often show lymphocytosis, reflecting an increase in reactive T cells responding to infected B cells.

Most EBV infections are self-limiting, lasting 2–4 weeks, though fatigue can persist longer. Severe complications are uncommon but can include hepatitis, splenic rupture, haemolytic anaemia or neurological involvement. Management is primarily supportive, focusing on rest, hydration and symptom relief. Understanding the interaction between EBV and the immune system helps explain the characteristic signs and guides safe management, including advising patients to avoid contact sports if splenomegaly is present.

Signs and symptoms

Most people who are infected with EBV are asymptomatic. The incubation period (this is the time from infection to the appearance of symptoms) ranges from 4 to 6 weeks. People with infectious mononucleosis can transmit the infection to others for a period of weeks. Once a person has had glandular fever, it is highly unlikely they will develop a second infection, as most people develop lifelong immunity to glandular fever after the primary infection.

Most people with infectious mononucleosis experience fatigue and prolonged malaise, which are the most common symptoms. A sore throat is also frequently reported. Many patients have a low-grade pyrexia, while joint and muscle aches (arthralgia and myalgia) may occur, but these are less common than in other viral infections. Nausea and reduced appetite are often present, typically without vomiting.

A number of other symptoms have been described in people with infectious mononucleosis (e.g. cough, ocular muscle pain, chest pain and photophobia). Splenomegaly may occur (see Figure 12.2).

Investigations

Infection with EBV provokes specific antibodies to EBV and also various unrelated non-EBV heterophile antibodies (antibodies against an antigen produced in one species that react against antigens from other species). These heterophile antibodies are not specific for the virus.

As the symptoms associated with infectious mononucleosis resemble those of many other viral infections, clinical examination alone is often insufficient for diagnosis. Blood tests are used to detect antibodies and confirm the presence of glandular fever. Common tests include the Paul–Bunnell test and the Monospot® test.

Positivity increases during the first 6 weeks of the illness and so the heterophile antibody test results may be negative early in the course of infectious mononucleosis and, as such, blood tests may need to be repeated.

Management

If there is suspected or confirmed splenic involvement, patients should avoid contact sports for at least three weeks due to the risk of splenic rupture. Symptomatic relief is the mainstay of treatment: paracetamol can be used for pain and pyrexia, and plenty of fluids are encouraged to help to prevent dehydration. There is no specific antiviral therapy available for EBV. In rare cases of severe tonsillar enlargement, a short course of corticosteroids may help to reduce swelling.

For infection prevention and control, patients should avoid kissing, close physical contact and sharing personal items such as cups or towels, and alcohol should be avoided. The majority of individuals will recover fully within 2–3 weeks, though fatigue, malaise, muscle aches and joint pains may persist for several weeks or months. Hospital admission may be necessary in severe cases; this may be to manage dehydration or provide intravenous fluids.

Potential complications

- Extreme tonsillar enlargement can cause upper airway obstruction
- Myocarditis and cardiac conduction abnormalities
- Splenic rupture
- Haemolytic anaemia and thrombocytopenia
- Acute interstitial nephritis and glomerulonephritis
- Neurological, including aseptic meningitis, encephalitis, cranial nerve palsies or Guillain–Barré syndrome
- Prolonged fatigue; depression
- Chronic fatigue
- Lymphoproliferative cancers.

Clinical considerations

Infectious mononucleosis is caused by Epstein–Barr virus (EBV), which is primarily transmitted through saliva. Typical symptoms include fatigue, fever, sore throat and swollen lymph nodes. Management is mainly supportive, with rest, adequate fluids and paracetamol; corticosteroids may be used in cases of severe tonsillar swelling. Patients should avoid contact sports if the spleen is enlarged and take precautions to prevent transmission, such as avoiding kissing, close contact or sharing utensils.

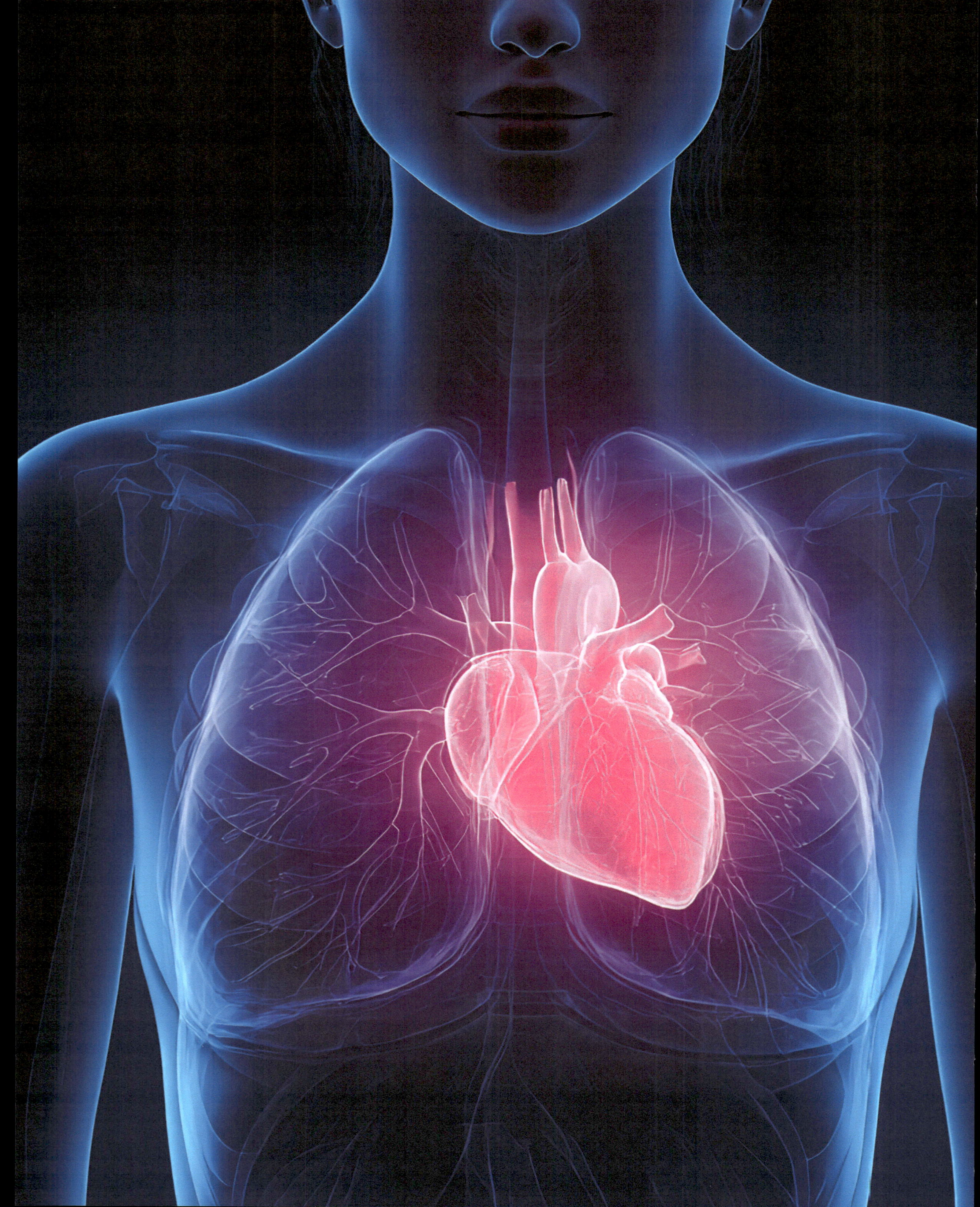

The nervous system

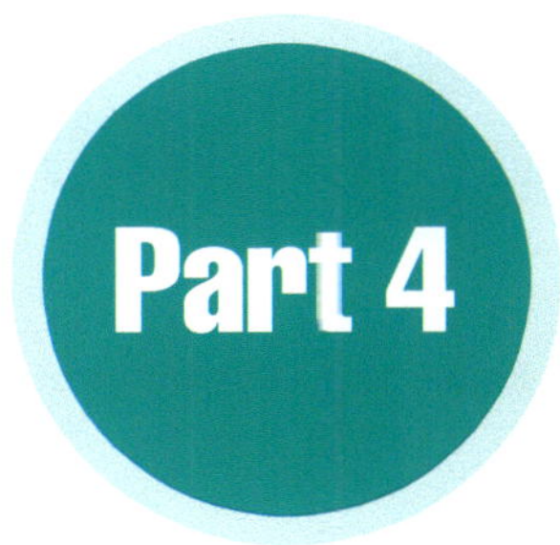

Chapters

13 Meningitis

Figure 13.1 Coverings of the brain.

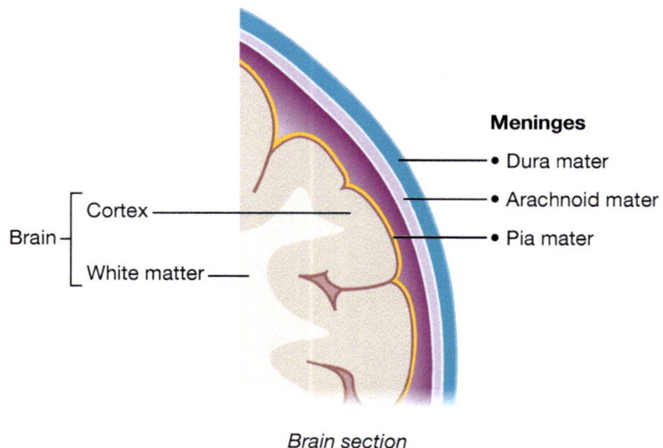

Figure 13.2 Brudzinski's and Kernig's signs.

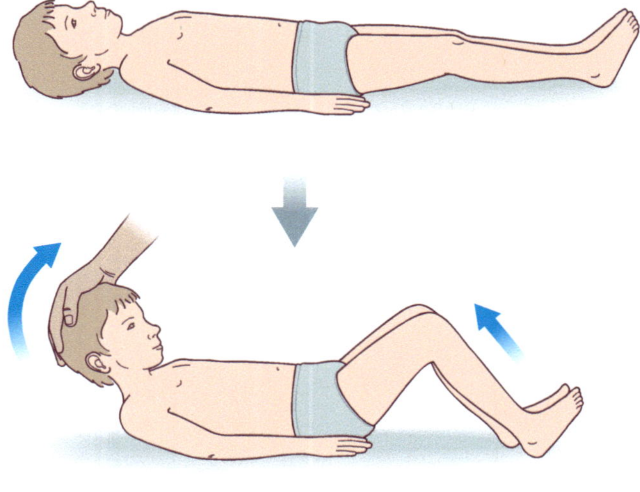

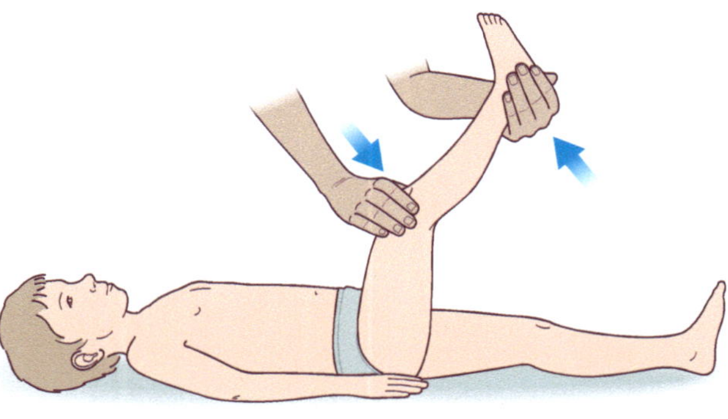

Overview of anatomy and physiology

The meninges are the protective coverings that envelop the brain (Figure 13.1). They serve a dual function: safeguarding the brain by enclosing a fluid-filled space and providing a supportive framework for the cerebral blood vessels. Structurally, the meninges consist of three distinct layers: the dura mater, the arachnoid mater and the pia mater.

The arachnoid mater is connected to the pia mater via delicate, web-like strands of connective tissue known as arachnoid trabeculae. The space between these two layers, termed the subarachnoid space, is occupied by cerebrospinal fluid (CSF), which cushions the brain and maintains a stable chemical environment. Within this space are several widened regions called cisterns, where CSF accumulates, functioning as reservoirs that facilitate circulation and cushioning of the central nervous system.

Pathophysiology

Meningitis is most commonly caused by bacterial or viral pathogens that reach the central nervous system via the bloodstream. In many cases, the infection originates elsewhere in the body, such as the respiratory tract or the pharynx, before spreading through tissues and entering the circulation.

Under normal conditions, the brain is protected by the blood–brain barrier (BBB), a specialised membrane that selectively restricts the passage of potentially harmful substances from the blood into the brain. However, there are several pathogens that can breach this barrier and cause infection of the meninges.

In response to infection, the body's immune system triggers an inflammatory cascade within the meninges. This involves the recruitment of immune cells, the release of inflammatory mediators and increased vascular permeability, all of which contribute to swelling or meningeal oedema. While this response is aimed at containing and eliminating the invading pathogens, the resultant inflammation can have unintended consequences. The swollen meninges can compress adjacent brain tissue and exert pressure on the spinal cord and cranial nerves, disrupting normal neural function. If severe or prolonged, this increased pressure can impair cerebral blood flow, compromise oxygen delivery to neural tissue, and lead to neurological deficits such as altered consciousness, seizures or focal neurological signs. Understanding this balance between protective inflammation and potential neural injury is essential for recognising the pathophysiology of meningitis and guiding timely clinical intervention.

In addition, pathogens may invade the CSF, the clear fluid that cushions and nourishes the brain and spinal cord. Infection of the CSF further amplifies meningeal inflammation and can increase intracranial pressure, the pressure within the skull, which may compress the brain and compromise its function. Understanding these mechanisms is critical for recognising the clinical features of meningitis and the potential complications associated with increased intracranial pressure.

Viral meningitis

Viral meningitis is the most frequently occurring form of meningitis; it is generally less severe than bacterial forms. It can be caused by a variety of viruses, including enteroviruses, the mumps virus and certain mosquito-borne viruses such as West Nile virus. Although symptoms can be uncomfortable and mimic those of more serious infections, viral meningitis is typically self-limiting, with most patients recovering fully without long-term complications. There is no specific treatment for this type of meningitis. In most cases, the illness resolves itself within a week without any complications.

Viral meningitis is most common in children and more widespread during the summer months.

Bacterial meningitis

Bacterial meningitis is generally a serious infection. It is caused by three types of bacteria: *Haemophilus influenzae* type B, *Neisseria meningitidis* and *Streptococcus pneumoniae*. Meningitis caused by *N. meningitidis* is known as meningococcal meningitis, while meningitis caused by *S. pneumoniae* is known as pneumococcal meningitis. Infection occurs when a person comes into close contact with respiratory secretions, such as saliva or nasal discharge, from someone who is infected.

The bacteria then cross the mucus layer and enter the bloodstream. If the body's immune response cannot clear the bacteria at this point, they may start to multiply uncontrollably in the bloodstream, causing severe damage to the lining of the blood vessels and resulting in septicaemia. Bacteria may also invade the CSF and the meninges, which leads to inflammation in this area, resulting in meningitis. A combination of the body's own immune response and toxins produced by the bacteria causes damage to the meninges.

Signs and symptoms

Meningitis is difficult to diagnose. It usually comes on suddenly and can easily be confused with the flu, as many of the symptoms are the same. In cases of suspected meningitis, treatment will usually begin before the diagnosis has been confirmed. This is because some of the tests can take several hours to complete and it could be dangerous to delay treatment for that amount of time.

The person with bacterial meningitis can present with restlessness, agitation, irritability, chills, pyrexia, photophobia, petechial rashes and seizures. Signs of meningeal irritation include stiff neck, positive Brudzinski's sign and positive Kernig's sign (Figure 13.2).

Management

Management of meningitis involves a combination of supportive care, targeted treatment of the causative organism and management of any complications, such as seizures or raised intracranial pressure. Supportive care may include adequate hydration, antipyretics, analgesics and antiemetics.

Viral meningitis is generally self-limiting and this often resolves within 1 to 2 weeks. Patients are usually advised to rest, stay well-hydrated and use analgesics for headache relief. Hospital admission is not always necessary for mild cases; such individuals can be managed at home with rest, symptomatic relief and antiemetics as needed. However, if the symptoms are severe and hospital admission is required, patients may initially receive empirical treatment similar to that for bacterial meningitis, including antibiotics. Once viral meningitis is confirmed, antibiotics are discontinued, and supportive therapy, particularly fluid management, is continued.

The most effective method of preventing meningitis is ensuring that vaccinations are kept up to date. Individuals who are eligible should receive the recommended vaccines, many of which are administered as part of the routine childhood immunisation programme.

Clinical considerations

Ensuring that vaccinations are up to date is the most effective method for preventing meningitis. Routine childhood immunisations, as well as vaccines for adolescents, adults and high-risk groups, protect against the most common bacterial and viral causes. Vaccination not only reduces the likelihood of severe illness and life-threatening complications but also helps prevent outbreaks in the community. While vaccines significantly lower risk, early recognition and prompt treatment remain essential for the rare cases that occur despite immunisation.

14 Multiple sclerosis

Figure 14.1 Neuronal cell with myelin sheath.

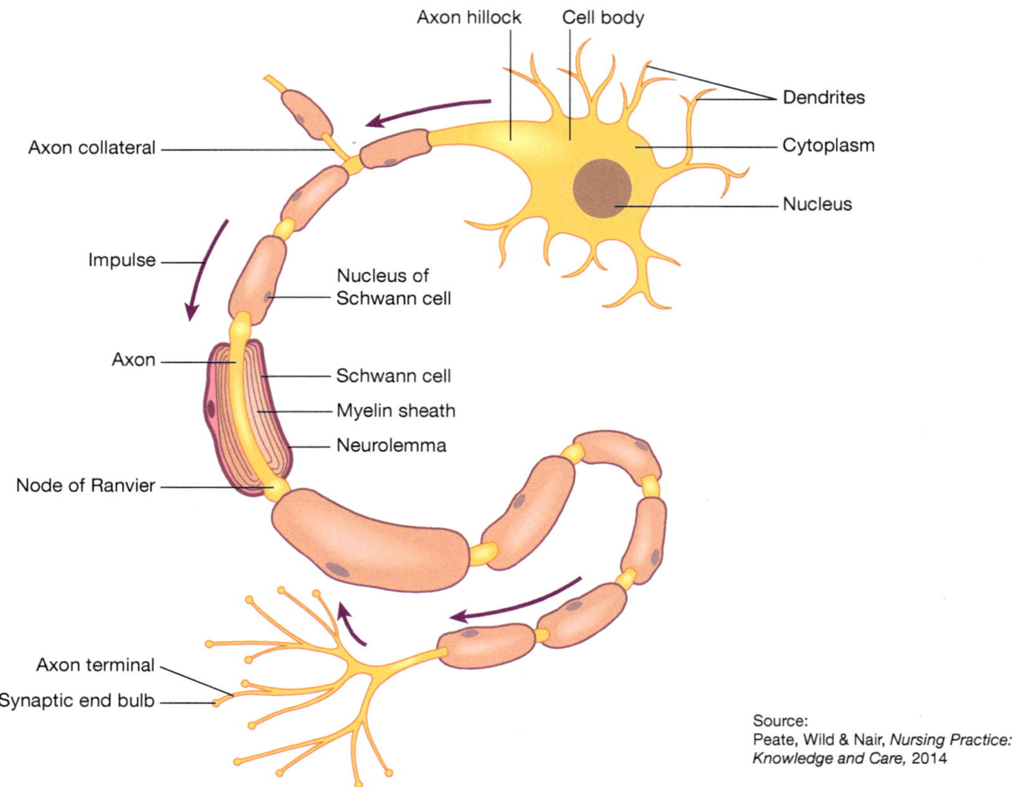

Source:
Peate, Wild & Nair, *Nursing Practice:
Knowledge and Care,* 2014

Figure 14.2 Normal nerve conduction along a myelinated fibre.

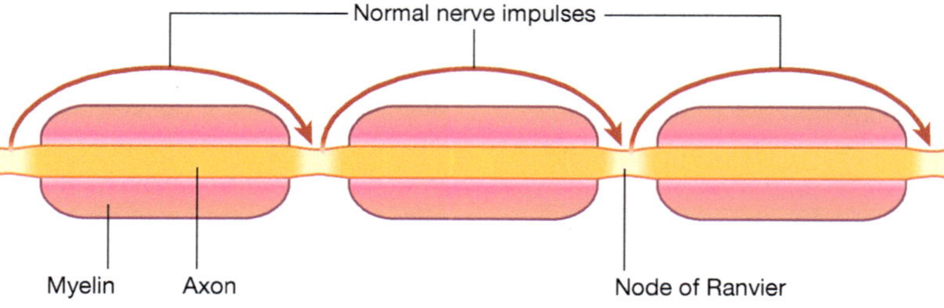

Figure 14.3 Nerve conduction in multiple sclerosis.

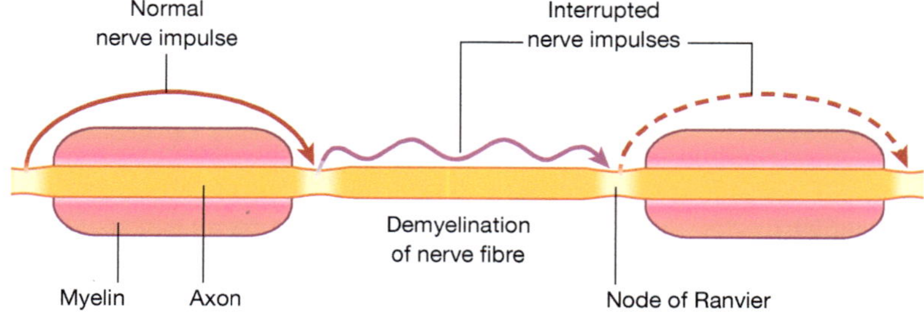

Overview of anatomy and physiology

Multiple sclerosis (MS) is a neurological disorder that affects the nerves of the brain and spinal cord, leading to difficulties with muscle movement, balance and vision. Each nerve fibre within the central nervous system is enveloped by a protective layer of protein that is known as myelin (Figure 14.1). This myelin sheath functions like insulation around an electrical wire, facilitating the efficient transmission of electrical signals, or impulses, from the brain to the rest of the body.

The brain and spinal cord contain thousands of interconnected nerve fibres that communicate through tiny electrical impulses. The myelin sheath is essential for these signals to travel quickly and accurately along each nerve fibre (Figure 14.2). In MS, the immune system mistakenly attacks the myelin, causing it to become damaged or lost. This demyelination disrupts the normal flow of electrical impulses, leading to the characteristic neurological symptoms of the disease, including impaired movement, loss of coordination and visual disturbances.

Pathophysiology

MS is considered an autoimmune disease, in which the body's immune system, which normally defends against infections, mistakenly attacks the central nervous system. During periods of disease activity, immune cells, particularly T cells, along with B cells and macrophages, target the myelin sheath surrounding nerve fibres in the brain and spinal cord. This immune attack leads to localised inflammation, disrupting the normal function of affected nerves and giving rise to neurological symptoms.

In some cases, the myelin sheath can repair itself through remyelination, allowing nerve fibres to regain function. However, repeated or severe bouts of inflammation can result in permanent damage. The affected areas develop small scars, known as sclerosis or plaques, where myelin and oligodendrocytes (the cells responsible for producing myelin) are destroyed. These plaques are typically scattered throughout the brain and spinal cord, and they vary in size and location, which contributes to the diversity of symptoms that are seen in MS.

Demyelination, together with plaque formation and glial scarring, impairs the conduction of electrical impulses along axons. Over time, this process can lead to axonal degeneration, which is a major contributor to the irreversible neurological deficits observed in those people with MS (Figure 14.3).

Signs and symptoms

MS causes a wide variety of symptoms. Many people experience only a few symptoms, and it is very unlikely that a person will develop all the symptoms that are described here. Symptoms of MS are usually unpredictable.

In some individuals, symptoms may progressively worsen over time. More commonly, symptoms come and go at different times. Periods when symptoms worsen are known as relapses. Periods when symptoms improve (or even disappear altogether) are called remissions.

Relapses can occur at any time, and symptoms may differ within each relapse. Although MS relapses often occur without an obvious cause, certain factors may trigger or exacerbate symptoms, including infections, physical exertion and exposure to heat. The symptoms that occur during a relapse depend on which part, or parts, of the brain or spinal cord are affected. Patients may have just one symptom in one part of the body or several symptoms in different parts of the body. The neurological symptoms of MS occur as a result of impaired nerve function, caused by damage to the myelin sheath and, in some cases, the underlying axons.

Diagnosis

Diagnosis of MS is challenging because the disease presents variably and there is no single definitive test available. Diagnosis is made based on a combination of clinical history, neurological examination, MRI evidence of demyelinating lesions, cerebrospinal fluid analysis for oligoclonal bands, and, in some cases, evoked potential testing, which may reveal delayed nerve conduction.

Management

Many individuals who are living with MS are able to manage their condition at home and maintain an active, independent life. Hospital admission is usually required only when the disease worsens or complications arise, such as respiratory infections or difficulties in daily self-care.

The disease process affects young adults; MS most commonly develops in young adults, typically between the ages of 20 and 40 years. The psychological and economic effects can be devastating for the patient and their relatives. Individuals with MS often need to adapt to changes in physical function while learning to manage the broader effects of the disease. The unpredictable course of MS demands that healthcare professionals remain flexible, vigilant and responsive to changes in symptoms, functional abilities and patient needs.

Interventions for individuals with MS are tailored to their coping strategies as well as those of their family or carers. Many nursing interventions focus on supporting the person with tasks of daily living that may be affected by the disease.

The person with MS may complain of fatigue with or without exertion. Fatigue affects every aspect of a person's life. Those offering care and support to people with MS can help the individual and their family to understand how to prevent fatigue and exacerbations. Daily routines for individuals with MS may incorporate periods of rest and activities that promote psychological relaxation. It is also important to advise patients to avoid extreme temperatures, as exposure to heat or cold can impair nerve conduction along demyelinated neurons, contributing to increased fatigue.

Maintaining mobility plays a large part in being independent. The person with MS may need assistance, depending on the advancement of the disease, in undertaking short walks, for example. Healthcare providers should work as a team with the patient at the centre of all that is done to encourage a positive outlook, while taking time to understand the patients and their relatives' fears and feelings.

Individuals with MS and their families should be educated on the importance of regular skin inspection to prevent pressure-related injuries. Particular attention should be paid to common pressure points, such as the sacrum and heels, looking for early signs of redness or blanching. If such changes are observed, the person should be encouraged to take measures to relieve pressure, such as repositioning, using cushions or pressure-relieving devices and ensuring that skin remains clean and dry. Regular monitoring and timely interventions can help prevent the development of pressure ulcers and associated complications.

15 Parkinson's disease

Figure 15.1 Anatomy of the brain showing the position of the substantia nigra.

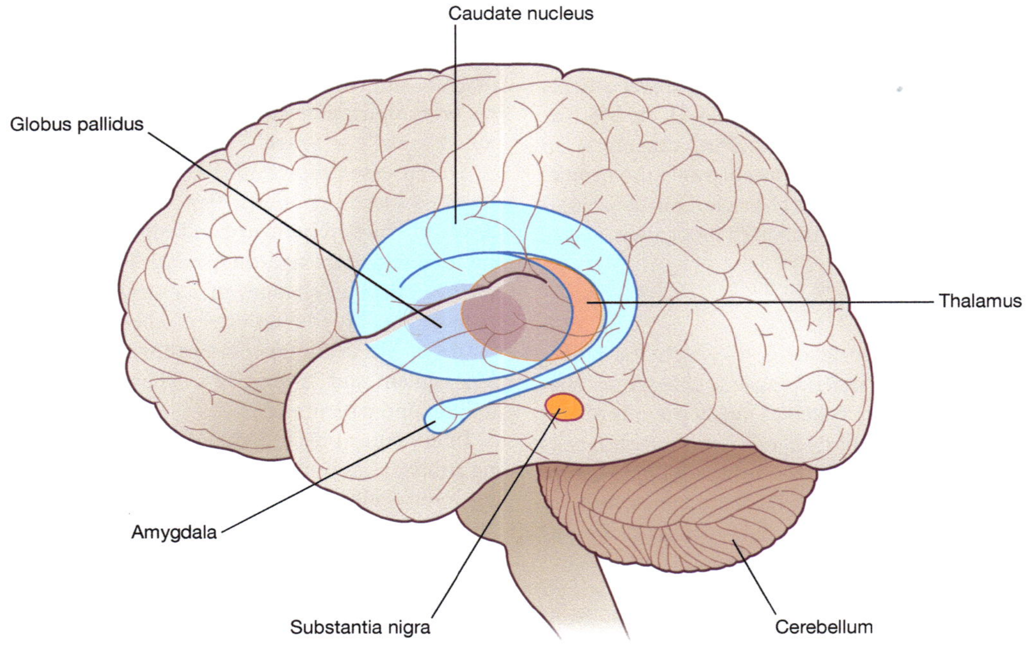

Table 15.1 Treatment modalities for Parkinson's disease.

Treatment type	Examples/approach	Purpose/effect
Medications	Levodopa/carbidopa, dopamine agonists, monoamine oxidase B inhibitors, catechol-O-methyltransferase inhibitors and anticholinergics	Replace or enhance dopamine, reduce motor symptoms such as bradykinesia, rigidity and tremor
Surgical treatments	Deep brain stimulation and lesioning procedures (e.g., pallidotomy and thalamotomy)	Improve motor control, reduce tremor, rigidity and medication-related fluctuations
Physiotherapy/exercise	Balance and gait training, strength exercises and stretching	Improve mobility, reduce stiffness and maintain independence
Occupational therapy	Task adaptation, use of assistive devices and home modifications	Support daily activities and maintain independence
Speech and language therapy	Voice exercises, swallowing strategies and communication aids	Improve speech clarity and address swallowing difficulties
Psychological/social support	Counselling, support groups and cognitive behavioural therapy	Address anxiety, depression and cognitive changes
Dietary/nutritional support	High-fibre diet, hydration and protein management with medications	Reduce constipation, maintain energy and optimise medication effectiveness

Overview of anatomy and physiology

Parkinson's disease is a chronic (persistent or long-term) disorder of part of the brain. It is named after the doctor who first described it. It mainly affects the way the brain coordinates the movements of the muscles in various parts of the body. A small part of the brain called the substantia nigra (Figure 15.1) is mainly affected. This area of the brain sends messages down nerves in the spinal cord, helping to control the muscles of the body. Messages are passed between brain cells, nerves and muscles by chemicals known as neurotransmitters. Dopamine is the main neurotransmitter made by the brain cells in the substantia nigra.

In Parkinson's disease, a number of cells in the substantia nigra become damaged, and they die. The exact cause of this is not known. Over time, more and more cells become damaged and die. As cells are damaged, the amount of dopamine that is produced is reduced. A combination of the reduction of cells and a low level of dopamine in the cells in this part of the brain causes nerve messages to the muscles to become slowed and to behave abnormally.

Pathophysiology

Dopamine is a crucial chemical messenger that facilitates communication between two key brain regions: the substantia nigra and the corpus striatum. This communication is essential for producing smooth and coordinated movement. In Parkinson's disease, the majority of movement-related symptoms have arisen from a deficiency of dopamine, caused by the gradual loss of dopamine-producing neurones in the substantia nigra. When dopamine levels fall, the signalling between the substantia nigra and corpus striatum becomes disrupted, leading to impaired movement. The severity of motor symptoms, such as tremor, rigidity and bradykinesia, generally correlates with the extent of dopamine loss.

Parkinson's disease also affects other brain cells, albeit to a lesser extent, and these changes may contribute to the non-motor symptoms of the condition, including cognitive decline, mood disturbances and autonomic dysfunction.

Although the link between dopamine deficiency and motor symptoms is well established, the precise reason why these neurones degenerate remains unclear. Research suggests that a combination of genetic vulnerabilities, cellular dysfunction, inflammation and oxidative stress may contribute to neuronal damage. Additionally, many affected neurones contain Lewy bodies, abnormal clumps composed primarily of the protein alpha-synuclein. The role of Lewy bodies in Parkinson's disease is not fully understood, but their presence is a hallmark of the condition.

Overall, it is thought that the progressive loss of dopamine results from a complex interplay of genetic and environmental factors rather than a single cause, highlighting the multifactorial nature of Parkinson's disease.

Signs and symptoms

The brain cells and nerves affected in Parkinson's disease normally help to produce smooth, coordinated movements of muscles. Therefore, three common Parkinson's symptoms that gradually develop are:

- **Slowness of movement** (bradykinesia). For example, the person may find it is becoming more of an effort to walk or to get up out of a chair. When this first develops, it may be mistaken for 'getting on in years', a normal consequence of old age. The diagnosis of Parkinson's disease may not become apparent unless other symptoms occur. In time, a typical walking pattern will often develop. This is a 'shuffling' type of walk with some difficulty in starting, stopping and turning easily.
- **Stiffness of muscles** (rigidity). Muscles become stiff and resistant to movement, often giving a tense feeling. This can affect the arms, legs and trunk and may reduce the natural arm swing while walking.
- **Shaking** (tremor) is common, but this does not always occur. It typically affects the fingers, thumbs, hands and arms but can affect other parts of the body. It is most noticeable when the person is resting. It may become worse when the individual is anxious or emotional. It tends to become less when the hand is being used to do something, such as picking up an object.

Symptoms usually progress slowly over time. However, the speed at which symptoms become worse will vary from person to person. It may take several years before they become bad enough to have much effect on daily life. At first, one side of the body may be more affected than the other.

Management

In the early stages of Parkinson's disease, many symptoms can be managed by primary care (GP) with support from family members and community care professionals. The disease progresses differently in each person, and most individuals can continue to live at home with appropriate care. Hospital admission is usually only required if complications develop, such as falls, infections or symptoms that cannot be safely managed in the community.

Nurses and other healthcare professionals, including physiotherapists, speech and language therapists and occupational therapists, can support patients and their families by providing practical advice and strategies to manage challenges that affect daily activities.

As Parkinson's disease progresses, mobility often becomes increasingly impaired. This may manifest as difficulty initiating or stopping walking, shuffling steps, unsteady or tottering gait, impaired balance and an increased risk of falls. Those who offer care and support should closely monitor individuals with Parkinson's disease and implement appropriate safety measures to minimise the risk of injury associated with impaired mobility.

Physiotherapy can help improve gait, balance and flexibility, aerobic activity and movement initiation, increase independence and provide advice about fall prevention and other safety information. Avoid walking frames (flow of movement is interrupted) unless fitted with wheels and a brake.

Occupational therapists may offer advice and help on maintaining all aspects relating to activities of daily living, both at work and at home, with the aim of maintaining work and family relationships, encouraging self-care where appropriate, assessing any safety issues, making cognitive assessments and arranging any appropriate interventions.

Speech therapy ensures methods of communication are available as the disease progresses and helps with swallowing difficulties (reducing the risk of aspiration).

Parkinson's disease management is multidisciplinary, combining medications, surgical options, rehabilitation therapies and psychosocial support to optimise quality of life and function (see Table 15.1).

Clinical considerations

Recent advances in Parkinson's disease focus on earlier detection through biomarkers and advanced imaging, as well as the development of disease-modifying therapies targeting neurodegeneration. Improvements in deep brain stimulation, continuous drug delivery and wearable monitoring devices are enhancing symptom management. There is a growing emphasis on personalised care tailored to an individual's genetics, symptoms and lifestyle, supported by multidisciplinary interventions, including physiotherapy, occupational therapy, speech therapy and mental health support.

16 Stroke

Figure 16.1 Blood flow through the brain.

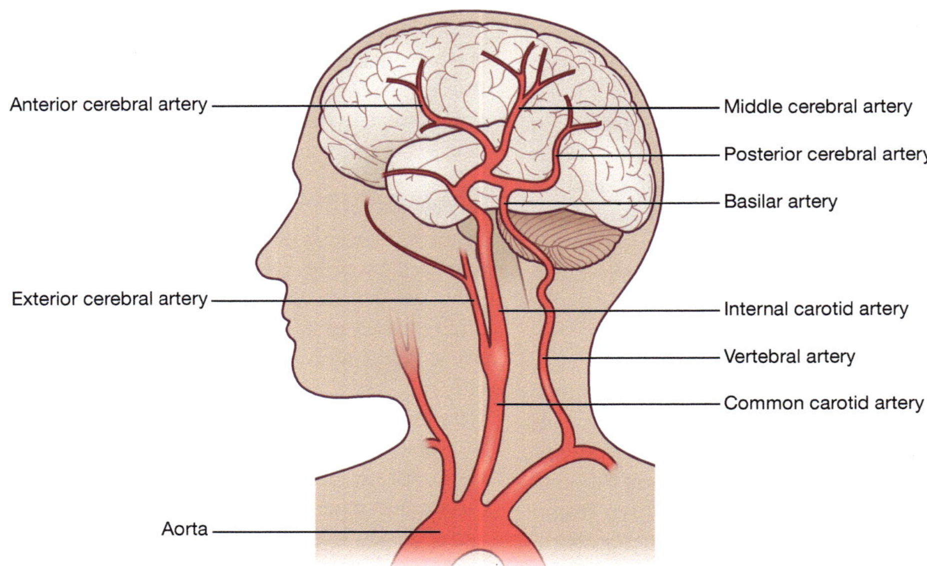

Figure 16.2 Ischaemia of brain tissue following vessel blockage.

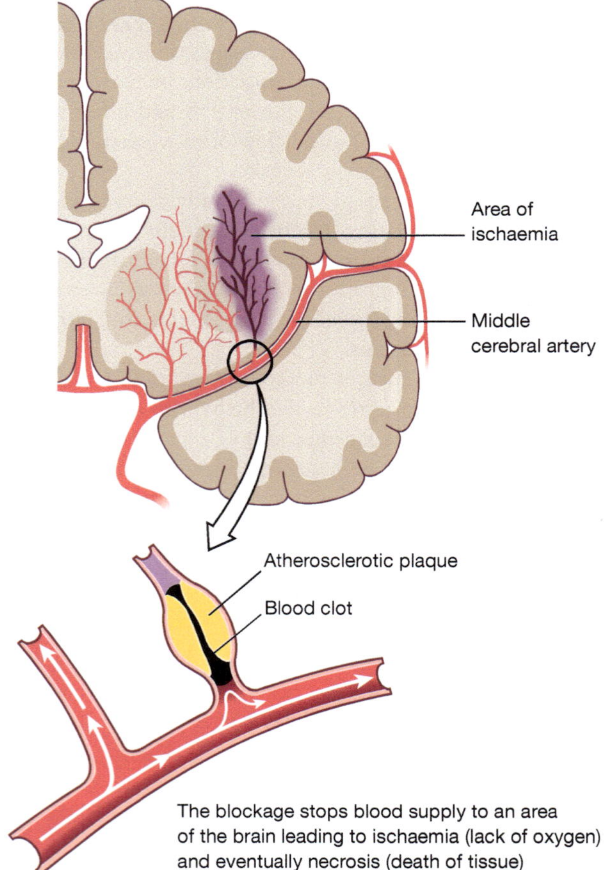

Figure 16.3 Haemorrhagic stroke.

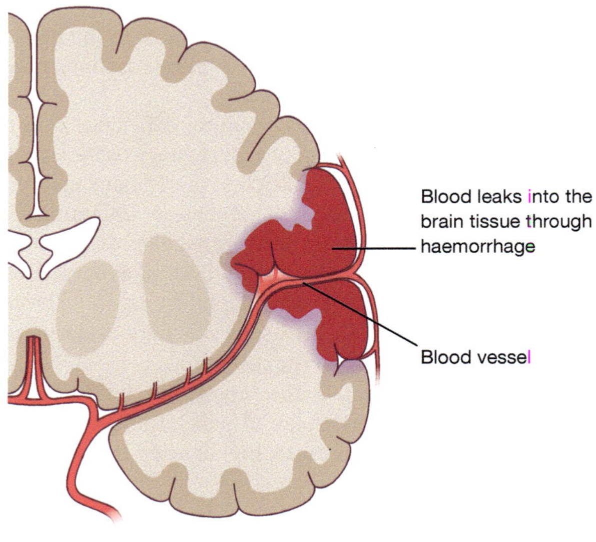

Overview of anatomy and physiology

Blood is supplied to the brain, face and scalp via two major sets of vessels: the right and left common carotid arteries and the right and left vertebral arteries (Figure 16.1).

In an adult, cerebral blood flow is typically 750 mL per minute or 15% of the cardiac output. This equates to 50–54 mL of blood per 100 g of brain tissue per minute. Too much blood (a condition known as hyperaemia) can raise intracranial pressure, which can compress and damage delicate brain tissue. Cerebral ischaemia occurs when blood flow to the brain falls below approximately 18–20 mL per 100 g of brain tissue per minute. Prolonged reduction below 10 mL per 100 g per minute can lead to irreversible neuronal injury and tissue death.

Cerebral blood flow is determined by a number of factors, such as the viscosity of blood, how dilated blood vessels are and the net pressure of the flow of blood into the brain, known as cerebral perfusion pressure, which is determined by the body's blood pressure. Cerebral blood vessels are able to change the flow of blood by altering diameters, in a process called autoregulation; they constrict when systemic blood pressure is raised and dilate when it is lowered. Arterioles also constrict and dilate in response to different chemical concentrations. For example, they dilate in response to higher levels of carbon dioxide in the blood.

Pathophysiology

A stroke, which may also be referred to as a cerebrovascular accident, occurs when there is a sudden interruption of blood flow to specific regions of the brain. This may result from an arterial blockage due to a thrombus or embolus, narrowing of the cerebral vessels, or rupture of a blood vessel. Strokes are broadly classified into two main types: ischaemic and haemorrhagic.

Ischaemic

This is the most common form of a stroke (80%), caused by blockage of blood flow to the brain by a blood clot (thrombus). Blood clots typically form in areas where the arteries have been narrowed or they are blocked by fatty cholesterol-containing deposits that are known as plaques (Figure 16.2).

Atrial fibrillation is a recognised cause of ischaemic stroke; this increases the risk of thrombus formation in the atria, which can dislodge and cause an ischaemic stroke.

Haemorrhagic

Haemorrhagic strokes (also known as cerebral haemorrhages or intracranial haemorrhages) usually occur when a blood vessel in the brain ruptures and bleeds into the brain (Figure 16.3). In about 5% of cases, the bleeding occurs on the surface of the brain (subarachnoid haemorrhage). Haemorrhagic stroke can also occur from the rupture of a balloon-like expansion of a blood vessel (aneurysm) and badly formed blood vessels in the brain.

Signs and symptoms

A stroke is the sudden onset of weakness, numbness, paralysis, slurred speech, aphasia, problems with vision and other manifestations of a sudden interruption of blood flow to a particular area of the brain. The ischaemic area involved determines the type of focal deficit that is seen in the patient. The FAST test is an easy way to remember the most common signs of stroke. Using the FAST test involves asking these simple questions:

F – Face: Ask the person to smile. Does one side of the face droop?
A – Arm: Ask the person to raise both arms. Does one arm drift downward?
S – Speech: Ask the person to repeat a simple phrase. Is the speech slurred or strange?
T – Time: If you see any of these signs, call 999 straight away.

Other symptoms may include motor deficits, depending on the brain region affected, resulting in hemiplegia or paralysis of one side of the body, hemiparesis, flaccidity or spasticity; behavioural changes; communication disorders; bladder and bowel dysfunction; and visual disturbances. Emotional and cognitive effects can include confusion, depression and impaired control or disinhibition.

Management

Management depends on the type of stroke. Treatment and care should take into account people's needs and preferences. People with acute stroke or transient ischaemic attack should have the opportunity, where possible, to make informed decisions about their care and treatment, in partnership with their healthcare professionals.

Effective communication between healthcare professionals and people with acute stroke or transient ischaemic attack, as well as their families and carers, is essential. It should be supported by evidence-based written information tailored to the person's needs. Treatment and care, and the information people are given about it, should be culturally appropriate.

Medication

This may include anticoagulants, antihypertensives and statin drugs. Heparin, warfarin and rivaroxaban are examples of anticoagulants. Medicines that are commonly used include thiazide diuretics, angiotensin-converting enzyme (ACE) inhibitors, calcium channel blockers and beta-blockers. Statins reduce the level of cholesterol in the blood.

Thrombolysis is a time-critical treatment for acute ischaemic stroke, aimed at dissolving the clot and restoring cerebral blood flow. Rapid recognition of stroke symptoms, such as sudden weakness, numbness, facial droop, speech difficulties or visual disturbances, is essential, as thrombolysis is most effective when administered within a narrow window from symptom onset, typically within 4.5 hours. Immediate activation of emergency protocols, prompt neuroimaging to confirm eligibility, and careful assessment of contraindications are vital. Early intervention with thrombolysis can significantly reduce neurological damage and improve functional outcomes, highlighting the importance of speed in both recognition and treatment.

Rehabilitation

After a stroke, the person may need to relearn skills and abilities or learn new ways of doing things to adapt to the damage a stroke has caused. This is known as stroke rehabilitation. It is difficult to predict the time it will take for someone to recover from a stroke, but the recovery can continue for a long time depending on the severity of the stroke.

Health professionals (e.g. physiotherapists, speech and language therapists, occupational therapists, ophthalmologists and psychologists, as well as doctors and nurses) will work out a rehabilitation programme.

Surgery

Surgery may be performed to prevent the occurrence of the stroke, to restore blood flow if the stroke has occurred and to repair vascular damage.

Prevention

Promoting a healthy lifestyle is fundamental for the prevention of cardiovascular and cerebrovascular disease. A diet low in saturated fats and rich in fibre is recommended, including at least five portions of fresh fruit and vegetables per day and incorporating whole grains. Regular physical activity, when combined with a balanced diet, is the most effective strategy for maintaining a healthy body weight. Achieving and sustaining a healthy weight helps reduce the risk of developing high blood pressure and other associated cardiovascular conditions.

Clinical considerations

Stroke is a medical emergency, and rapid recognition and intervention are essential to improve outcomes. Early signs may include sudden weakness or numbness on one side of the body, facial droop, speech difficulties, visual disturbances or severe headache. Timely treatment, such as thrombolysis or thrombectomy, is most effective when initiated within hours of symptom onset. Immediate action involves activating emergency protocols, ensuring basic life support and expediting neuroimaging. Continuous monitoring of neurological status, vital signs and early management of complications is critical for optimal patient care.

The blood

Chapters

17 Anaemia

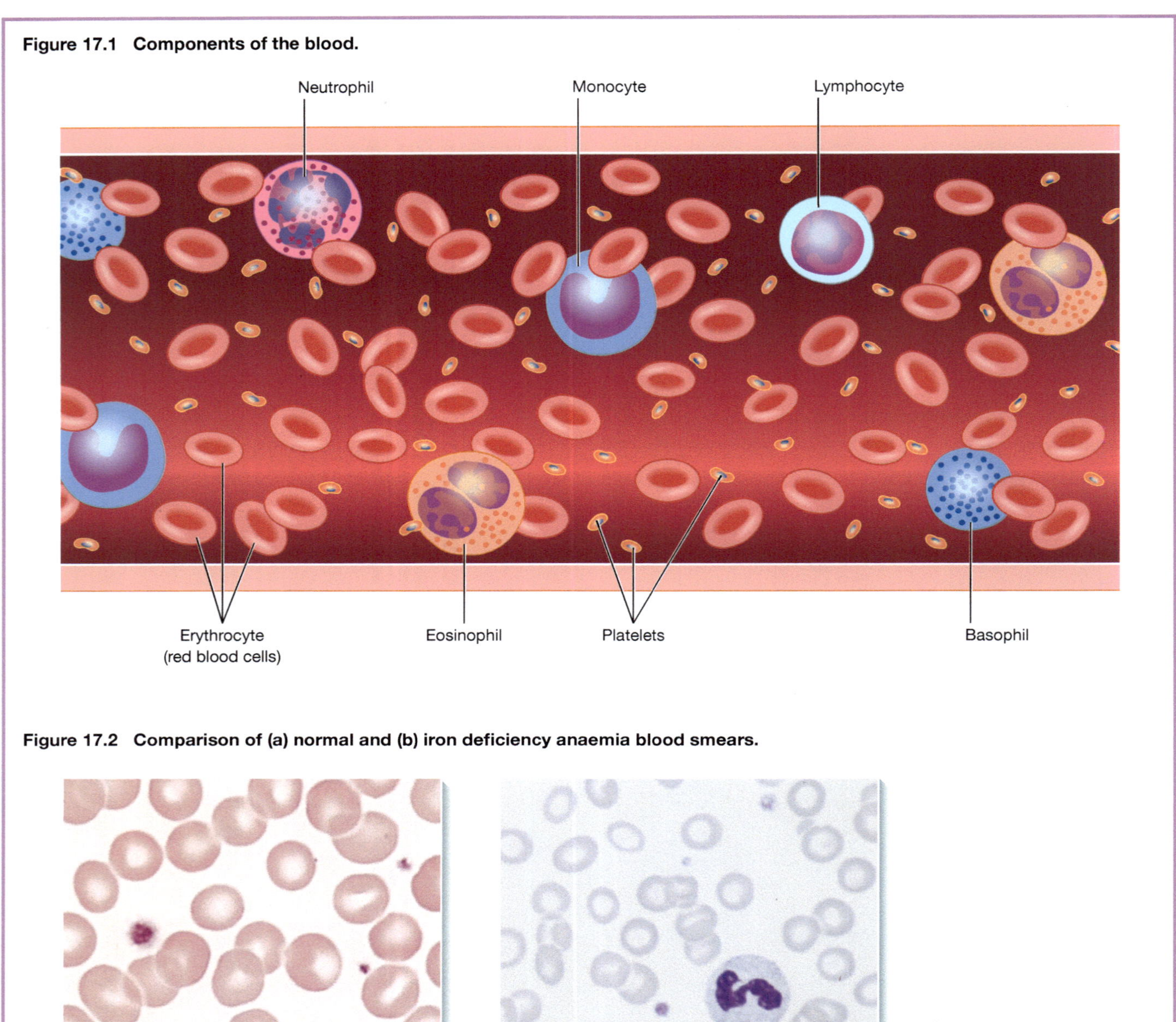

Figure 17.1 Components of the blood.

Figure 17.2 Comparison of (a) normal and (b) iron deficiency anaemia blood smears.

Overview of anatomy and physiology

Blood consists of plasma and various cellular components. The cellular elements include erythrocytes (red blood cells), leukocytes (white blood cells) and thrombocytes (platelets), all of which are suspended within the plasma along with other particulate matter (Figure 17.1). Plasma is a clear, straw-coloured fluid that accounts for more than half of the total blood volume. The viscosity of blood (related to its thickness), which ranges from 3.5 to 5.5 compared with 1.000 for water (meaning blood is 3.5 to 5.5 times more viscous than water), is primarily influenced by the presence of red blood cells and plasma proteins. When there is an increase in the concentration of these components, this results in higher viscosity along with a slower rate of blood flow.

Plasma, which is the liquid part of the blood, is composed of water (91%), protein (8%) (albumin, globulin, prothrombin and fibrinogen), salts (0.9%) (sodium chloride, sodium bicarbonate and others), and the remaining 0.1% is made up of a range of organic materials (e.g. fats, glucose, urea, uric acid, cholesterol and amino acids). These dissolved substances give plasma a greater density and viscosity than water.

Plasma proteins make up 7% of the plasma and these proteins stay in the blood vessel, as they are too large to diffuse through capillaries and are responsible for creating the osmotic pressure of blood. When plasma proteins are lost, as occurs in patients with severe burns, fluid shifts from the bloodstream into the surrounding tissues by osmosis, leading to the development of oedema.

Pathophysiology

Anaemia is a condition in which the haemoglobin concentration in the blood is below the normal range, or when the number of red blood cells is reduced. There are several types of anaemia, each has its own distinct cause. The most common form is iron-deficiency anaemia, while other types include vitamin B_{12} deficiency anaemia and aplastic anaemia.

Iron deficiency anaemia

Iron-deficiency anaemia develops when the body lacks sufficient iron, leading to a reduced number of red blood cells (Figure 17.2). Iron is present in foods such as red meat, poultry, lentils, beans and leafy green vegetables. The body uses iron in order to produce haemoglobin, which enables the red blood cells to carry and store oxygen. Any excess iron is stored in the liver, spleen and muscle tissue, where it can be mobilised for red blood cell production as required. Certain conditions, including inflammatory bowel disease or coeliac disease, can impair iron absorption from the gastrointestinal tract, thereby affecting red blood cell synthesis.

Vitamin B_{12}/Folate deficiency anaemia

Pernicious anaemia is the most common cause of vitamin B_{12} deficiency in the UK. Pernicious anaemia is an autoimmune condition that affects the stomach, impairing the production of intrinsic factor, which is essential for vitamin B_{12} absorption. An autoimmune condition means the immune system (the body's natural defence system that protects against illness and infection) attacks the body's healthy cells. In pernicious anaemia, the immune system attacks the stomach cells responsible for producing intrinsic factor. This means the body cannot absorb vitamin B_{12}, which causes a deficiency.

Vitamin B_{12} and folate work together, supporting red blood cell production. Vitamin B_{12} is also essential for maintaining a healthy nervous system, including the brain, nerves and spinal cord. Folate is particularly important during pregnancy, as it helps reduce the risk of birth defects in the developing baby.

Aplastic anaemia

Aplastic anaemia is a rare, potentially life-threatening failure of haematopoiesis (the process by which the body produces blood cells), characterised by pancytopaenia (a reduction in all three major types of blood cells) and a hypocellular bone marrow. Aplastic anaemia is diagnosed when the bone marrow is underpopulated and the blood shows low counts of all cell types, but there is no cancer, infection or scarring causing the problem.

Most cases are acquired and immune-mediated, although inherited forms also exist. Environmental triggers include certain drugs, viruses and toxins, but many cases remain idiopathic (cause unknown). Drugs associated with aplastic anaemia include some antiepileptics (e.g. carbamazepine), non-steroidal anti-inflammatory drugs (e.g. ibuprofen) and chemotherapy agents. Exposure to chemicals such as benzene can also increase the risk.

In aplastic anaemia, the person may experience increasing fatigue, weakness and shortness of breath. Bleeding, easy bruising and small red or purple spots on the skin (petechiae) may be observed. Frequent infections, such as sore throats, can also occur. Pyrexia that is accompanied by shivering is a serious symptom that requires immediate medical attention.

Signs and symptoms of anaemia

The symptoms of anaemia vary depending on its underlying cause. However, some general symptoms are common to most types, including fatigue, shortness of breath, lethargy, dizziness or fainting, tinnitus, headache, hair loss (alopecia), constipation and reduced appetite.

Management

The management of anaemia will depend on the type. Iron-deficiency anaemia is usually treated with oral iron supplements, and in less common cases, iron may be given parenterally (by injection). Common preparations include ferrous gluconate and ferrous sulphate. Before giving iron, checks should be made to ensure it will not interfere with other medicines that the patient is taking and that other medicines will not reduce the effectiveness of the iron, such as antacids, certain antibiotics (e.g. tetracyclines) and thyroid medications. Liquid iron preparations can stain the teeth; patients should be informed of this. Side effects of iron tablets may include constipation, passing black stools and dysphagia; laxatives may be required to help manage constipation.

Folic acid supplements are used to restore folate levels and are generally taken for about four months. Patients should also receive guidance on iron-rich foods, such as red meat, leafy green vegetables and fortified cereals. Polyphenols in tea and coffee can reduce iron absorption, so patients should be advised to limit these beverages until iron levels are restored.

Those patients who are unable to obtain adequate vitamin B_{12} from their diet, such as vegans, may require lifelong supplementation to prevent deficiency.

18 Venous thromboembolism

Figure 18.1   A normal vein with blood flow and a vein with a thrombus.

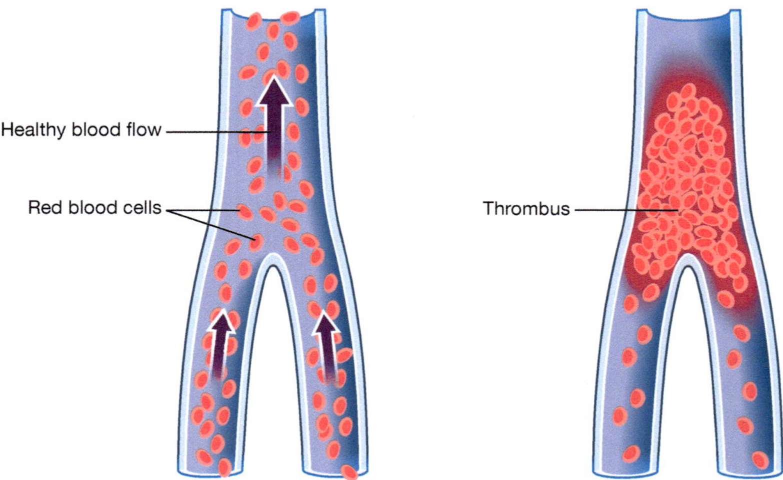

Figure 18.2   Capillaries.

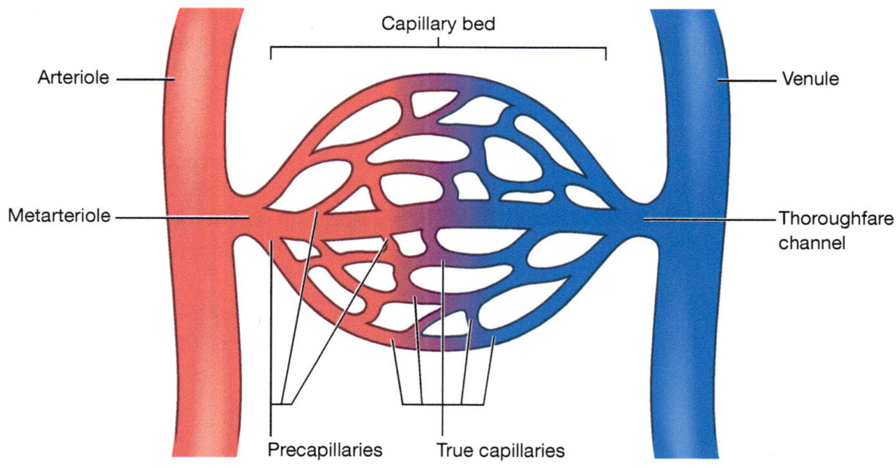

Figure 18.3   Smear of blood with platelet.

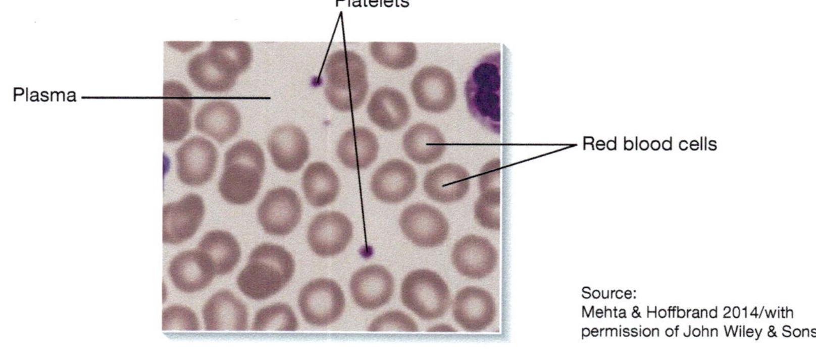

Source:
Mehta & Hoffbrand 2014/with
permission of John Wiley & Sons

Overview of anatomy and physiology

Venous thromboembolism (VTE) is a condition characterised by the formation of a blood clot in the venous system, most commonly in the legs, but it can also occur in the arms or other veins. VTE encompasses deep vein thrombosis (DVT) and pulmonary embolism (PE), which represent different manifestations of the same pathological process. A serious complication occurs when part of a thrombus dislodges and travels to the lungs, resulting in PE, which can be life-threatening (see Figure 18.1).

Blood circulates through the body in a closed-loop system, pumped by the heart. In the pulmonary circulation, the right side of the heart sends deoxygenated blood to the lungs for oxygenation, while in the systemic circulation, the left side of the heart distributes oxygenated blood to the body's tissues. Both sides of the heart circulate an equivalent volume of blood per minute, known as cardiac output.

In systemic circulation, blood leaves the left ventricle via the aorta, which branches into progressively smaller arteries and arterioles, eventually reaching the capillaries. Capillaries, which are the smallest and most numerous blood vessels in the human body (ranging from 5 to 10 μm in diameter and numbering around 10 billion), are also the thinnest-walled vessels; an inner diameter of 5 μm is just wide enough for an erythrocyte to squeeze through (Figure 18.2). After exchanging gases, nutrients and waste products with tissues, blood returns to the heart via venules and veins.

This venous return is particularly important in the context of VTE, as blood flow in veins is slower than in arteries and is influenced by gravity, especially in the lower limbs. Slow or stagnant blood flow, combined with vein valve structure and immobility, can contribute to venous stasis, a key factor in the formation of venous thrombi. Understanding this normal circulation helps explain why clots commonly form in the deep veins of the legs and how they can travel to the lungs, causing PE.

Pathophysiology

The mechanism of thrombus formation in veins is described by **Virchow's triad**, first proposed in the mid-19th century. This triad identifies three interrelated factors:

1 **Endothelial injury** – damage to the vein wall from trauma, surgery or inflammation exposes subendothelial collagen and triggers platelet adhesion.
2 **Venous stasis** – slowed or stagnant blood flow, often due to immobility or prolonged bed rest, allows clotting factors to accumulate.
3 **Hypercoagulability** – changes in blood composition, such as elevated clotting factors or reduced natural anticoagulants, increase the risk of spontaneous clot formation.

Thrombi form when platelets adhere to exposed collagen and release chemical mediators such as adenosine diphosphate (ADP) and thromboxane, which promote further platelet aggregation (see Figure 18.3). Fibrin then traps red blood cells, causing the clot to grow. A thrombus can develop in the superficial or deep veins of the legs. The blood flow is sluggish in the affected vessels and clotting cascade takes place. Platelets aggregate at the site of injury to the vessel wall or where there is venous stasis. Clots may remain stable in the vein or embolise, potentially causing PE, a serious and sometimes fatal complication.

Signs and symptoms

Most of the time, VTE may not present with any symptoms. The person may present with swelling of the limb, which is often unilateral. There may be localised tenderness or pain, especially in the calf or thigh. Warmth, redness or a feeling of heaviness in the affected limb can occur. Occasionally, the patient may present with low-grade pyrexia. PE often presents in a more dramatic manner; see Chapter 27 of this book.

Early recognition is critical to reduce morbidity and mortality. Clinical assessment tools such as the Wells Score can help quantify pre-test probability, while D-dimer testing and imaging (ultrasound for DVT, CT pulmonary angiography for PE) confirm the diagnosis.

Management

Contemporary management of VTE integrates anticoagulation, mechanical support and lifestyle measures. Anticoagulant medicines prevent a blood clot from getting bigger; they remain the cornerstone of therapy. Anticoagulation can also help stop part of the blood clot from breaking off and becoming lodged in another part of the bloodstream (an embolism). Although they are often referred to as 'blood-thinning' medicines, anticoagulants do not actually thin the blood. They alter chemicals within it, which prevents the clots from forming so easily.

There are different types of anticoagulants that are used to treat VTE: heparin, warfarin and long-term direct oral anticoagulant therapy. Heparin is usually prescribed first, as it works immediately to prevent further clot extension. After this initial treatment, the patient may also need to take long-term therapy to prevent another blood clot from forming.

Warfarin is taken as a tablet. It may be taken after an initial heparin treatment to prevent further blood clots from occurring. It is usually recommended that warfarin be taken for 3–6 months. In some cases, warfarin may need to be taken for longer, even for life.

Graduated compression stockings may help prevent calf pain and swelling and lower the risk of ulcers developing after having a DVT. They can also help prevent post-thrombotic syndrome – damage to the tissue of the calf caused by the increase in venous pressure that occurs when a vein is blocked (by a clot) and blood is diverted to the outer veins. The person wearing them must be assessed fully before wearing the stockings. Intermittent pneumatic compression devices can be used for those patients with contraindications to pharmacological prophylaxis.

VTE is a complex, multifactorial condition with potentially serious consequences. Contemporary practice emphasises the importance of early recognition through careful risk assessment and clinical vigilance; timely identification can prevent progression and complications. Management includes prompt anticoagulation using low molecular weight heparin, direct oral anticoagulants or warfarin, as appropriate, alongside the use of mechanical support and encouragement of mobility to reduce the risk of recurrence. Equally important is patient information and ongoing monitoring for complications, including post-thrombotic syndrome and recurrent VTE.

Clinical considerations

Careful risk assessment is essential to identify patients at increased risk of VTE, such as those who are immobile, recovering from surgery or have underlying hypercoagulable conditions. Encouraging early mobilisation and leg exercises can reduce venous stasis, while pharmacological prophylaxis with anticoagulants, such as low molecular weight heparin or direct oral anticoagulants, should be administered according to clinical guidelines for at-risk patients. For those who cannot receive anticoagulation, mechanical measures, including graduated compression stockings or intermittent pneumatic compression devices, are valuable in reducing the risk of thrombus formation. Providing patients with information is also critical, ensuring individuals understand the signs and symptoms of DVT and pulmonary embolism, the importance of adhering to prophylaxis measures, and the need for ongoing monitoring of anticoagulant therapy to detect complications early and optimise outcomes.

19 Leukaemia

Figure 19.1   Development of blood cells from the bone marrow.

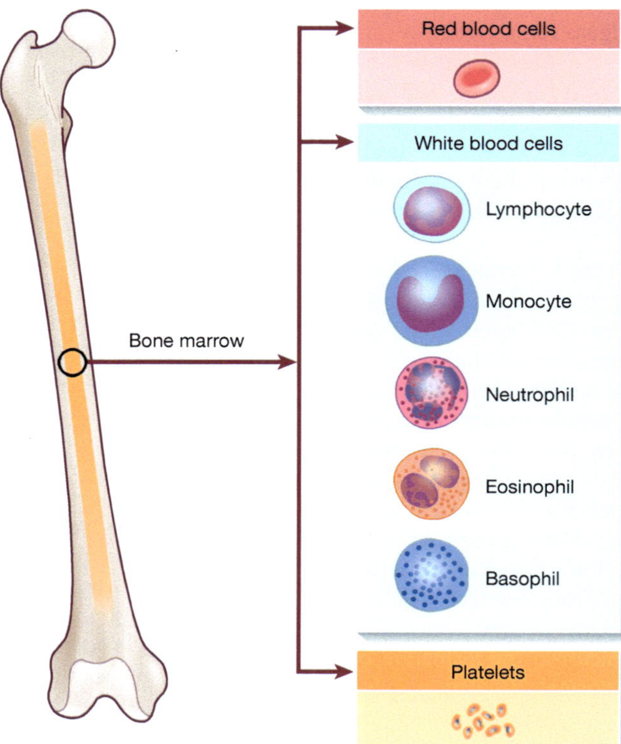

Figure 19.2   Division of stem cells into blood cells.

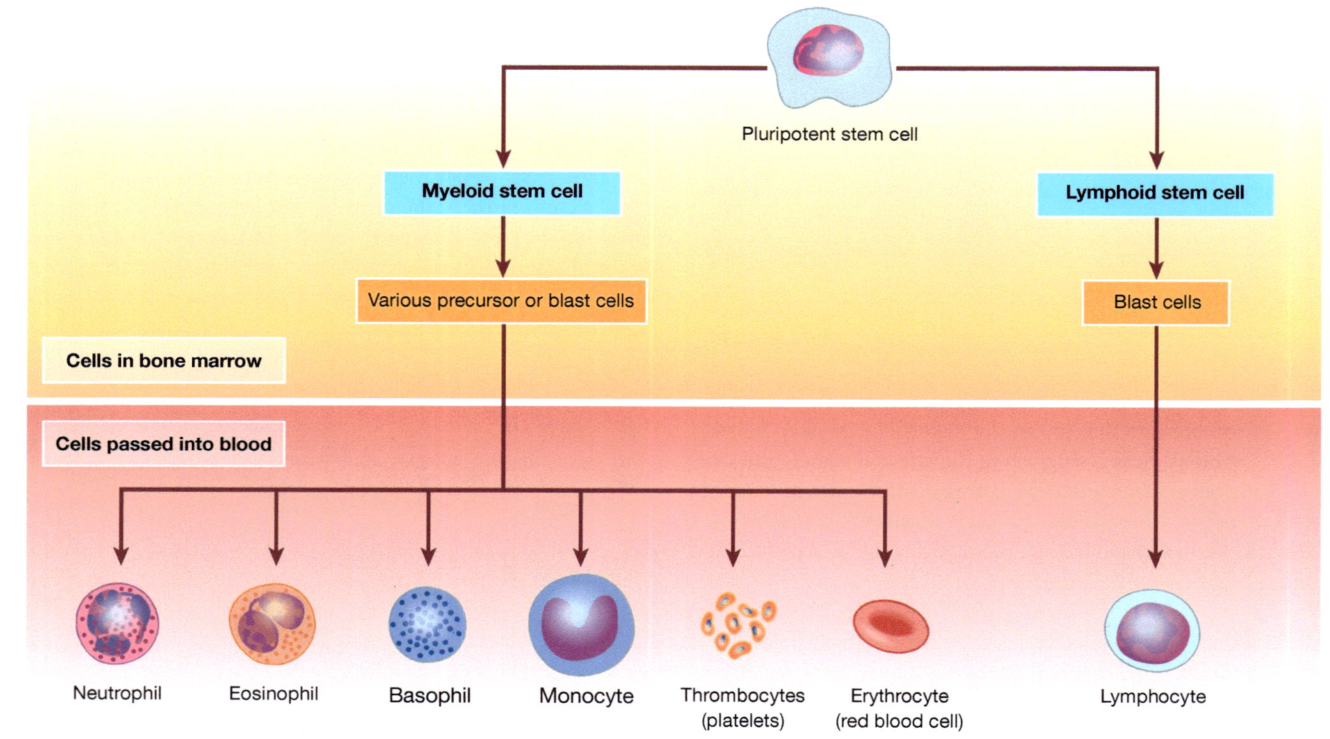

Leukaemia: Overview

Leukaemia is a cancer of the bone marrow, the tissue responsible for producing blood cells. It is a malignant disorder characterised by the abnormal proliferation of immature white blood cells. In the UK, leukaemia is the twelfth most common cancer in adults and affects slightly more men than women.

All blood cells are produced by the bone marrow, a spongy tissue found inside bones (see Figure 19.1). Bone marrow contains haematopoietic stem cells, which are pluripotent cells capable of giving rise to all the specialised blood cells in the body (see Figure 19.2). There are two main stem cell lineages in the bone marrow: myeloid and lymphoid, both derived from pluripotent stem cells. Stem cells continuously divide, producing some cells that remain as stem cells and others that mature through precursor stages into fully functional blood cells. Mature blood cells are then released into the bloodstream.

The largest reservoirs of bone marrow are found in the large flat bones, such as the pelvis and sternum. Healthy bone marrow function relies on adequate nutrition, including iron, folate and certain vitamins, to support the production of blood cells.

In acute leukaemia, the bone marrow releases large numbers of immature white blood cells that are called blast cells; they accumulate rapidly and interfere with normal blood cell production. Leukaemia is broadly classified into acute and chronic forms. Acute leukaemias are subdivided into acute lymphoblastic leukaemia (ALL) and acute myeloid leukaemia (AML), while chronic leukaemias include chronic lymphocytic leukaemia (CLL) and chronic myeloid leukaemia (CML). Chronic leukaemias involve a slower accumulation of more mature, but functionally abnormal, white blood cells.

Risk factors

Men are more likely than women to develop CML, CLL and AML. The risk of most leukaemias, with the exception of ALL, generally increases with age. Those patients who have previously undergone chemotherapy or radiotherapy for other cancers have an increased risk of developing certain types of leukaemia. Similarly, individuals who are exposed to very high levels of ionising radiation, such as survivors of nuclear accidents, are at increased risk. Exposure to specific chemicals, particularly benzene, which is found in petrol and some industrial processes, is also associated with a higher risk of certain leukaemias, most notably AML.

Pathophysiology

Acute leukaemia

Acute leukaemia is an aggressive form of cancer that develops rapidly. Symptoms appear quickly, and if it remains untreated, the condition can become life-threatening. In acute leukaemia, the bone marrow produces large numbers of immature, poorly differentiated white blood cells that proliferate rapidly; these cells have a prolonged lifespan and do not function normally. The overproduction of these immature cells crowds out healthy blood cells; it impairs the bone marrow's ability to produce normal red cells, white cells and platelets.

Acute leukaemias are classified according to the type of cell involved: AML involves the overproduction of immature myeloid cells, while ALL involves immature lymphoid cells (lymphoblasts).

ALL is the most common form of leukaemia in children, whereas AML occurs more frequently in adults. In both types, the immature cells reproduce quickly and fail to mature sufficiently to carry out their normal immune functions; understanding can help to explain the clinical consequences of acute leukaemia and underpins why patients may develop the symptoms and complications that are associated with the disease.

Chronic leukaemia

Chronic leukaemia is an uncommon type of cancer. About 800 people in the UK are diagnosed with CML each year. CML can affect people of any age, but it is more common in people aged 40–60. There is no evidence that it runs in families.

Chronic leukaemia is characterised by the excessive accumulation of relatively mature, yet abnormal, white blood cells. The disease usually progresses slowly over months or years. Although the affected cells are produced at a higher rate than normal, these cells are functionally impaired. Unlike acute leukaemia, which requires urgent treatment, some chronic leukaemias, particularly in their early stages, may be carefully monitored before therapy is initiated to ensure that treatment is optimally timed. Chronic leukaemia most commonly occurs in older adults, although it can occasionally develop in younger individuals.

Signs and symptoms

Symptoms of leukaemia vary depending on the specific type and stage of the disease. Common presenting features include fatigue and breathlessness due to anaemia, easy bruising (petechiae) or abnormal bleeding (including from the gums or nose), abdominal discomfort caused by an enlarged spleen or liver, unexplained weight loss and swollen lymph nodes in areas such as the neck (cervical), underarms (axilla) or groin (inguinal).

Management

Patients with leukaemia require a comprehensive assessment of pain, activity tolerance, vital signs, nutritional status and signs of bleeding or infection to enable the planning of high-quality care. It is important to minimise the risk of trauma, such as by avoiding shaving with a straight-edge razor, taking precautions when mobilising after medications that may cause dizziness or low blood pressure, and using care with sharp utensils. Patients should be encouraged to maintain adequate hydration and nutrition and to take frequent rest periods, as fatigue is a common and significant symptom.

Those who offer care and support must follow local policies and protocols for the care of patients with leukaemia, including strict hand hygiene before and after patient contact and advising on the limitation of unnecessary visitors to reduce the risk of infection.

Treatment options

A combination of medications and therapies is aimed at controlling the disease, managing symptoms and supporting recovery. Cytotoxic drugs (chemotherapy) remain a mainstay for many leukaemias, often administered in risk-adapted combination regimens tailored to the type and stage of disease. Pain management is an important component of supportive care, with opioids and non-opioid strategies used according to patient needs.

Radiotherapy is used selectively, primarily for specific complications such as central nervous system involvement or as part of preparative regimens for haematopoietic stem cell transplant (bone marrow transplant).

Targeted therapies and immunotherapies have transformed contemporary leukaemia care. These therapies have revolutionised the treatment of blood cancers by offering more precise and personalised approaches to combat the disease.

Some patients with acute promyelocytic leukaemia (APL) may be treated with all-trans retinoic acid (ATRA), often in combination with arsenic trioxide (ATO). ATRA works by promoting the maturation of immature blast cells into functional blood cells, rapidly reducing the number of abnormal cells and improving symptoms.

Clinical considerations

Caring for patients with leukaemia requires a holistic approach that addresses medical and psychosocial needs. Monitor patients for infection, bleeding, anaemia and treatment side effects and provide clear information about the condition, treatment options and potential complications. Supporting emotional well-being is essential, including recognising anxiety, fatigue and fear, and referring patients or families to counselling or support services when needed. Encouraging self-care, such as adequate nutrition, hydration, rest and gentle physical activity, is important, as is involving family members in care, helping them understand infection prevention, symptom monitoring and ways to support the patient at home.

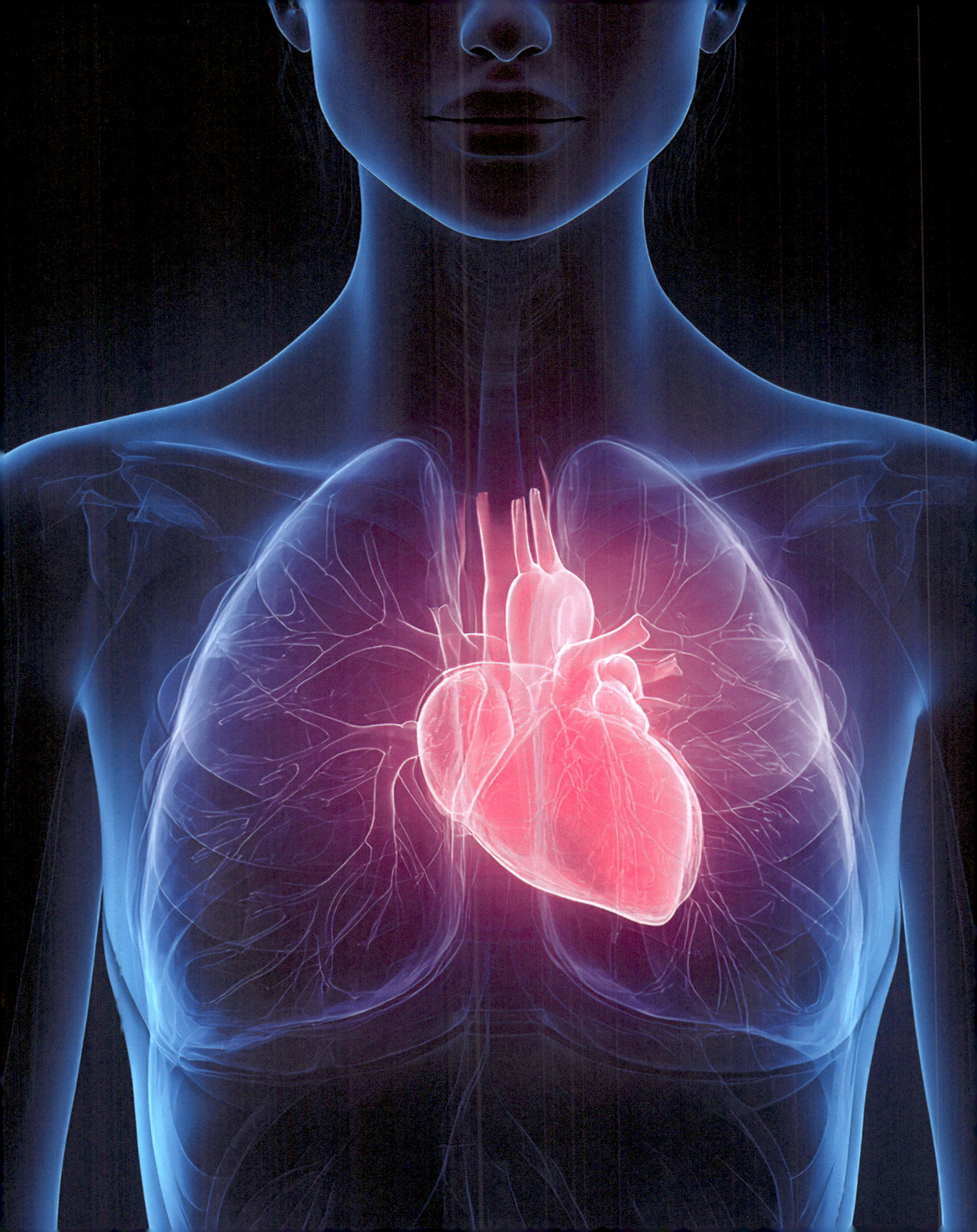

20 Thrombocytopenia

Figure 20.1 Blood cells.

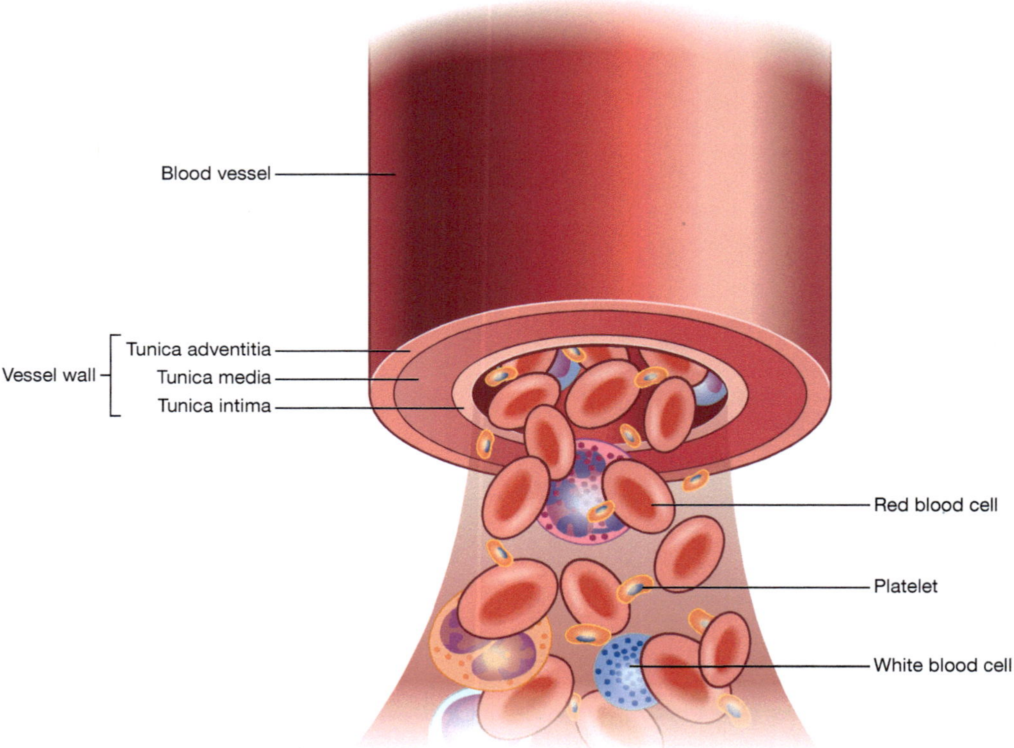

Table 20.1 The function of platelets.

Function	Description
Clot formation	Platelets adhere to damaged vessels and each other to form a plug that stops bleeding.
Maintain vessel integrity	Platelets help prevent leakage of blood from small vessels.
Release of chemicals	Platelets release substances that help more platelets stick together (aggregation) and support clotting.
Support healing	Platelets release growth factors that aid tissue repair and wound healing.

Thrombocytopenia refers to a condition in which the number of platelets (thrombocytes) in the blood is abnormally low. This occurs when platelets are removed from the circulation faster than the bone marrow can produce them, or when their production is impaired. Platelets play a crucial role in blood clotting and maintaining vascular integrity, so a reduced platelet count increases the risk of bleeding, bruising and difficulty controlling haemorrhage. Thrombocytopenia can result from a variety of causes, including bone marrow disorders, certain medications, autoimmune conditions, infections or as a complication of other diseases such as leukaemia.

What are platelets?

Platelets are tiny cells (Figure 20.1) that circulate in the blood and whose function is to take part in the clotting process. Each platelet contains numerous granules that store compounds essential for promoting platelet adhesion, both to one another and to the damaged lining of blood vessels, thereby supporting the formation of a stable blood clot.

The normal platelet count in circulating blood ranges from 150,000 to 400,000 platelets per microlitre (μL). Newborn babies may have slightly lower counts at birth, but these typically reach the adult range by around 2–3 months of age.

Platelets, like red and most white cells, are produced in the bone marrow. They originate from megakaryocytes, very large bone marrow cells that release platelets through a process of fragmentation, with each megakaryocyte generating over 1,000 platelets. The primary hormone regulating the development and maturation of megakaryocytes is thrombopoietin.

Function of platelets

Platelets are essential for the formation of blood clots, helping to prevent haemorrhage following injury to blood vessels. An adequate number of normally functioning platelets is also necessary to maintain vascular integrity and to prevent the leakage of red blood cells from apparently uninjured vessels (see Table 20.1).

In the event of bleeding, muscles in the vessel wall contract and reduce blood flow. The platelets then stick to each other (aggregation) and hold on to the vessel wall (primary haemostasis). The coagulation factors are then activated, resulting in normally liquid blood becoming an insoluble clot.

Pathophysiology

The three distinct types of thrombocytopenia are immune thrombocytopenic purpura (ITP), thrombotic thrombocytopenic purpura (TTP) and haemolytic uraemic syndrome (HUS).

ITP is an autoimmune disorder in which antibodies target platelets, marking them for destruction by the spleen. The spleen is part of the reticuloendothelial system (also called the mononuclear phagocyte system) and is responsible for the detection and destruction of aged, damaged or antibody-coated blood cells, including red blood cells and platelets. Although the bone marrow increases platelet production, it cannot keep up with the rate of destruction. Acute ITP is more common in children, often resolving spontaneously without treatment, while chronic ITP is more common in adults and may require monitoring rather than immediate therapy, depending on platelet count, bleeding risk and lifestyle factors such as contact sports or manual work.

TTP is a rare condition in which small blood clots form throughout the microvasculature. This widespread clotting consumes large numbers of platelets, leading to thrombocytopenia (platelet numbers are abnormally low). TTP is often associated with a deficiency or inhibition of the enzyme ADAMTS13, which normally regulates von Willebrand factor activity (essential for normal blood clotting).

HUS is a rare disorder characterised by thrombocytopenia, destruction of red blood cells (haemolytic anaemia) and kidney injury. HUS most commonly occurs after infection with Shiga toxin-producing Escherichia coli (STEC), which releases toxins that damage blood vessel linings and trigger platelet activation.

Drug-induced thrombocytopenia

Although allergic reactions to medications can occur in susceptible individuals, they are relatively rare. Certain drugs can also trigger serious immune-mediated reactions involving blood platelets. In these cases, the drug binds to the surface of the platelet, forming a drug-platelet complex that is recognised by the immune system as foreign. This triggers the production of antibodies against the complex, resulting in the destruction of the platelets and potentially leading to thrombocytopenia.

Signs and symptoms

Symptoms of thrombocytopenia may include easy or excessive bruising, small red, purple or dark spots on the skin (petechiae), often appearing on the lower legs, prolonged bleeding from cuts, spontaneous bleeding from the gums or nose, blood in the urine or stools, unusually heavy menstrual periods and excessive bleeding during surgery or dental procedures. In individuals with darker skin pigmentation, petechiae and bruising may appear brown, purple or bluish and may be more easily detected on palms, soles, mucous membranes or conjunctiva.

Management

Patients with thrombocytopenia are at an increased risk of bleeding, particularly from the gums and mucous membranes, making early detection essential to prevent significant blood loss. The provision of care focuses on prevention, early recognition and management of complications. This includes minimising the risk of injury, preventing falls, maintaining skin integrity and monitoring for infection, especially in patients receiving corticosteroids, which can increase susceptibility to bruising and skin breakdown. The patient should also be assessed for signs of microvascular complications, such as ischaemia of the extremities or organ dysfunction. Fluid balance should be monitored and stool tested for occult blood to detect early hypovolaemia. Psychosocial support is important, particularly for patients who require isolation, to address emotional and practical needs. The provision of information for patients and families is essential, including guidance on injury prevention, recognising early signs of bleeding, infection or ischaemia and understanding the support needed for activities of living.

Clinical considerations

Pharmacological interventions for thrombocytopenia are tailored to the underlying cause and severity of the condition. Corticosteroids are commonly used to suppress immune-mediated platelet destruction. In acute or severe cases, intravenous immunoglobulin (IVIG) may be administered to rapidly increase platelet counts. For patients with chronic or refractory thrombocytopenia, thrombopoietin receptor agonists (such as eltrombopag or romiplostim) can stimulate platelet production in the bone marrow, while immunosuppressive drugs or monoclonal antibodies (e.g. rituximab) may be employed to reduce autoimmune-mediated platelet destruction. In drug-induced thrombocytopenia, discontinuation of the offending medication is essential. Platelet transfusions may be indicated in severe thrombocytopenia or active bleeding, providing immediate haemostatic support.

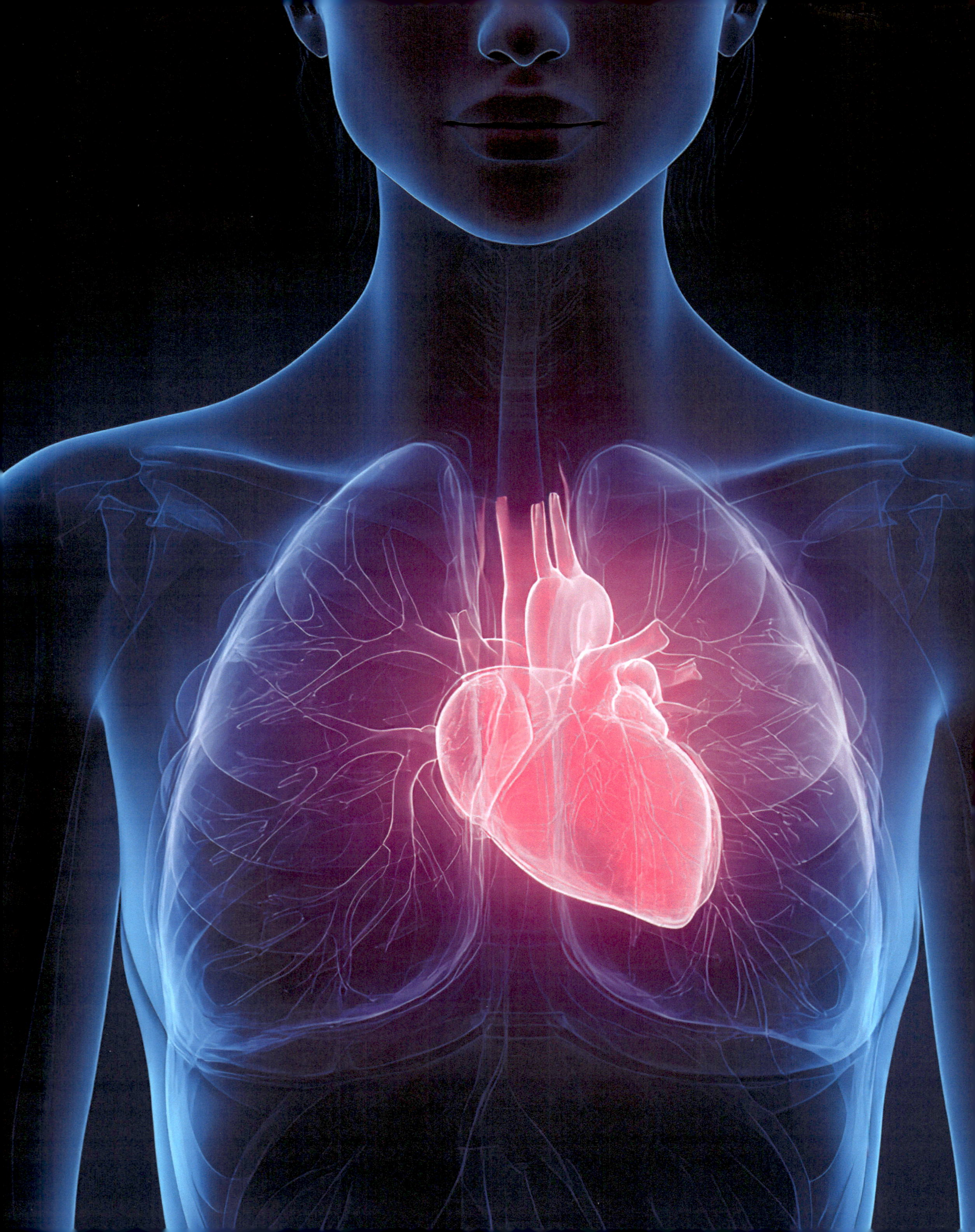

The cardiovascular system

Chapters

21 Heart failure

Figure 21.1   Chambers of the heart.

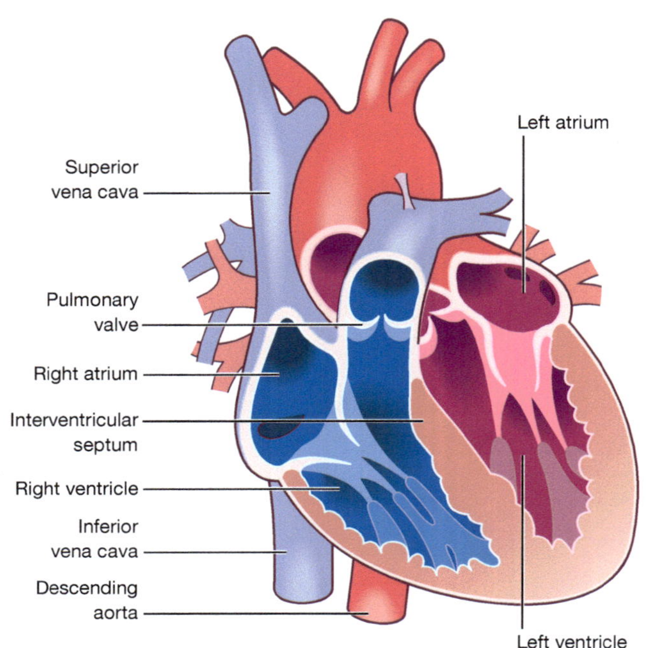

Source:
Peate, Wild & Nair, *Nursing Practice: Knowledge and Care,* 2014

Figure 21.2   Conducting system of the heart.

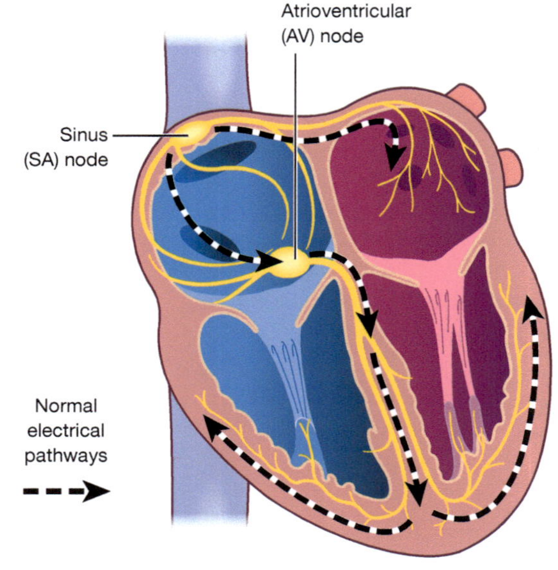

Source:
Peate, Wild & Nair, *Nursing Practice: Knowledge and Care,* 2014

Figure 21.3   Enlarged left ventricle in heart failure.

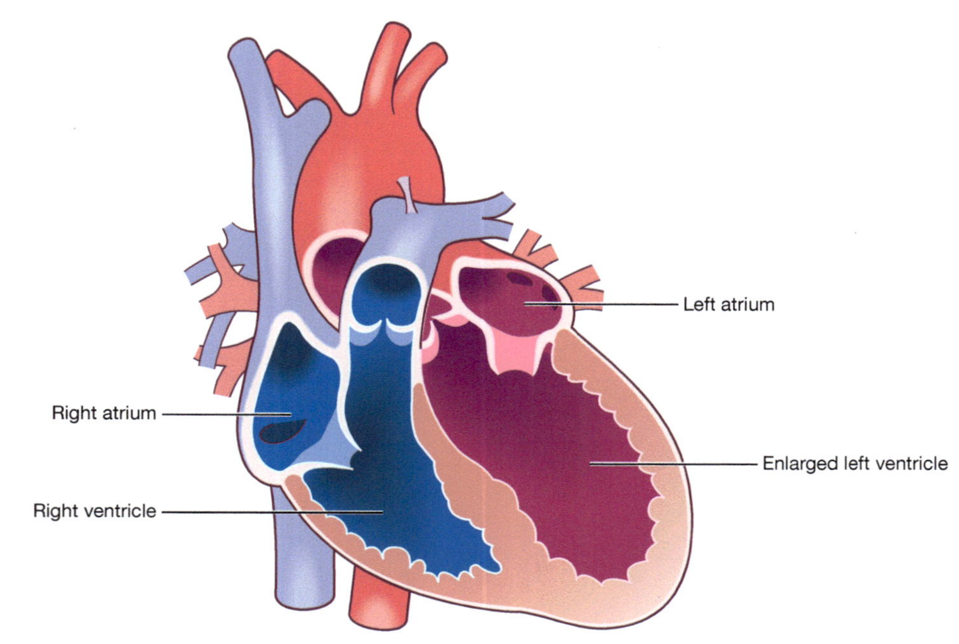

The heart

Heart failure is a condition in which the heart is unable to pump blood effectively to meet the body's metabolic needs. The most common cause is damage to the heart muscle, often following a myocardial infarction. Other important causes include ischaemic heart disease, chronic hypertension, valvular heart disease and cardiomyopathies (these are a group of diseases that affect the heart muscle). Heart failure may present with symptoms such as breathlessness, fatigue and fluid retention, and management should follow evidence-based guidelines, including optimisation of pharmacological therapy, lifestyle interventions and regular monitoring.

The heart has four chambers, two atria and two ventricles (Figure 21.1). The walls of the heart chambers are made mainly of special heart muscle. Each heartbeat starts with a tiny electrical impulse near the top of the heart, which spreads through the heart muscle and makes it contract (squeeze) (Figure 21.2).

The electrical impulse originates in the sinoatrial (SA) node and spreads through the atria, causing them to contract and push blood into the ventricles. The impulse then reaches the atrioventricular (AV) node, travels down the Bundle of His and Purkinje fibres and spreads through the ventricular walls, causing the ventricles to contract and eject blood into the arteries.

Pathophysiology

Heart failure is a condition in which the heart is unable to pump blood effectively to meet the metabolic needs of the body. It arises from damage to the myocardium or conditions that increase the workload of the heart. Common causes of this condition include myocardial infarction, which results in loss of functional heart muscle due to ischaemia; chronic hypertension, causing an increase of the force required to eject blood; valvular heart disease, which can cause obstruction or allow backward flow of blood; and cardiomyopathies or infiltrative conditions such as amyloidosis, resulting in stiffening of the heart walls and impaired filling. Over time, these stresses lead to structural changes, including ventricular dilation, wall remodelling and alterations to heart shape, (see Figure 21.3) which further reduce the heart's mechanical efficiency.

In a healthy heart, increased ventricular filling enhances contraction through the Frank–Starling mechanism, resulting in a rise in cardiac output. In heart failure, the overstretched myocardial fibres contract less effectively, leading to reduced stroke volume and also increased end-systolic volume. Ventricular enlargement and changes in shape and structure exacerbate this inefficiency, resulting in reduced cardiac output along with an accompanying increased cardiac workload.

In chronic heart failure, the body responds to the heart's reduced pumping ability by activating hormonal and nervous system mechanisms that help maintain blood flow and blood pressure.

When the person's blood pressure drops, sensors in the arteries (the baroreceptors) detect it, and this triggers the nervous system to release hormones that will tighten the blood vessels (vasoconstriction), helping to maintain circulation.

Simultaneously, reduced renal perfusion stimulates renin release, leading to the production of angiotensin II, which causes constriction of the blood vessels and promotes aldosterone secretion, increasing sodium and water retention. While these responses temporarily maintain perfusion, they also contribute to ventricular remodelling, fluid overload and progression of heart failure – meaning, the body's attempts to compensate help at first, but over time they strain the heart, cause fluid buildup and make heart failure worse.

Overall, heart failure leads to reduced cardiac output, elevated ventricular pressures and congestion in both the systemic and pulmonary circulation; this results in symptoms such as breathlessness, fatigue, fluid retention and reduced exercise tolerance. A clear understanding of the interplay between myocardial dysfunction, structural changes and neurohormonal compensatory mechanisms is essential for effective management and improving patient outcomes.

Signs and symptoms

The symptoms of heart failure can vary between individuals. The main features include breathlessness, fatigue and peripheral oedema; this typically presents as swelling of the ankles, which may extend up the legs. This swelling is often less pronounced in the morning and worsens throughout the day as a result of fluid accumulation.

Other common symptoms may include cough, wheezing, nausea, weight changes, palpitations (tachycardia) and reduced exercise tolerance. In severe cases, pulmonary congestion or pulmonary oedema may occur, causing marked breathlessness, difficulty lying flat (orthopnoea) or sudden nighttime breathlessness (paroxysmal nocturnal dyspnoea).

Management

To provide high-quality care, healthcare professionals should undertake a comprehensive assessment and develop an individualised care plan with the patient (when able), addressing all of the identified problems. Vital signs should be monitored frequently, with observation intervals guided by clinical stability. In acute heart failure or unstable patients, continuous ECG monitoring is often performed to allow early detection of life-threatening events. Early detection of changes in vital signs and prompt intervention may be lifesaving.

Lifestyle modification is an important aspect of care. Patients who smoke should be supported with smoking cessation strategies, and advice on healthy nutrition and weight management should be provided, particularly for those who are overweight or obese. Patients should be positioned upright in bed, supported by pillows, unless contraindicated, to reduce breathlessness.

Alcohol can act as a negative inotrope (reducing the strength of the heart's contractions), increase blood pressure and raise the risk of arrhythmias. Patients should limit alcohol intake or abstain entirely if alcohol-induced cardiomyopathy is present. In patients with severe heart failure, particularly those with hyponatraemia, sensible fluid restriction may be necessary, taking care to avoid dehydration, especially in elderly patients on high-dose diuretics.

Pharmacological treatment

Angiotensin-converting enzyme (ACE) inhibitors are the first-line treatment for heart failure with reduced ejection fraction (HFrEF). They dilate blood vessels, lower blood pressure and reduce cardiac workload. Angiotensin II receptor blockers (ARBs) are alternatives for patients who are intolerant of ACE inhibitors. Angiotensin receptor–neprilysin inhibitors (ARNIs), such as sacubitril/valsartan, combine neprilysin inhibition with angiotensin receptor blockade and offer further reductions in mortality and hospitalisation compared with ACE inhibitors.

Evidence-based beta-blockers (bisoprolol, carvedilol, nebivolol and metoprolol succinate) reduce sympathetic overactivity, improve ventricular function and lower mortality. Introduce gradually and titrate to the maximum tolerated dose.

Mineralocorticoid receptor antagonists (spironolactone and eplerenone) improve survival and reduce hospitalisation while helping to prevent cardiac remodelling. Regularly monitor renal function and potassium levels.

Sodium-glucose cotransporter-2 (SGLT2) inhibitors such as dapagliflozin and empagliflozin reduce mortality and hospitalisation and improve symptoms regardless of diabetes status.

Loop diuretics (e.g. furosemide) provide symptomatic relief from fluid overload, but do not improve survival. Digoxin can improve symptoms and reduce hospitalisation, particularly in atrial fibrillation, but requires careful monitoring for toxicity.

Inotropes (e.g. dobutamine and milrinone), reserved for acute or advanced heart failure to support cardiac output, carry a risk of arrhythmia and increased mortality with prolonged use.

Clinical considerations

Lifestyle changes are essential in managing heart failure and improving quality of life. Support patients to stop smoking and limit alcohol intake. A balanced, low-sodium diet helps control fluid retention; fluid intake may need to be moderated in advanced cases. Regular, gentle exercise, tailored to ability, can enhance fitness and mood. Daily weight monitoring aids early detection of fluid overload. With the patient, address psychosocial needs, encourage medication concordance and involve family members in supporting long-term lifestyle adjustments.

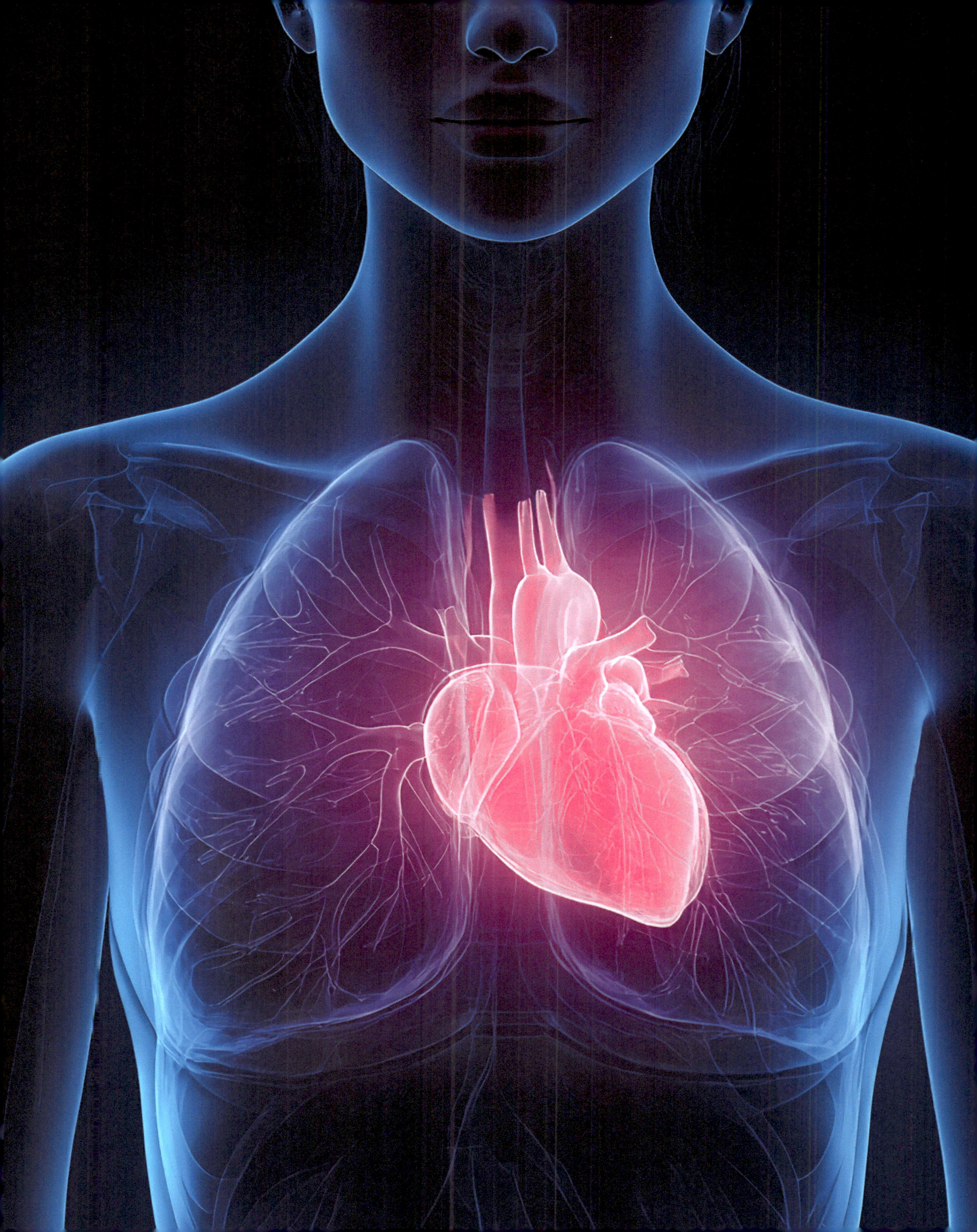

22 Myocardial infarction

Figure 22.1 Blood vessels of the heart.

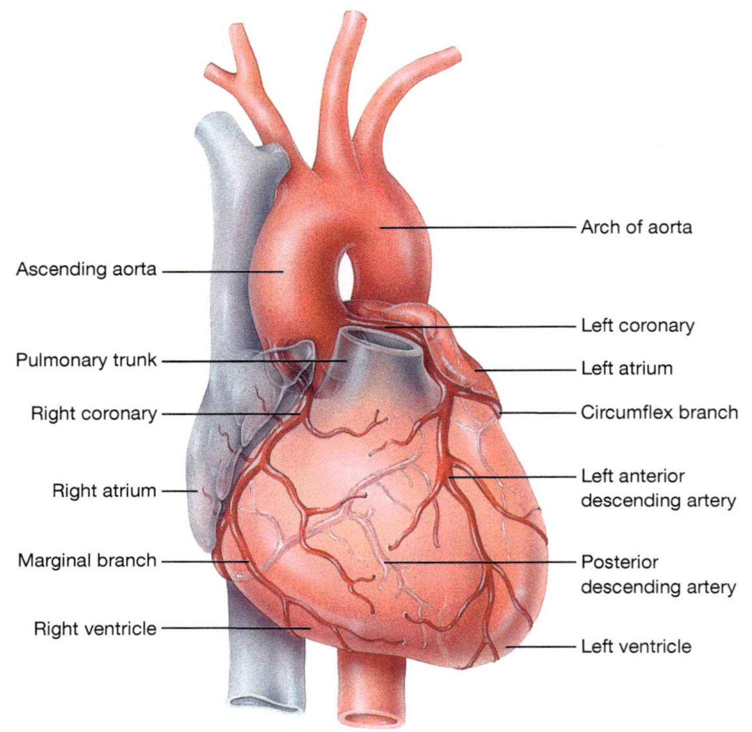

Source:
Peate et al. 2014/with permission of John Wiley & Sons

Figure 22.2 Atheroma in a blood vessel.

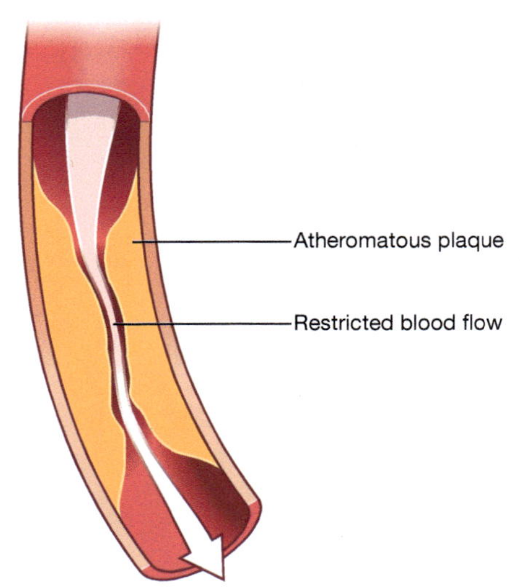

Figure 22.3 Damaged myocardium from myocardial interaction.

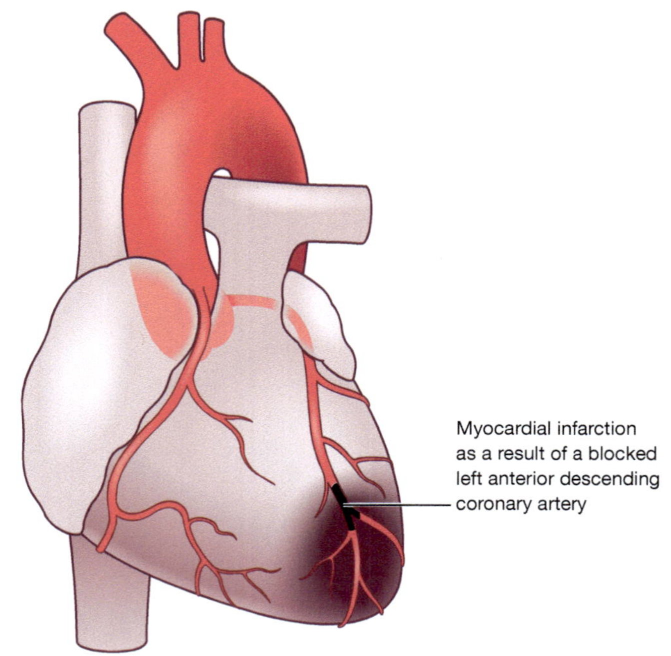

Figure 22.4 Areas where pain may be felt in MI.

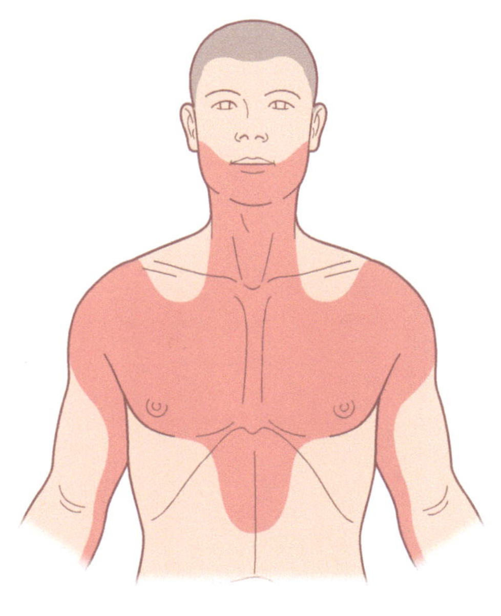

Source:
Peate, Wild & Nair, *Nursing Practice: Knowledge and Care*, 2014

The heart

The heart is primarily composed of specialised muscle, the myocardium, which contracts to pump blood into the arteries, delivering it to all parts of the body. The myocardium requires a continuous supply of oxygen and nutrients, which is provided by the coronary arteries. These arteries branch from the aorta and divide into smaller branches to supply all regions of the heart muscle (Figure 22.1).

Any reduction in coronary blood flow, from atherosclerosis or a coronary thrombosis, can cause myocardial damage, impairing cardiac contraction. This may lead to myocardial infarction (MI) and contribute to the development of heart failure, as the damaged heart muscle struggles to maintain adequate cardiac output.

Pathophysiology

MI occurs when blood flow to a portion of the heart muscle is abruptly blocked, leading to ischaemia and necrosis of the myocardium. The most common cause is thrombosis forming at the site of a ruptured or eroded atherosclerotic plaque in a coronary artery (see Figure 22.2). Atherosclerosis is a chronic condition in which fatty deposits, or plaques, develop within the arterial wall over the years. Plaques consist of a lipid-rich core covered by a fibrous cap; their rupture exposes pro-thrombotic material to the bloodstream, triggering platelet aggregation and activation of the coagulation cascade, forming an occlusive thrombus.

MI is a major subset of acute coronary syndromes (ACS), which also include unstable angina and non-ST-elevation myocardial infarction (NSTEMI). When the thrombus fully occludes the artery and reduces blood flow below a critical threshold, myocardial cells are deprived of oxygen and nutrients. Necrosis begins within 20–40 minutes of sustained ischaemia, although the extent of injury depends on the duration of occlusion, the size of the affected artery and the presence of collateral circulation (see Figure 22.3).

The location of the infarction is determined by the coronary artery involved. Occlusion of the left main coronary artery typically causes a large anterolateral infarct, while the left anterior descending artery affects the anterior wall. Blockage of the right coronary artery often results in an inferior infarct and can affect the cardiac conduction system. Damaged myocardium is replaced over time by fibrous scar tissue, which lacks contractility, contributing to ventricular remodelling, reduced cardiac output and impaired systolic function.

Necrotic tissue also conducts electrical impulses more slowly than healthy myocardium, increasing the risk of arrhythmias, including potentially life-threatening ventricular tachycardia or fibrillation. The resultant reduction in effective cardiac output may lead to systemic hypoperfusion, pulmonary congestion and the development of heart failure.

Current understanding emphasises the importance of rapid reperfusion therapy, including percutaneous coronary intervention (PCI) or thrombolysis, to restore blood flow and limit myocardial damage. Early intervention not only preserves myocardial function but also reduces the risk of complications such as ventricular remodelling, cardiogenic shock and sudden cardiac death.

Understanding the interplay between atherosclerotic plaque instability, thrombus formation, myocardial necrosis and subsequent remodelling is essential for effective clinical management, guiding the use of antiplatelet therapy, anticoagulation and interventions to improve survival and long-term outcomes.

Signs and symptoms

A person having an acute MI usually has sudden chest pain that is felt behind the breastbone and sometimes travels to the left arm or the left side of the neck (Figure 22.4). Additionally, the person may have shortness of breath, sweating, nausea, vomiting, abnormal heartbeats and anxiety. Rapid, irregular pulse, hypotension and dyspnoea (shortness of breath) may all present as symptoms. The anxiety is often described as a 'sense of impending doom'. Dyspnoea occurs when the damage to the heart limits the output of the left ventricle, causing left ventricular failure and consequent pulmonary oedema.

Women experience fewer of these symptoms than men but usually have shortness of breath, weakness, a feeling of indigestion and fatigue. Atypical presentations are more common in women, older adults and people with diabetes. In many cases, in some estimates as high as 64%, the person does not have chest pain or other symptoms. These are called 'silent' MIs.

Management

Patients experiencing an acute MI require prompt, coordinated care to stabilise cardiac function, relieve symptoms and prevent complications. Initial assessment should include vital signs, ECG monitoring, oxygen saturation and pain evaluation. Continuous cardiac monitoring is essential due to the high risk of arrhythmias, heart block or sudden cardiac arrest.

Patients should initially limit physical activity to reduce myocardial oxygen demand. Complete bed rest is generally not prolonged; early mobilisation is encouraged once clinically safe to reduce the risk of venous thromboembolism, muscle deconditioning and pulmonary complications. Patients should be positioned upright or semi-upright to aid breathing and reduce cardiac workload, unless contraindicated.

Relief of ischaemic pain is a priority, both for comfort and to reduce sympathetic activation. Intravenous morphine is commonly used, titrated to effect and administered alongside an antiemetic to prevent opioid-induced nausea or vomiting. Morphine also helps alleviate anxiety, which can exacerbate tachycardia and myocardial oxygen demand. Persistent chest pain may be treated with sublingual nitrates, provided blood pressure is adequate, while beta-blockers may be administered early if not contraindicated to reduce heart rate, myocardial workload and arrhythmia risk.

The administration of dual antiplatelet therapy (e.g. aspirin plus a P2Y12 inhibitor – clopidogrel) and anticoagulation per protocol to prevent further thrombosis may be required. Oxygen therapy is administered only if oxygen saturation is below recommended thresholds. Adjunctive medications, such as statins, ACE inhibitors or ARNI therapy (valsartan), may be started according to local protocols once the patient is stable.

Monitoring and ongoing assessment: Vital signs, ECG, urine output and fluid balance should be observed frequently. Pain levels, symptom progression and potential complications, such as heart failure, cardiogenic shock or bleeding, should be continuously assessed.

Patient and family support: Anxiety and fear are common during AMI. Clear explanations about interventions, reassurance and emotional support are essential. Education should also focus on lifestyle factors, smoking cessation, dietary advice and understanding of medications and follow-up care.

Overall goal: The aim of nursing management is to stabilise the patient, relieve pain, prevent complications and support recovery, while preparing the patient and family for post-AMI care, rehabilitation and secondary prevention.

Pharmacological and non-pharmacological treatment

Anticoagulant therapy is initiated promptly to reduce the risk of further thrombus formation. Where primary PCI is not immediately available, thrombolytic agents such as reteplase, alteplase or tenecteplase may be administered as soon as possible to restore blood flow and limit myocardial damage. Emergency PCI is the preferred reperfusion strategy in most settings. This involves inserting a catheter via the radial or femoral artery into the blocked coronary artery. A balloon is inflated briefly to open the vessel, and a stent is usually deployed to maintain arterial patency and improve blood flow to the myocardium.

Clinical considerations

Percutaneous coronary intervention (PCI) is indicated for patients with acute myocardial infarction, unstable angina or high-risk NSTEMI who require rapid reperfusion. Before the procedure, assess for allergies to contrast agents, evaluate renal function and coagulation status, obtain informed consent, establish intravenous access and ensure continuous cardiac monitoring.

During PCI, a catheter is inserted via the radial or femoral artery and guided to the blocked coronary vessel. Balloon angioplasty is performed to open the artery, and a stent is usually deployed to maintain vessel patency.

Following the procedure, close monitoring is essential. Vital signs and ECG should be observed, the access site checked for bleeding or haematoma, and patients monitored for signs of reperfusion arrhythmias. Dual antiplatelet therapy, often aspirin plus a P2Y12 inhibitor, is prescribed alongside anticoagulation as per protocol to reduce the risk of further clot formation.

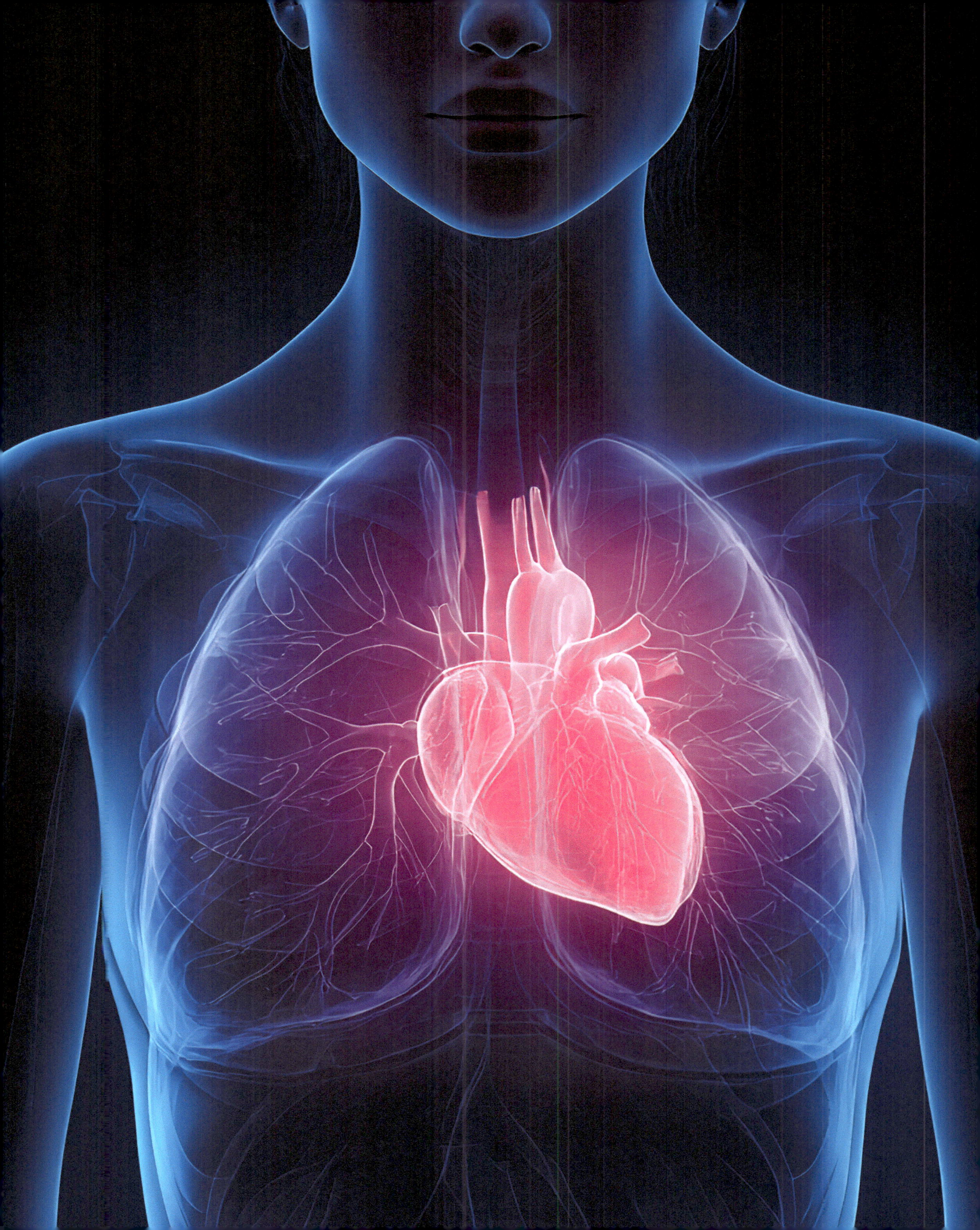

23 Peripheral arterial disease

Figure 23.1   An artery.

Figure 23.2   A vein.

Source:
Peate, Wild & Nair, *Nursing Practice: Knowledge and Care,* 2014

Source:
Peate, Wild & Nair, *Nursing Practice: Knowledge and Care,* 2014

Figure 23.3   An artery with an atheroma.

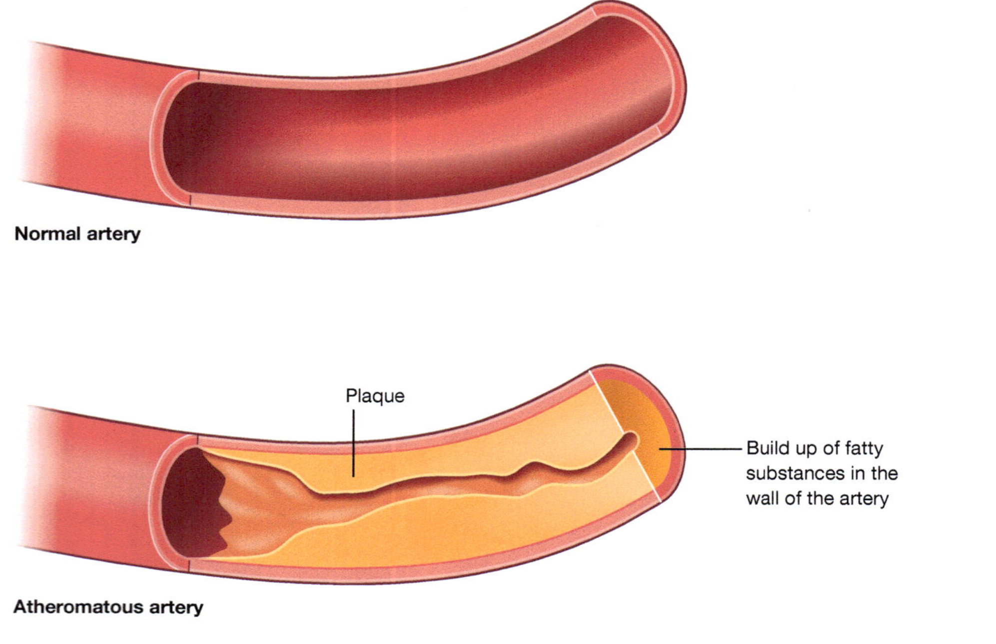

Arteries and veins

Arteries and veins have the same layers of tissues in their walls, but the proportions of these layers differ. Lining the core of each is a thin layer of endothelium, and covering each is a sheath of connective tissue, but an artery has thick intermediate layers of elastic and muscular fibre, while in the vein these are much thinner and less developed. With the exception of pulmonary and umbilical veins and arteries, arteries carry oxygenated blood from the heart, while veins return deoxygenated blood to the heart.

The thicker and more muscular walls of arteries (Figure 23.1) help them to withstand and absorb the pressure waves which begin in the heart and are transmitted by the blood. The arterial wall expands and swells with the force of each contraction of the heart, then snaps back to push the blood forward as the heart rests. From the arteries, blood enters smaller branches of arteries called arterioles and then the capillary network.

Just as arterioles are smaller branches of arteries, so venules are smaller branches of veins. Venules receive blood from the capillaries and branch into veins that return blood to the heart. They do not need the strength and elasticity of the arteries, so the walls of the veins are thin and almost floppy. To make up for this, many veins are located in the skeletal muscles, and the least movement of a limb squeezes the vein and drives the blood toward the heart. One-way valves ensure flow in the right direction (Figure 23.2).

Pathophysiology

PAD is a common condition in which the arteries supplying the legs become narrowed due to a build-up of fatty deposits that are known as atheroma (see Figure 23.3) (the condition affects legs most commonly). This restricts blood flow to the leg muscles and can lead to symptoms such as pain on walking (intermittent claudication) or, in advanced cases, critical limb ischaemia. Atheroma consists of cholesterol, lipids and other cellular debris and develops gradually within the arterial wall, progressively causing a reduction in the vessel's diameter.

Atherosclerosis is a progressive process that begins early in life and develops over many years, often without symptoms until blood flow becomes significantly restricted. Atherosclerosis is the underlying cause of many cardiovascular diseases, including coronary artery disease, stroke and PAD.

Damage to the endothelium occurs due to high blood pressure, smoking, high levels of cholesterol or raised blood glucose in diabetes. Once the endothelium is damaged, low-density lipoprotein (LDL) cholesterol particles can penetrate the arterial wall and become oxidised. This triggers an inflammatory response. Macrophages engulf the oxidised LDL and become foam cells, forming what are known as fatty streaks, the earliest visible sign of atherosclerosis.

Atherosclerosis is more likely to develop in people who smoke, have high cholesterol, hypertension, diabetes, obesity or a sedentary lifestyle. Age, genetic predisposition and poor diet are also contributing factors. The process is slow and often silent, highlighting the importance of preventive care, healthy lifestyle choices and early risk assessment to reduce cardiovascular complications.

PAD is a manifestation of systemic atherosclerosis, meaning that affected patients are also at increased risk of coronary artery disease and stroke. Risk factors include smoking, diabetes, hypertension, dyslipidaemia and older age.

Signs and symptoms

The typical symptom is pain, which develops in one or both calves during walking or exercise and is relieved after resting for a few minutes. This pain varies between cases, and there may be aching, cramping or tiredness in the legs. This is called intermittent claudication. It is due to the narrowing of one (or more) of the arteries in the leg. The most common artery affected is the femoral artery.

When a person walks, the muscles in the calves require an increased supply of blood and oxygen to meet the demands of movement. However, if the arteries supplying the legs are narrowed, such as in PAD, this additional blood flow cannot be delivered effectively. As a result, the muscles become deprived of oxygen, leading to pain known as intermittent claudication. This discomfort typically appears during physical activity, particularly when walking uphill or climbing stairs, as these actions place greater demands on the muscles. The pain usually subsides with rest, when the oxygen requirement decreases. If the narrowing occurs in arteries higher up the circulatory pathway, such as the iliac arteries or the aorta, the reduced blood flow can affect the thighs or buttocks, causing pain in these areas during walking rather than in the calves.

If the blood supply is very much reduced, then the person may develop pain even at rest, particularly at night when the legs are raised in bed. Typically, rest pain first develops in the toes and feet rather than in the calves. Ulcers (sores) may develop on the skin of the feet or lower leg if the blood supply to the skin is poor. In a small number of cases, gangrene (death of tissue) of a foot may result.

Management

Pain management is an important aspect of care for patients with arterial insufficiency. If pain occurs during exercise, patients should walk to the point of moderate pain, rest and then continue, rather than avoiding activity altogether. They should be encouraged to undertake regular, moderate exercise within their limits, as this can help improve collateral circulation and walking distance over time. Walking programmes that gradually increase duration and intensity are particularly beneficial in PAD.

Patients should be advised to keep warm, especially in cold weather, but to avoid tight-fitting clothing that may restrict circulation. They should also be encouraged to stop smoking, as smoking significantly worsens arterial insufficiency. In addition, patients should avoid exposure to cold temperatures and sitting with legs crossed for long periods, as these can further reduce blood flow.

Pharmacological management may include antiplatelet agents (such as aspirin or clopidogrel) to reduce cardiovascular risk and lipid-lowering therapy (such as statins) to manage atherosclerosis. Naftidrofuryl oxalate may be considered, in accordance with national guidance, for the treatment of intermittent claudication in PAD when lifestyle modification alone is insufficient. It works by improving cellular oxygen utilisation and blood flow. Beta blockers are generally not first-line for PAD and should be used with caution, as they may potentially worsen peripheral circulation. Anticoagulants are not routinely indicated unless there is another coexisting condition (such as atrial fibrillation) that requires them.

Surgery

There are two main types of surgical treatment for PAD. Angioplasty involves widening a narrowed or blocked artery by inflating a small balloon inside the vessel, often followed by placement of a stent to keep it open. Bypass grafting involves creating a detour around the blocked artery using a vein from another part of the body, such as the saphenous vein, or occasionally a synthetic graft.

Clinical considerations

Encourage regular, tolerable walking to improve circulation, avoid smoking, tight clothing and prolonged cold exposure. If indicated, use antiplatelets and statins to reduce cardiovascular risk, with naftidrofuryl oxalate for intermittent claudication if needed. Severe or persistent symptoms may require angioplasty or bypass grafting. Monitor symptom progression and functional ability regularly.

24 Angina

Figure 24.1 Blockage of the coronary artery.

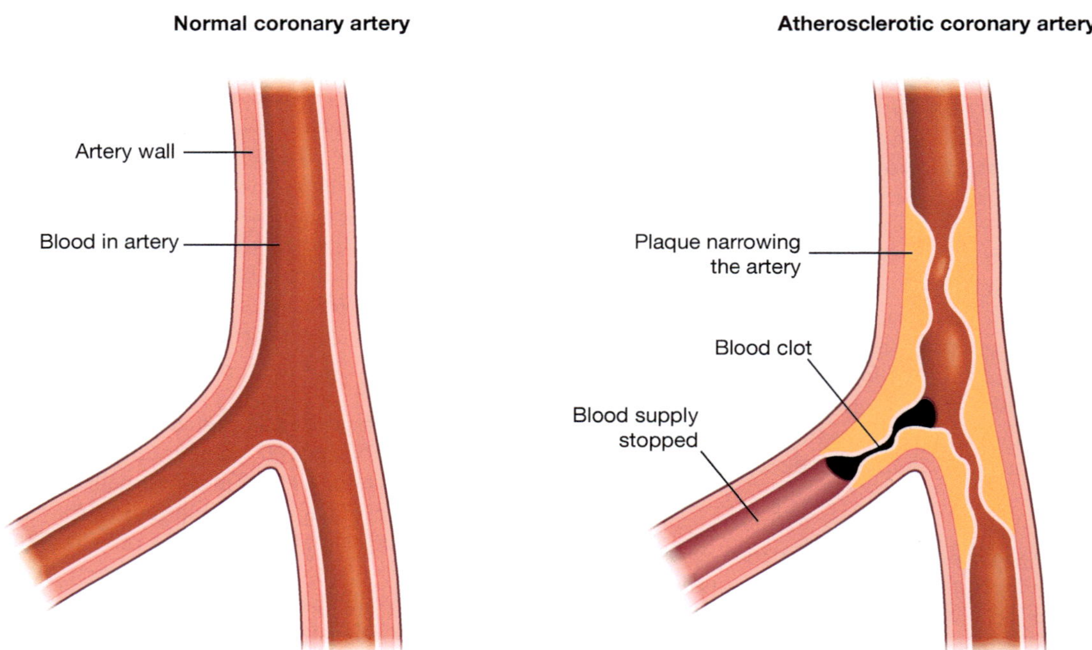

Figure 24.2 Coronary artery disease showing healthy heart, angina pectoris and myocardial infarction.

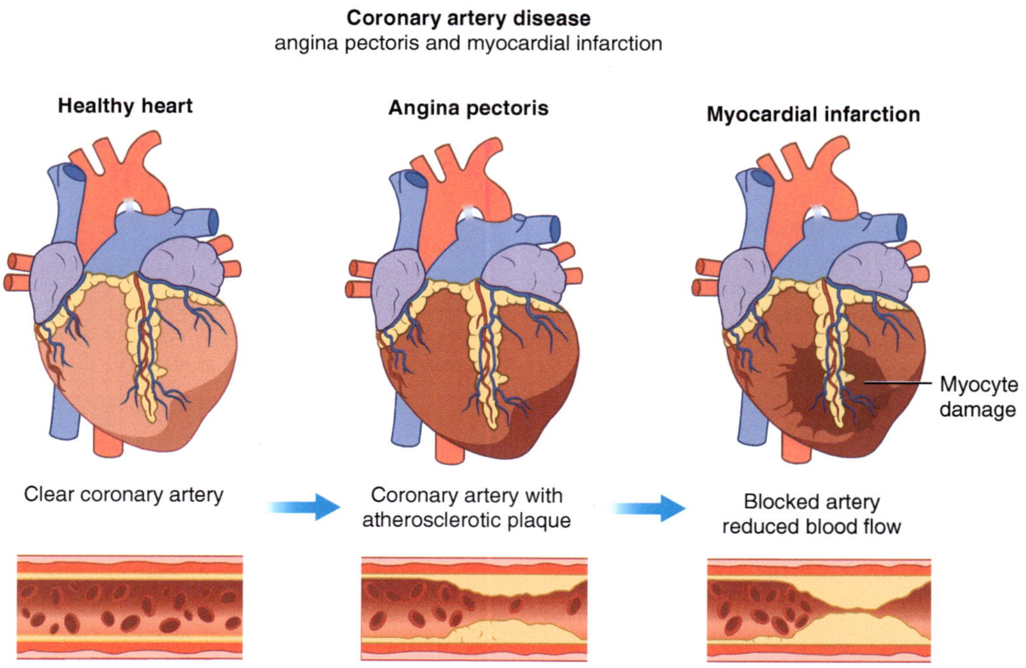

Overview

Angina is chest pain that originates from the heart, usually caused by narrowing of the coronary arteries, which supply blood to the heart muscle (Figures 24.1 and 24.2). The heart is made of specialised muscle that requires a constant blood supply to function effectively. The coronary arteries branch off the aorta, the main artery carrying blood from the heart to the rest of the body. In angina, one or more coronary arteries are narrowed, often due to atherosclerosis, reducing blood flow to part of the heart muscle and causing pain. Usual treatment includes statins to lower cholesterol, low-dose aspirin to reduce the risk of heart attack and beta blockers to decrease the heart's workload and help prevent angina episodes.

Pathophysiology

Angina pain closely resembles the signs and symptoms of MI; thus, it is vital to be able to differentiate between the two conditions, as the treatment differs in both cases. If a patient has pain associated with angina, this is usually relieved by vasodilators (e.g. glyceryl trinitrate [GTN]). Stable anginal pain is rarely fatal, but worsening or angina occurring at rest may indicate a more serious condition requiring urgent attention.

Angina results from reduced blood flow through the coronary arteries, usually due to atherosclerotic narrowing. At rest, oxygen supply to the heart muscle may be adequate, but during exertion, increased heart rate and contractility raise myocardial oxygen demand. When blood flow cannot meet this demand, myocardial ischaemia occurs, leading to the accumulation of metabolic by-products such as lactic acid, which stimulate nerve endings and produce chest pain. Angina pain is typically relieved by vasodilators, such as GTN, which reduce cardiac workload and improve oxygen delivery. Clinically, patients may present with pallor, dyspnoea, cyanosis, diaphoresis and tachycardia. In patients with darker skin, reliance on skin colour alone can be misleading. Clinicians should assess mucous membranes, nail beds, vital signs and patient-reported symptoms to detect signs of ischaemia or acute coronary events.

Types of angina
Stable angina

This is the most common type of angina. Pain is usually triggered by physical exertion or emotional stress, which increases heart rate and oxygen demand. It is called 'stable' because the attacks follow a regular pattern and occur with similar triggers. Patients can often predict when an attack will happen. Episodes typically last 5–10 minutes and are usually relieved by rest or by taking short-acting nitrates such as GTN.

Unstable angina

This type does not follow a predictable pattern. Attacks can occur with minimal exertion or even at rest and tend to be more severe, longer-lasting (typically 10–20 minutes), and more frequent than stable angina. Stable angina can progress to unstable angina, which is considered an acute coronary syndrome and requires urgent medical attention.

Variant (prinzmetal) angina

A rare form of angina caused by coronary artery spasm, which temporarily reduces blood flow to the heart muscle. Variant angina is often severe, occurs at rest and frequently happens at night or in the early morning. It is usually relieved by nitrates or calcium channel blockers.

Signs and symptoms

Angina is characterised by chest pain or discomfort, often described as pressure, heaviness or tightness, which may radiate to the neck, jaw, shoulder, arm, back or upper abdomen. Associated symptoms can include breathlessness, sweating, nausea, dizziness or palpitations. Pain develops when the oxygen demand of the heart exceeds the supply from the coronary arteries, commonly triggered by physical exertion, emotional stress, cold or after meals. In stable angina, attacks are usually predictable, brief (less than 10 minutes) and relieved by rest or short-acting nitrates. Unstable angina occurs at rest or with minimal exertion, is more severe and prolonged, and signals a higher risk of myocardial infarction, while variant angina results from coronary artery spasm, often at rest or during the night. Recognising the pattern and triggers of angina is essential for timely assessment and management.

Management

Healthcare professionals play a crucial role in the management and care of patients with angina. A thorough assessment must document the location, duration and intensity of chest pain and identify any cardiovascular risk factors that can be used to guide care. Management includes relieving symptoms, reducing anxiety and providing patients with information and advice about risk factors and lifestyle measures that can help to lower cardiovascular risk.

The main goals of treatment in angina are to relieve symptoms, slow disease progression and reduce the risk of future events, particularly myocardial infarction and premature death. Smoking cessation is especially important, as it reduces acute cardiovascular stress and helps slow the progression of atherosclerosis, lowering the risk of angina, myocardial infarction and other complications. Healthcare professionals should offer support to patients to quit smoking and actively support them in achieving this goal.

Pharmacological interventions

Pharmacological management depends on the patient's comorbidities, contraindications and preferences.

First-line medications are taken regularly to reduce the frequency and severity of angina attacks. These include beta blockers, which lower heart rate and myocardial oxygen demand, and rate-limiting calcium channel blockers, such as verapamil or diltiazem, which reduce heart rate and relax coronary arteries. Long-acting nitrates may be added when symptoms are not adequately controlled or if first-line drugs are unsuitable.

For immediate relief, patients are prescribed short-acting GTN, usually in sublingual tablet or spray form. GTN dilates the coronary arteries, reducing the workload of the heart. GTN does not reduce long-term cardiovascular risk, which must be addressed separately.

Coronary revascularisation

Coronary revascularisation is indicated for patients at high risk or those whose symptoms are not adequately controlled with optimal medical therapy. Following revascularisation, a cardiac rehabilitation programme should be arranged to support recovery and reduce future cardiovascular risk. Coronary artery bypass grafting (CABG) and percutaneous coronary intervention (PCI) have specific indications: CABG is generally preferred for multi-vessel or left main disease, while PCI is often used for single-vessel or focal lesions. For low-risk patients with stable angina, medical management remains the initial strategy of choice, as it carries the lowest procedural risk.

Clinical considerations

Using the PQRST pain assessment approach for angina:

P = What provokes the pain? What activity were you doing?
Q = Describe the quality – is it burning, dull, pressure, heavy or stabbing?
R = Does the pain radiate to any other body part?
S = How severe is your pain, graded on a pain scale of 1–10?
T = How long does it last, what makes it worse and what relieves it?

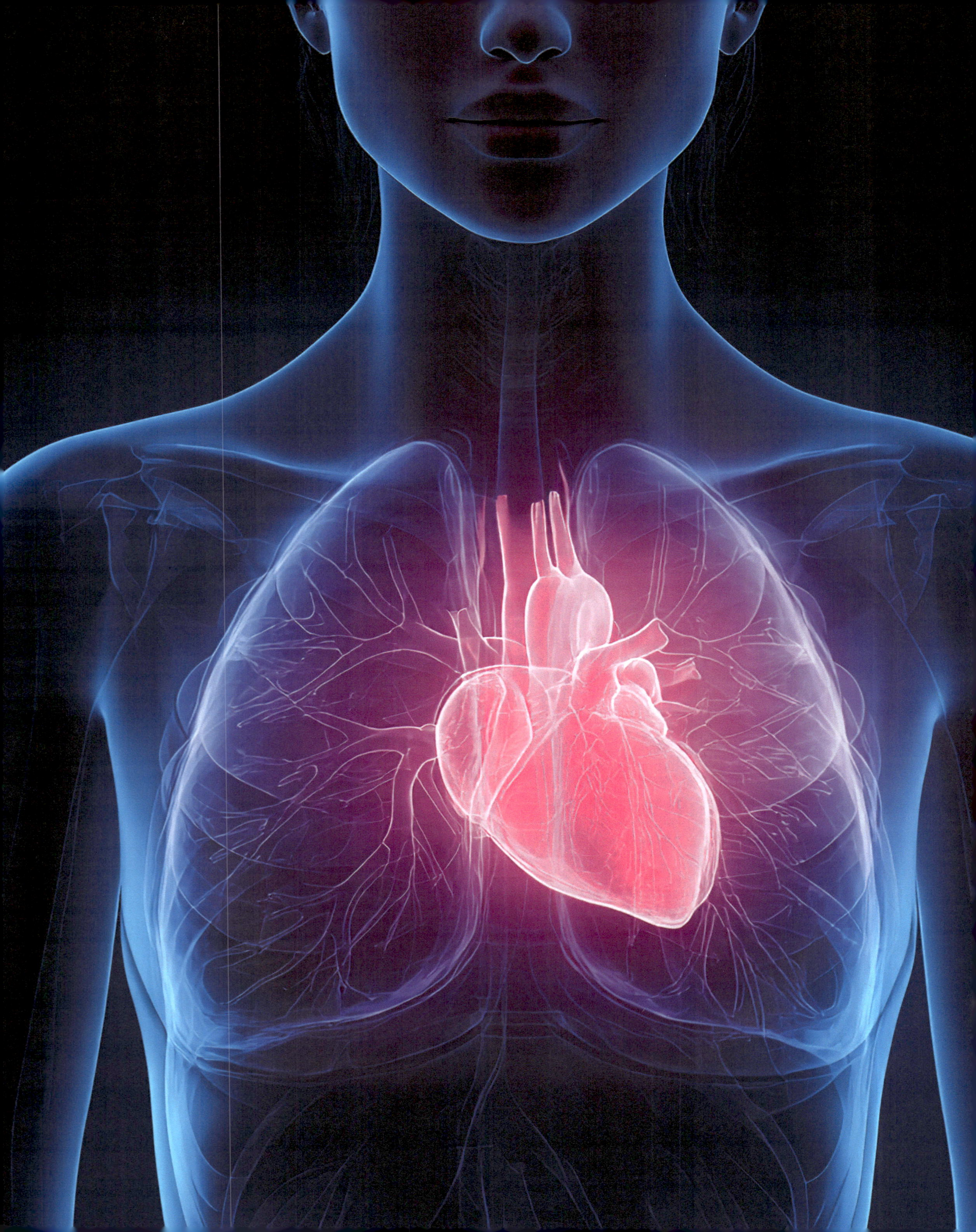

The respiratory system

Chapters

25 Asthma

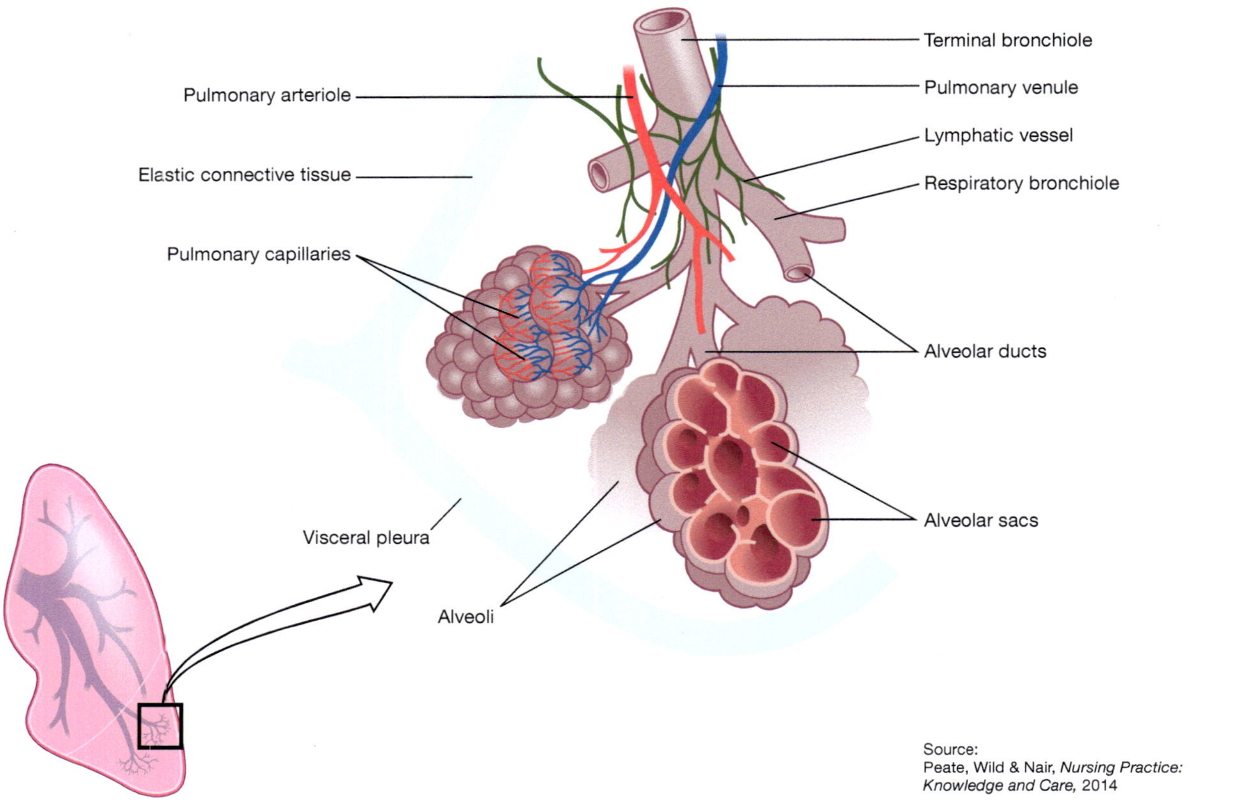

Figure 25.1 Bronchial tree.

Source:
Peate, Wild & Nair, *Nursing Practice: Knowledge and Care,* 2014

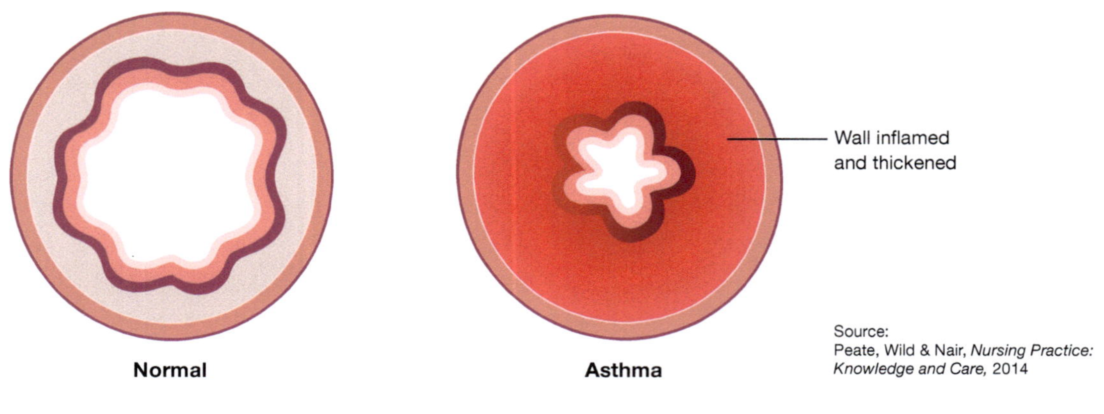

Figure 25.2 Changes in the bronchioles in asthma.

Source:
Peate, Wild & Nair, *Nursing Practice: Knowledge and Care,* 2014

The airways

Asthma is a chronic inflammatory disease of the airways, affecting both the bronchi and bronchioles, which carry air to and from the lungs (see Figure 25.1). In asthma, these airways can become inflamed, hyperresponsive and prone to narrowing, leading to variable airflow obstruction. The conducting airways consist of cartilaginous bronchi, which branch into smaller membranous bronchi and then into bronchioles. The smallest non-gas-exchanging airways, the terminal bronchioles, are approximately 0.5 mm in diameter, while airways less than 2 mm are classified as small and contribute significantly to airway resistance. Gas exchange occurs in the respiratory bronchioles, alveolar ducts and alveoli.

Asthma involves a complex interplay of cellular and molecular mechanisms. Mast cells release histamine (a chemical messenger) and other mediators, while eosinophils, basophils, neutrophils and macrophages contribute to both early- and late-phase inflammatory responses. Sensory stretch and irritant receptors, along with cholinergic motor nerves, regulate airway smooth muscle and glandular activity. In asthma, airway smooth muscle contraction is exaggerated, mucus secretion is increased, and the airway wall becomes oedematous, all of which amplify airflow limitation. These changes vary in distribution and severity, accounting for the episodic nature of asthma symptoms such as wheeze, breathlessness and cough.

Pathophysiology

Asthma is characterised by chronic airway inflammation, hyperresponsiveness and variable airflow obstruction. The inflammatory process involves multiple cell types. T lymphocytes play a key role by releasing cytokines that regulate the inflammatory response, while fibroblasts, endothelial cells and epithelial cells contribute to the persistence and chronicity of the disease. Adhesion molecules, such as selectins and integrins, direct the movement and activation of inflammatory cells, and cell-derived mediators influence smooth muscle tone, mucus secretion and structural remodelling of the airway wall.

Airway hyperresponsiveness, or bronchial hyperreactivity, refers to an exaggerated constrictive response to a wide range of stimuli. This may occur through direct stimulation of airway smooth muscle or indirectly via mediators released from mast cells and non-myelinated sensory neurones. The severity of hyperresponsiveness generally correlates with clinical severity.

The resulting airway obstruction increases resistance to airflow and reduces expiratory flow rates, impairing the ability to fully expel air and potentially leading to hyperinflation. Although hyperinflation may temporarily maintain airway patency, it alters pulmonary mechanics and increases the work of breathing. Chronic inflammation and repeated obstruction can also lead to structural changes, including smooth muscle hypertrophy and subepithelial fibrosis, which further contribute to airflow limitation and the persistence of asthma symptoms (see Figure 25.2).

Bronchial hyperresponsiveness

The lungs may become overinflated; this is done in an attempt to help overcome airflow obstruction, but this compensation becomes ineffective when each breath (known as tidal volume) mostly fills non-functional areas of the lung (this is the pulmonary dead space), leading to reduced ventilation of the alveoli. Uneven changes in airflow resistance, the resulting uneven distribution of air and alterations in circulation from increased intra-alveolar pressure due to hyperinflation all lead to ventilation–perfusion mismatch (this mismatch occurs when air and blood do not meet properly in the lungs, so oxygen cannot efficiently get into the blood). Vasoconstriction due to alveolar hypoxia also contributes to this mismatch. Vasoconstriction is also considered an adaptive response to ventilation/perfusion mismatch.

Signs and symptoms

The symptoms of asthma can range from mild to severe. When symptoms worsen significantly, this is referred to as an asthma attack. Common symptoms include breathlessness, chest tightness (often described as a band tightening around the chest), wheezing (a whistling sound during breathing) and coughing, which is frequently worse at night or in the early morning. Attacks may be triggered by exercise, allergens, respiratory infections or other irritants.

Severe asthma attacks often develop gradually over 6–48 hours, but in some individuals, the symptoms can worsen rapidly and they will require urgent medical attention.

Causes of asthma symptoms

Asthma symptoms can be triggered or worsened by various factors, and identifying individual triggers is important for management. Common triggers include allergens such as dust, animal fur, cockroaches, mould and pollen. Irritants such as cigarette smoke, air pollution, workplace dust or chemicals and sprays (e.g. hairspray) can also provoke symptoms. Certain medications, including aspirin, other non-steroidal anti-inflammatory drugs and non-selective beta blockers, may trigger attacks. Viral infections, such as colds, often worsen asthma and some food or drink chemicals can contribute. Avoiding or reducing exposure to these triggers helps prevent asthma flare-ups.

Management

The primary aim of asthma treatment is to achieve and maintain control, allowing patients to lead full and unrestricted lives. With effective therapy, most people with asthma can be largely symptom-free and maintain normal daily activities. Long-term management focuses on avoiding triggers, adhering to prescribed medications, stopping smoking and maintaining a healthy weight, as these measures can help to reduce the frequency and severity of asthma attacks.

In acute or severe asthma exacerbations, careful monitoring and timely intervention are essential aspects of care provision. Continuous observation of vital signs, alongside the safe administration of oxygen and prescribed medications, helps stabilise the patient. Peak expiratory flow rate (PEFR) is a useful tool for assessing the severity of an attack and the effectiveness of treatment. PEFR should be measured frequently depending on the person's condition, and pre- and post-bronchodilator measurements are important to guide therapy and assess the efficacy of care interventions.

Overall, asthma management combines preventive strategies to minimise exacerbations with prompt treatment of acute attacks. Patient education, self-monitoring and adherence to prescribed therapy are essential components that empower patients to maintain control, reduce complications and live healthy, active lives.

26 Chronic bronchitis

Figure 26.1 Respiratory system.

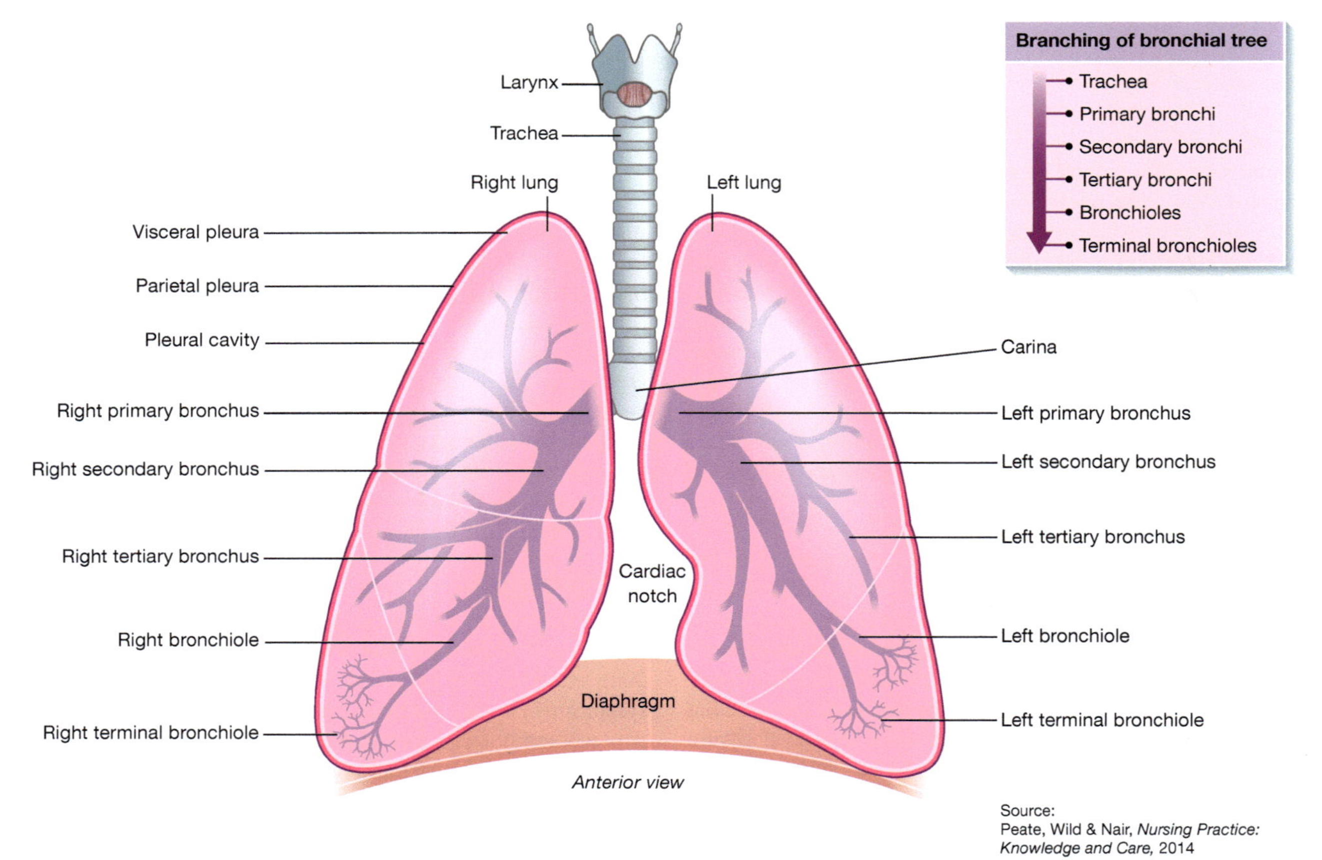

Figure 26.2 Narrowing of the inflamed bronchial tube.

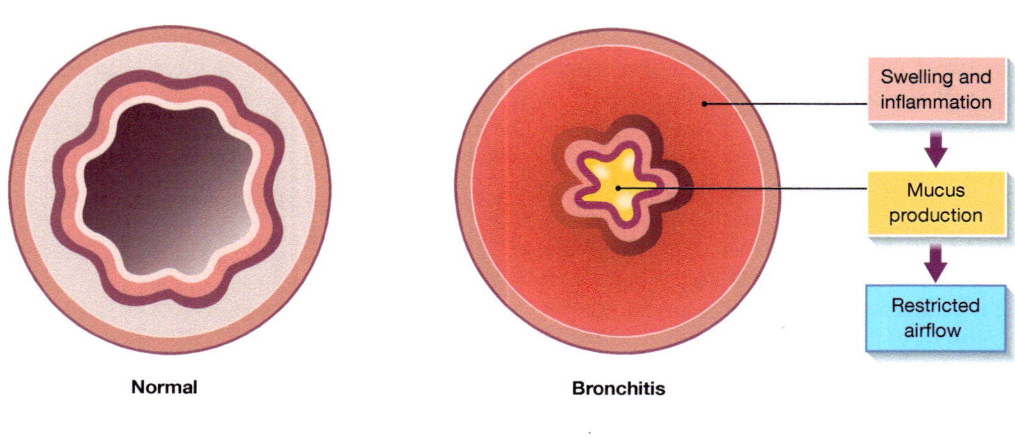

Respiratory tract

The upper respiratory tract is formed of the oral cavity (mouth), the nasal cavity (the nose), the pharynx and the larynx. As well as providing smell and speech, the upper respiratory tract ensures that the air entering the lower respiratory tract is warm, moist and clean.

The lower respiratory tract includes the trachea, the right and left primary bronchi and the constituents of both lungs (Figure 26.1). The trachea (or windpipe) is a tubular vessel that transports air from the larynx downwards towards the lungs. The trachea is lined with pseudostratified ciliated columnar epithelium. This helps to ensure that any inhaled debris is trapped and propelled upwards towards the oesophagus and pharynx to be swallowed or expectorated. The trachea and the bronchi also contain irritant receptors, which stimulate coughs, forcing larger invading particles upwards.

The bronchi are the main airways in the lungs, which branch off on either side of the trachea. They lead to smaller and smaller airways inside the lungs that are known as bronchioles (Figure 26.1). The bronchial walls secrete mucus; these secretions also play a part in helping to trap dust and other particles, preventing them from causing irritation.

The nasal cavity, also lined with a mucous membrane, is composed of pseudostratified ciliated columnar epithelium, which contains an extensive capillary network along with numerous mucus-secreting goblet cells.

Pathophysiology

Chronic bronchitis is a clinical phenotype of chronic obstructive pulmonary disease (COPD), defined by a productive cough lasting for at least 3 months in 2 consecutive years. It primarily affects the conducting airways, particularly the bronchi, which develop chronic inflammation, mucosal swelling and excessive mucus production.

In a healthy respiratory tract, the epithelium produces mucus to trap inhaled particles, including dust, bacteria and viruses. Tiny hair-like projections that are called cilia move this mucus upward toward the throat; this process is known as mucociliary clearance. This mechanism keeps the airways clear of debris and pathogens; in doing this, optimal airflow and gas exchange are maintained. In chronic bronchitis, the persistent inflammation disrupts this defence system (see Figure 26.2). Ciliated epithelial cells are gradually lost, and they are replaced by mucus-secreting goblet cells and, in some areas, metaplastic squamous cells. The loss of functional cilia impairs mucus clearance, which then allows the secretions to accumulate within the airways.

In chronic bronchitis, the inflammation is predominantly neutrophilic. The neutrophils release proteolytic enzymes and inflammatory mediators, which damage the airway epithelium and stimulate further mucus production. The retained mucus creates a warm, nutrient-rich environment that promotes bacterial growth; this predisposes the patient to recurrent infections. This establishes a self-perpetuating cycle of inflammation, infection and mucus hypersecretion.

Airway narrowing results from the combination of mucosal oedema, excessive mucus and smooth muscle contraction, also known as bronchospasm. Both large and small airways are affected, contributing to airflow obstruction. This obstruction, together with mucus plugging, leads to ventilation–perfusion mismatch, impaired gas exchange and clinical symptoms including dyspnoea, wheezing and chronic productive cough.

With ongoing disease, structural changes or airway remodelling develop. The small airways become fibrotic, the bronchial walls thicken and elastic recoil is reduced. These changes contribute to persistent airflow limitation. The continued overproduction of mucus, coupled with dysfunctional cilia, further impedes clearance, increasing susceptibility to bacterial colonisation and exacerbations.

Clinically, chronic bronchitis presents with persistent cough and sputum production, reflecting the combined effects of chronic airway inflammation, impaired mucociliary clearance, airway narrowing and recurrent infection. The condition exemplifies how repeated injury and inflammation in the airways can progressively compromise respiratory function and quality of life.

Signs and symptoms

Cough and sputum production are the hallmark symptoms of chronic bronchitis. These typically persist for at least 3 months and occur on most days, often varying in intensity and the volume of sputum from one patient to another. The sputum may be clear, yellowish, greenish or occasionally blood-tinged, reflecting ongoing airway inflammation or secondary infection.

Cigarette smoking is the leading cause of chronic bronchitis; many patients present with the classic 'smoker's cough'. This is characterised by a cough that is often worse on rising in the morning, accompanied by expectoration of discoloured mucus, which gradually diminishes as the day progresses. The morning predominance occurs because mucus accumulates in the airways overnight, while mucociliary clearance is less effective.

Patients may also experience wheezing, a high-pitched whistling sound during breathing, due to partial airway obstruction. Dyspnoea is common and may initially be exertional but can progress to occur at rest as the disease advances and airflow limitation becomes more severe.

The combination of persistent coughing, sputum production and laboured breathing can be physically exhausting. Frequent coughing requires repeated contraction of respiratory muscles, increasing energy expenditure. Additionally, impaired gas exchange from narrowed, mucus-filled airways reduces oxygen delivery to tissues, which contributes to fatigue. Night-time symptoms, including coughing that interrupts sleep, further exacerbate tiredness and can lead to reduced concentration, decreased exercise tolerance and overall diminished quality of life.

Management

The cornerstone of managing chronic bronchitis is avoiding triggers that exacerbate symptoms, particularly cigarette smoke, environmental pollutants and respiratory irritants. Smoking cessation is essential, tobacco smoke damages the airway epithelium, impairs ciliary function and increases susceptibility to respiratory infections.

During acute exacerbations, short-acting bronchodilators, either β_2-agonists (salbutamol and terbutaline) or anticholinergics (ipratropium bromide), should be administered to relieve bronchoconstriction. In selected patients, a short course of systemic corticosteroids (usually 5–7 days) may be prescribed. Antibiotics may be indicated if a bacterial infection is suspected.

Annual influenza vaccination is recommended unless contraindicated, and pneumococcal vaccination should be considered in patients with significant respiratory comorbidity. Patients should be advised on supportive self-care measures, including adequate rest, maintaining hydration, avoiding smoke and irritant fumes, and optimising concordance to prescribed inhaled medications.

Overall, the management of chronic bronchitis combines trigger avoidance, pharmacological therapy during exacerbations, preventive vaccination and lifestyle support, with a strong emphasis on smoking cessation.

Clinical considerations

Definition: productive cough 3 months or more in 2 consecutive years; COPD phenotype.

Symptoms: daily cough, sputum, wheeze, dyspnoea; worse in mornings.

Exacerbations: infections or irritants; treated with short-acting bronchodilators ± short-course corticosteroids.

Key risk factors: smoking, air pollution, occupational exposures and recurrent infections.

Pathophysiology: neutrophilic inflammation, ciliary dysfunction, goblet cell hyperplasia, mucus hypersecretion and airway narrowing.

Management: trigger avoidance, inhaled bronchodilators, corticosteroids for exacerbations, vaccinations and supportive care.

Complications: recurrent infections, progressive airflow limitation, hypoxia, fatigue and COPD progression.

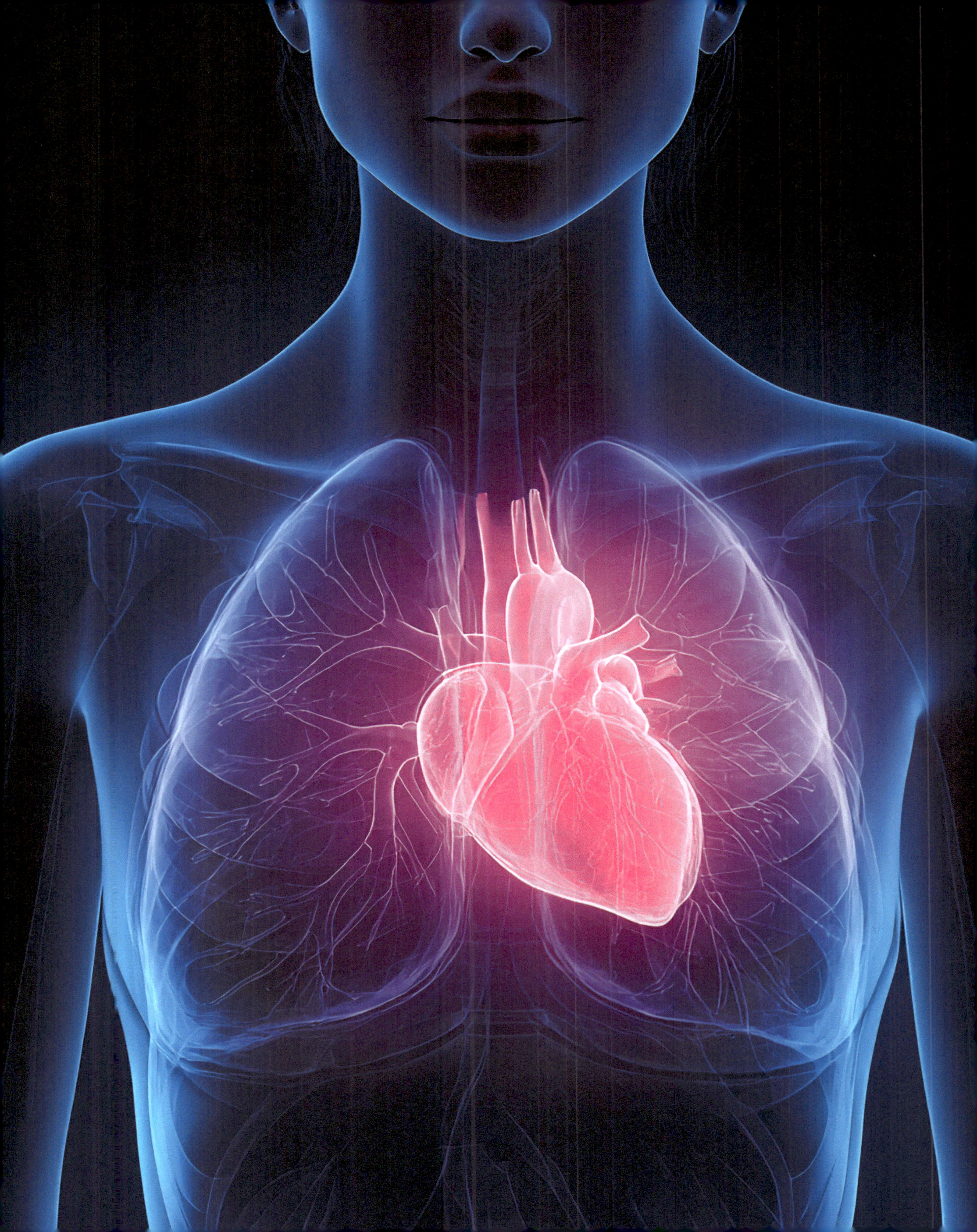

27 Pulmonary embolism

Figure 27.1 Formation of a pulmonary embolism: a blood clot from the leg vein, travels to the heart and then becomes lodged in a blood vessel (artery) in the lungs.

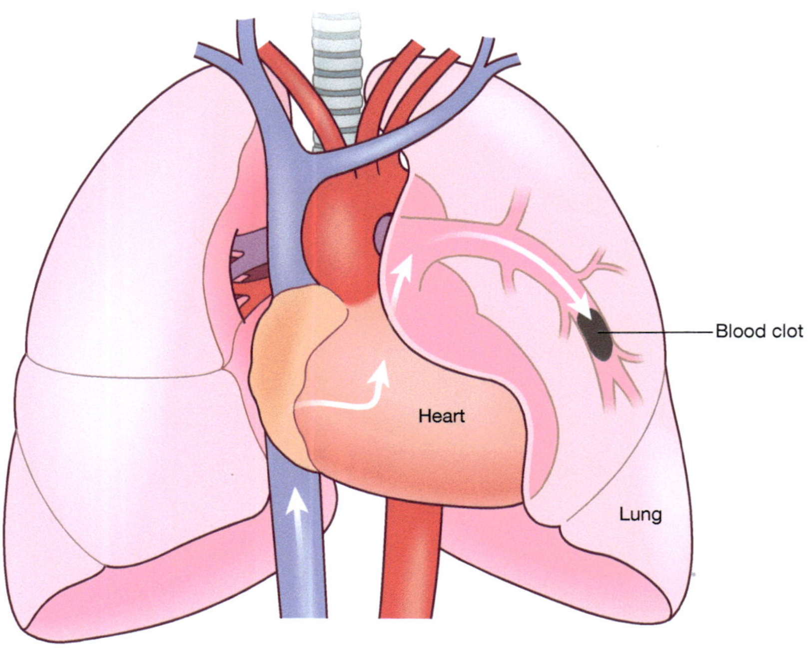

Figure 27.2 Normal blood flow, deep vein thrombosis and embolus.

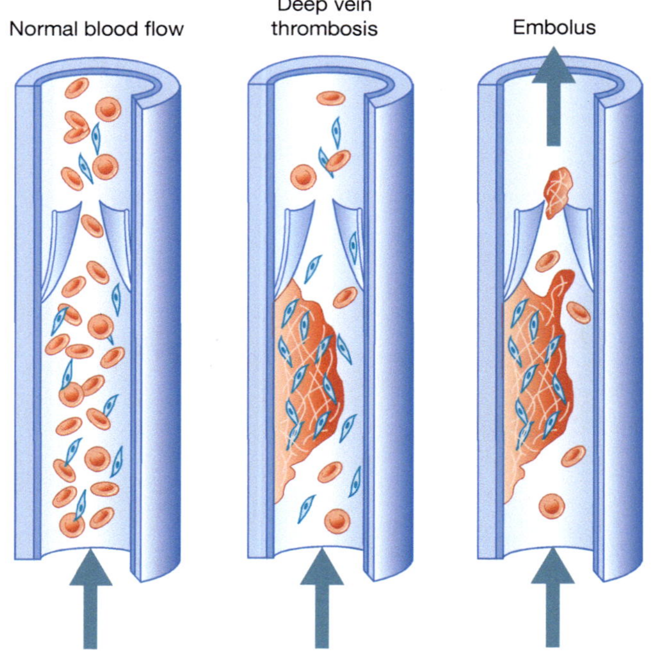

Overview

Pulmonary embolism (PE) occurs when a thrombus or other material obstructs blood flow in the pulmonary arteries. Small emboli (microemboli) may be clinically silent, causing no noticeable symptoms. Moderate-sized emboli often present with a sudden onset of dyspnoea, tachypnoea and sometimes chest discomfort. Large emboli that significantly impede pulmonary blood flow can lead to hypotension, syncope, cardiovascular collapse or sudden death (see Figure 27.1). The majority of PEs originate from thrombi in the deep veins of the lower extremities, a condition known as deep vein thrombosis (DVT), which embolise to the lungs (see Figure 27.2). Pulmonary infarction may occur if blood flow obstruction leads to tissue necrosis, presenting as sharp, pleuritic chest pain that worsens with respiration and may be accompanied by haemoptysis. Additional signs can include tachycardia, low-grade fever and anxiety. Early recognition and treatment are essential to prevent morbidity and mortality, with anticoagulation forming the mainstay of therapy.

Pathophysiology

A PE happens when a blood clot, usually from the deep veins of the legs or pelvis, travels through the veins and lodges in the arteries of the lungs. This can block blood flow and affect both the heart and lungs. PE is part of a group of conditions called venous thromboembolism, which also includes DVT.

Slowed blood flow can occur after long periods of immobility, such as after surgery or during long travel. Vessel injury can happen from trauma, surgery or medical devices. Blood may clot more easily in conditions such as cancer, pregnancy or certain inherited disorders.

When a clot breaks off, it becomes an embolus and it then travels to the lungs. The embolus blocks part of the pulmonary circulation; this then increases pressure in the pulmonary arteries. The right side of the heart has to work harder to push blood through, which can cause it to stretch and fail if the obstruction is large. This can reduce blood flow to the rest of the body, leading to low blood pressure, collapse or even shock.

Blocked blood flow also causes problems with oxygen exchange in the lungs. Areas of the lung that receive air but not blood cannot transfer oxygen efficiently, causing shortness of breath and low oxygen levels.

Some areas of the lung may undergo tissue death, known as pulmonary infarction, which can cause sharp, pleuritic chest pain or coughing up blood (haemoptysis). This is uncommon because the lungs have a dual blood supply from both the pulmonary and bronchial arteries.

Many clots are gradually broken down by the body's natural clot-dissolving system, but some may persist, leading to chronic problems such as pulmonary hypertension or long-term shortness of breath.

Understanding the pathophysiology of PE helps in the recognition of symptoms early, assessing risk and providing timely treatment, including anticoagulation, supportive care or interventions to remove the clot.

Blood vessel damage

If a blood vessel is damaged, the inner lining, which is the endothelium, can become disrupted, which may cause the vessel to narrow or become blocked, promoting the formation of a blood clot. Blood vessels can be damaged by injuries such as fractures or severe muscle trauma. Surgical procedures, particularly those involving lower body, may also injure vessels and increase the risk of clot formation. Certain conditions, such as vasculitis, and some medications, including chemotherapy agents, can similarly damage blood vessels and contribute to clot development.

Diagnosis

Because the severity of PE varies and its symptoms are common in other conditions, making a diagnosis can be challenging. A range of tests and investigations may be used to help confirm the diagnosis. These include ultrasound of the legs to detect DVT, a blood test for D-dimer to indicate clot formation, a ventilation–perfusion (V/Q) scan to assess blood flow in the lungs, and a CT pulmonary angiography (CTPA) scan to visualise clots in the pulmonary arteries.

Management

Management of PE follows NICE guidelines and is based on the severity of the embolism, patient risk factors and comorbidities; local policy and protocol will also be in place. The first step is risk assessment. High-risk or 'massive' PE presents with sustained hypotension, shock or cardiac arrest and requires urgent intervention. Intermediate-risk ('submassive') PE refers to patients who are normotensive but show right ventricular dysfunction or raised cardiac biomarkers. Low-risk PE patients are haemodynamically stable without evidence of right heart strain. Risk stratification guides treatment intensity and monitoring.

Immediate management aims to stabilise the patient. Oxygen is administered if hypoxaemia is present, and intravenous fluids support blood pressure cautiously. In high-risk PE, thrombolytic therapy such as intravenous alteplase is used to rapidly dissolve clots, ideally in a high-dependency setting. If thrombolysis is contraindicated or unsuccessful, surgical or catheter-directed thrombectomy may be considered.

For most patients, anticoagulation forms the basis of treatment. In the acute phase, patients are commonly started on low-molecular-weight heparin (LMWH), such as enoxaparin, due to its rapid onset of action and predictable dosing. LMWH is administered subcutaneously and continues until a longer-term anticoagulant is established. In many cases, patients are transitioned to direct oral anticoagulants (DOACs) like apixaban or rivaroxaban for ease of use and consistent anticoagulant effect. Warfarin remains an alternative for patients with contraindications to DOACs or specific conditions such as mechanical heart valves. Anticoagulation is usually continued for at least three months, with longer durations considered for persistent risk factors or unprovoked PE.

Mechanical prophylaxis is also important, particularly for patients at high risk of clot formation who cannot take anticoagulants. Graduated compression stockings may improve venous return in the legs, while intermittent pneumatic compression (IPC) devices mimic muscle contractions to reduce venous stasis.

Monitoring and follow-up include observation of vital signs, oxygenation and right ventricular function. Patients are offered information and advice on mobility, hydration and recognising DVT symptoms. Long-term follow-up screens for chronic thromboembolic pulmonary hypertension and ensure safe anticoagulant use.

Contemporary practice emphasises early diagnosis, risk-stratified treatment, initial LMWH therapy, transition to DOACs, mechanical prophylaxis and structured follow-up, supported by a multidisciplinary team to optimise outcomes and minimise complications.

Clinical considerations

Safe anticoagulant use requires checking for contraindications such as active bleeding, recent major surgery, or uncontrolled hypertension and assessing kidney and liver function for dose adjustment. Patients should be monitored for signs of bleeding, educated on adherence, symptom recognition and drug interactions, and have therapy adjusted if invasive procedures are planned. Regular follow-up ensures treatment remains safe and effective.

28 Chronic obstructive pulmonary disease

Figure 28.1 Emphysema.

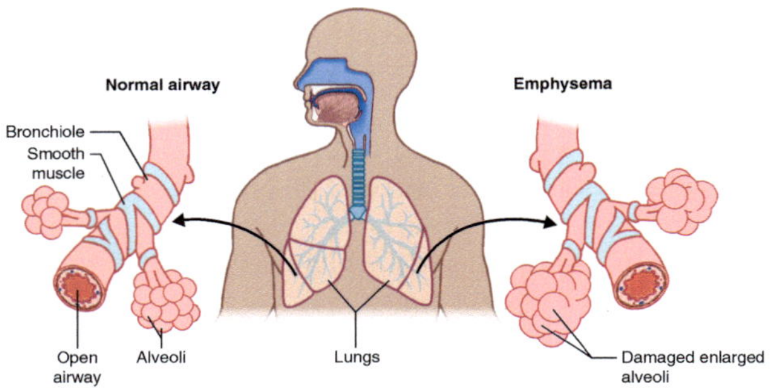

Source:
Felner, K. Schneider,
M. 2008/John Wiley & Sons

Figure 28.2 Bronchitis.

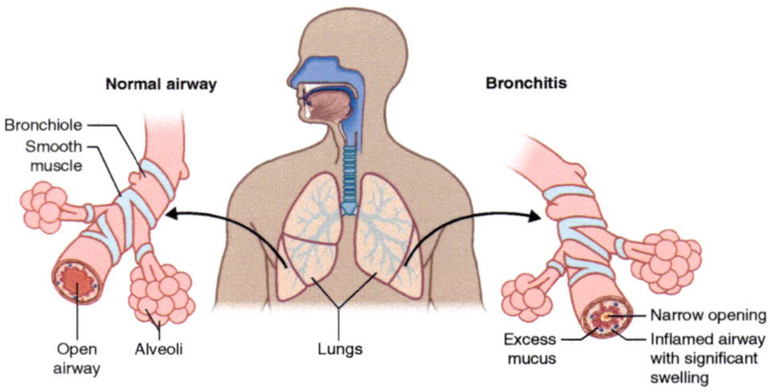

Source:
Felner, K. Schneider,
M. 2008/John Wiley & Sons

Figure 28.3 Normal lung and a lung with bronchial stricture (arrowed).

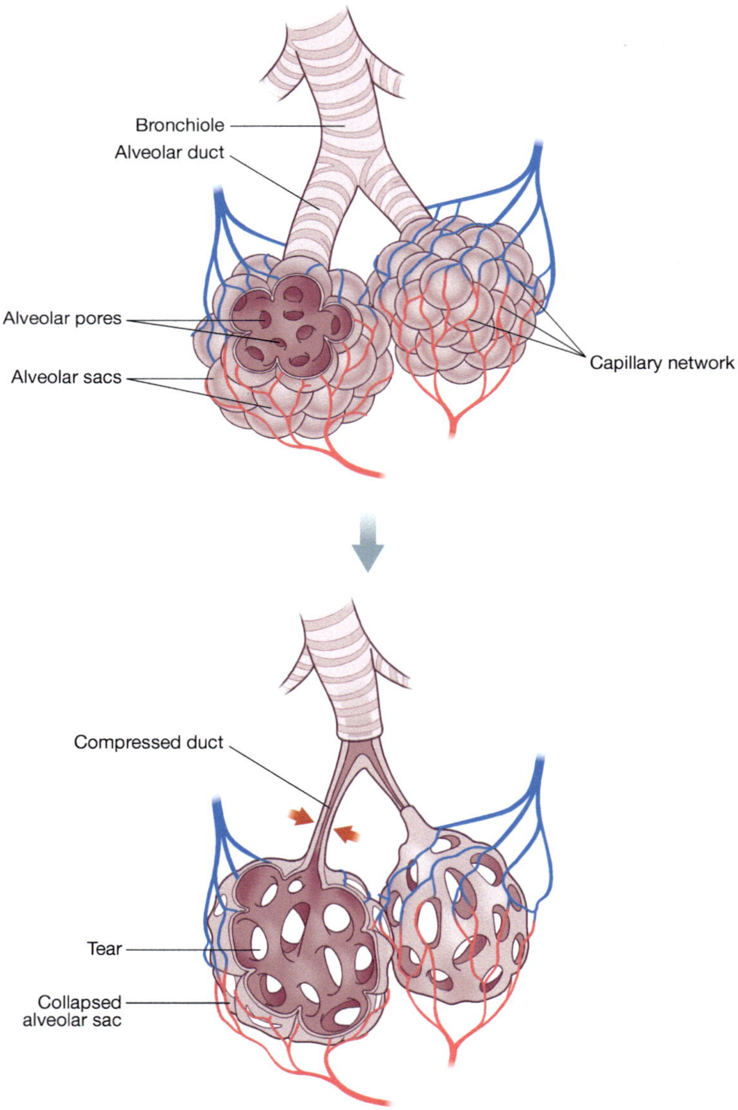

Overview

The lungs are the primary organs of the respiratory system. Their main function is to bring oxygen (O_2) into the body and remove carbon dioxide (CO_2), a waste product of metabolism. The lungs also help maintain acid-base balance by regulating CO_2 levels, which influence blood pH. They play a role in filtering small blood clots and particles, protecting the heart and circulation. Other functions include vocalisation, as air moving through the vocal cords produces sound, and immune defence, as the lungs trap pathogens and particulates with mucus and cilia.

Pathophysiology

COPD is a progressive lung condition that includes chronic bronchitis, emphysema and chronic obstructive airways disease (see Figures 28.1 and 28.2). It is characterised by persistent airflow limitation that is usually not fully reversible, causing increasing difficulty in breathing. The disease develops slowly over many years, often affecting middle-aged and older adults, and is closely associated with smoking and environmental exposures.

The underlying pathophysiology of COPD involves chronic inflammation of the airways and structural damage to the lung tissue. The most consistent change is hypertrophy and an increased number of mucus-secreting goblet cells in the bronchial tree, particularly in the larger airways. This leads to excess mucus production, contributing to airway obstruction and cough. The small airways are affected early, with inflammation initially reversible, which explains why lung function can improve if smoking is stopped early. As the disease progresses, chronic inflammation persists even if smoking ceases, and fibrosis and squamous cell metaplasia develop in the bronchial walls.

Airflow limitation in COPD results from a combination of narrowed, inflamed airways and destruction of alveolar walls (emphysema) (see Figure 28.3). Loss of elastic recoil causes the small airways to collapse during expiration, further impairing airflow and making it increasingly difficult to breathe out. Over time, these changes lead to progressive breathlessness, reduced exercise tolerance and recurrent respiratory infections.

Smoking is the main cause of COPD; chemicals in tobacco smoke trigger airway inflammation, increase mucus production and damage alveoli. Other environmental factors include occupational exposure to dusts and chemicals, such as grains, cadmium, coal dust or isocyanates (a group of chemicals commonly used in industrial processes, e.g. paints, varnishes, adhesives, foams and plastics) and air pollution, which can contribute even in non-smokers.

A rare genetic factor, alpha-1 antitrypsin deficiency, predisposes some individuals to COPD at a younger age, often under 35 years. Alpha-1 antitrypsin is a protein that protects lung tissue from damaging enzymes. Without it, even normal physiological processes can cause lung damage, accelerating the development of COPD.

In summary, COPD is a chronic, progressive disease that is caused by a combination of inflammation, structural lung damage and airway remodelling, with airflow limitation worsened by emphysema. The disease is primarily driven by smoking, but environmental exposures and genetic predisposition can also contribute. Understanding the pathophysiology is essential for healthcare professionals to identify risk factors, recognise symptoms and implement interventions such as smoking cessation, pulmonary rehabilitation and pharmacological therapy to slow disease progression and improve quality of life.

Signs and symptoms

COPD develops gradually, so patients may not initially recognise their symptoms. Common symptoms include progressive breathlessness on exertion, persistent cough with sputum production, wheezing (typically this is an expiratory wheeze) and frequent chest infections, particularly during the winter. Exacerbations, or 'flare-ups', occur when symptoms suddenly worsen; these are often triggered by bacterial or viral infections and are a common reason for a person to be admitted to hospital. During flare-ups, patients may produce more sputum, which can become yellow or green, and they can also experience increased breathlessness and wheeze.

Other features of COPD include extreme fatigue, weight loss and swelling of the ankles, which may reflect systemic effects or right heart strain.

When assessing patients, it is important to consider skin pigmentation, as some signs may be less visible in people with darker skin. Cyanosis, or a bluish tint, may be subtle and is better assessed in the lips, tongue, nail beds or conjunctiva. Pallor should be checked in the mucous membranes rather than relying solely on skin tone. Clubbing of fingers, oedema and overall respiratory effort are detectable regardless of skin colour, and they provide important clinical information.

Overall, a careful combination of patient-reported symptoms, observation of breathing and assessment of visible physiological signs ensures accurate recognition of COPD in all patients, regardless of skin pigmentation. Early detection and monitoring of symptoms and exacerbations are key to improving outcomes and reducing complications.

Management

There is currently no cure for COPD, but treatment can slow disease progression, relieve symptoms and improve quality of life. The most important intervention is smoking cessation, which prevents further lung damage and can improve outcomes even in established disease. Avoiding environmental pollutants and occupational exposures is also important.

Pharmacological management is tailored to symptom severity and frequency of exacerbations. Short-acting bronchodilators provide rapid relief and include beta-2 agonists (e.g. salbutamol and terbutaline) and antimuscarinics (e.g. ipratropium). Long-acting bronchodilators (LABAs, such as salmeterol or formoterol; LAMAs, e.g. tiotropium) are used for maintenance therapy. Inhaled corticosteroids (ICS) reduce airway inflammation and are often combined with LABAs for moderate-to-severe COPD or frequent exacerbations. For patients with persistent symptoms or repeated exacerbations, triple therapy (LABA + LAMA + ICS) may be prescribed to optimise symptom control and reduce exacerbation risk.

Pulmonary rehabilitation combines exercise training, education and breathing techniques to improve functional ability and reduce breathlessness. Vaccinations are recommended to prevent respiratory infections. Self-management plans empower patients to recognise early signs of exacerbations, adjust treatment when appropriate and seek timely medical review, helping to reduce hospital admissions. Nutritional support may be needed for weight loss or muscle wasting; physiotherapy can assist with mucus clearance.

For patients with chronic hypoxaemia, long-term oxygen therapy improves survival and quality of life. In acute exacerbations or advanced disease with hypercapnia, non-invasive ventilation (NIV) can support breathing and prevent respiratory failure.

Regular monitoring is vital to assess symptom control, lung function, treatment adherence and overall quality of life. Providing patients with information about recognising changes in breathlessness, sputum colour or volume is key to prompt management of exacerbations.

Clinical considerations

The MRC dyspnoea scale assesses the severity of breathlessness in daily activities, from Grade 1 (breathless on strenuous exercise) to Grade 5 (too breathless to leave the house). It helps evaluate functional impact, monitor disease progression and guide treatment and can be combined with lung function tests for a fuller assessment.

The gastrointestinal system

Chapters

29 Peritonitis

Figure 29.1 Location of the parietal and visceral peritoneum.

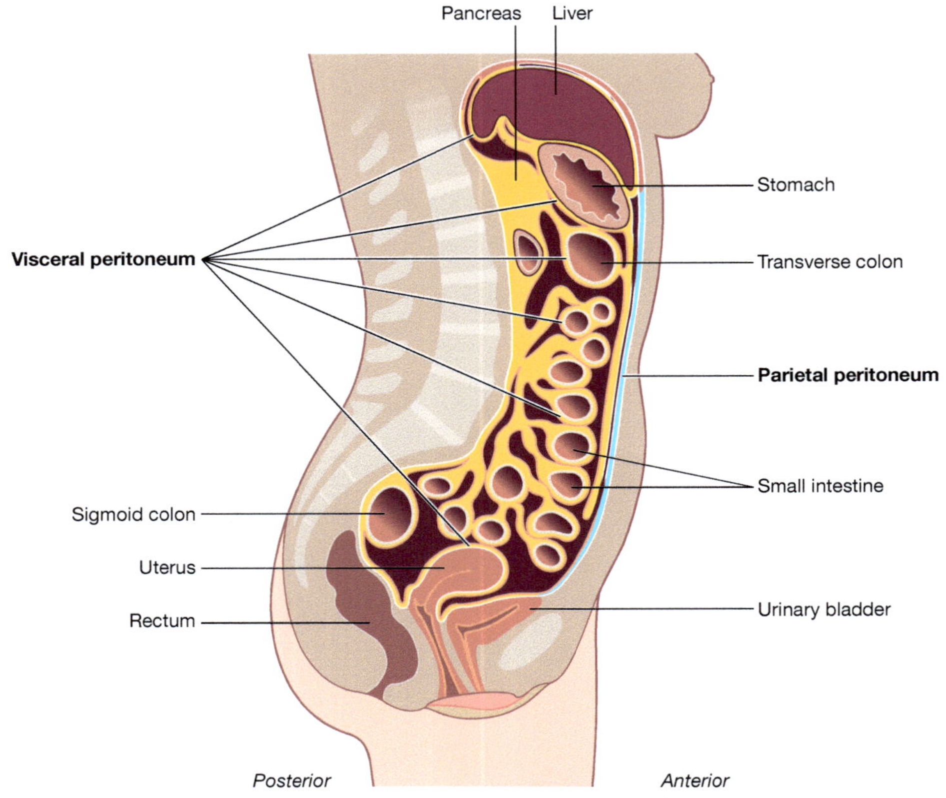

Figure 29.2 Peritonitis: Inflammation of the peritoneum.

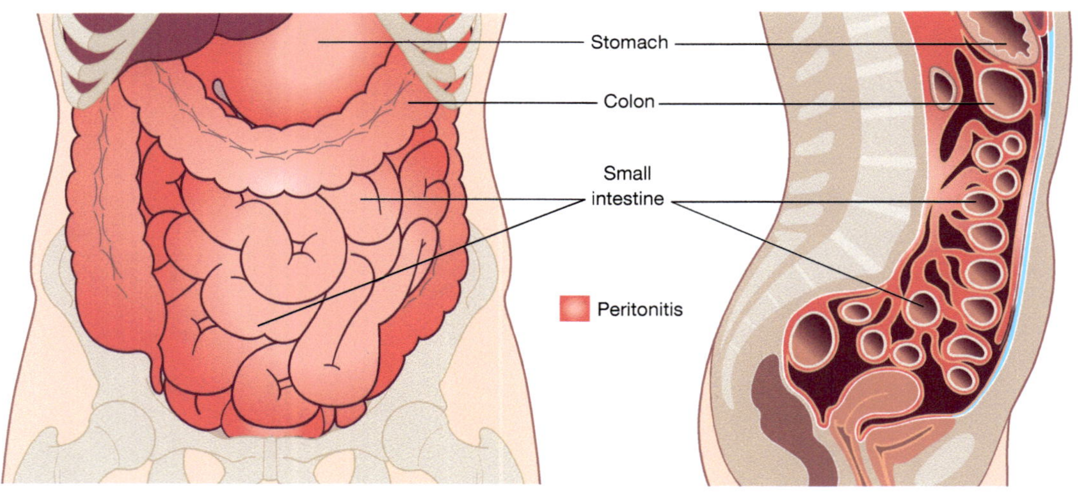

The peritoneum

The peritoneum is a smooth, transparent serous membrane that lines the abdominal cavity and folds over the abdominal and pelvic organs. It consists of two layers: the parietal peritoneum, which lines the abdominal wall, and the visceral peritoneum, which covers the organs (Figure 29.1). Between these layers lies the peritoneal cavity, a potential space containing a small amount of serous fluid. This fluid, secreted by mesothelial cells and partly as a transudate allows the layers to slide smoothly over each other, reducing friction during movements such as peristalsis, and coats organ surfaces to facilitate frictionless motion.

Peritoneal fluid is in dynamic equilibrium with plasma, but unlike plasma, it contains very little fibrinogen under normal conditions. When injury, surgery or inflammation occurs, plasma proteins, including fibrinogen, can leak into the cavity, leading to fibrin deposition. The peritoneum has high local fibrinolytic activity, which breaks down fibrin and helps prevent the formation of adhesions between organs.

The peritoneal folds and mesentery provide a pathway for blood vessels, lymphatics and nerves to reach the abdominal organs. The large surface area of the peritoneum also allows rapid absorption of substances, which is useful for intraperitoneal drug delivery, but it also means that bacterial toxins can quickly provoke peritonitis. Overall, the peritoneum maintains organ mobility, supports homeostasis and protects against adhesion formation, while allowing efficient vascular and neural connections to the viscera.

Pathophysiology

Peritonitis occurs when the normally sterile peritoneal cavity becomes contaminated by infection or chemical irritants (see Figure 29.2). Chemical peritonitis often precedes bacterial infection and can result from leakage of gastric juices, such as hydrochloric acid and pepsin, or bile following perforation of a peptic ulcer or rupture of the gallbladder. These substances can trigger an acute inflammatory response.

Bacterial peritonitis usually arises from gut bacteria, which include *Escherichia coli*, *Klebsiella*, *Proteus* or *Pseudomonas*. Once bacteria enter the peritoneal space, local immune and inflammatory mechanisms are then activated. Mast cells release histamine and other vasoactive substances, which causes capillary dilation and increased permeability, allowing immune cells and plasma proteins to reach the site of infection. Polymorphonuclear leukocytes (a type of white blood cell) migrate into the peritoneum to phagocytose bacteria and debris, while fibrin-rich exudate forms to localise and contain the infection. This process helps the host to eliminate bacteria and limit damage.

If contamination is massive or if it is ongoing, these defences may be overwhelmed, leading to generalised inflammation of the peritoneal cavity. Fluid shifts into the peritoneal space (third spacing), reducing circulating blood volume and potentially causing hypovolaemia. Bacteria or their toxins may enter the bloodstream, resulting in septicaemia.

Spontaneous bacterial peritonitis can occur without abdominal rupture; this occurs usually in those patients with advanced liver disease and ascites. The accumulated fluid provides a medium that is susceptible to bacterial growth, increasing the risk of infection.

Overall, peritonitis involves a complex interplay of chemical irritation, bacterial invasion, immune response and inflammatory processes, with potential systemic consequences if the infection is not controlled. Prompt recognition and treatment are essential to prevent severe complications such as shock, organ failure or death.

Signs and symptoms

Those people with peritonitis present with a range of abdominal and systemic signs, which vary depending on severity, extent and the patient's overall health. The most prominent feature is acute abdominal pain; this is often sudden, diffuse and severe, but sometimes localises to the area of greatest inflammation. When the patient moves, this can worsen the pain and patients may adopt a guarded posture to minimise discomfort.

On examination, the abdomen is often tender and rigid, with involuntary muscle guarding that may feel board-like. Rebound tenderness is frequently observed (this is pain felt when pressure on the abdomen is released, rather than when applied). Bowel sounds may be reduced or absent in peritonitis due to paralytic ileus, but their presence or absence cannot be used alone to rule in or out the condition. They should always be interpreted alongside other clinical signs, such as abdominal tenderness, guarding, distention and systemic symptoms. Abdominal distension, nausea and vomiting are common.

Systemic signs reflect the body's inflammatory and fluid response. Patients may exhibit pyrexia, malaise, tachycardia and rapid breathing, and some may become restless or disoriented. In severe cases, oliguria, dehydration and hypotensive shock may develop due to fluid shifts into the peritoneal cavity.

Clinical assessment relies on careful history, physical examination and monitoring of vital signs. Early recognition of these signs is essential to promptly initiate treatment, prevent progression to sepsis or organ failure, and improve patient outcomes.

Most instances of peritonitis are caused by an infection that spreads to the peritoneum. Common causes of secondary peritonitis include perforations from stomach ulcers, perforated appendix, Crohn's disease and diverticulitis.

Management

Peritonitis is a medical emergency that requires rapid assessment and treatment to prevent life-threatening complications. The first step is to identify and manage the underlying cause of the inflammation. Vital signs are closely monitored, often hourly, in the early stages. Blood cultures are obtained before starting antibiotics to help identify the causative organism.

Patients are often kept nil by mouth (nothing to eat or drink) to rest the gastrointestinal tract, especially if nausea or vomiting is present. Intravenous fluids are given to maintain hydration and correct electrolyte imbalances. Broad-spectrum intravenous antibiotics are initiated promptly to control infection, and analgesics are administered to relieve pain.

If the peritonitis has a surgical cause, operative management is essential. For example, an appendicectomy is performed in cases of perforated appendicitis, and the peritoneal cavity is thoroughly irrigated (lavaged) with warm saline to remove pus, debris and bacteria. Drains may be inserted to prevent fluid accumulation. Other procedures may include repair of a perforated peptic ulcer, resection of necrotic bowel or drainage of abscesses.

Some patients may have difficulty digesting food, so enteral nutrition via a nasogastric or surgically placed feeding tube may be needed. If enteral feeding is not possible, parenteral nutrition (nutrition through a vein) may be used temporarily.

Early recognition, prompt antibiotic therapy and appropriate surgical intervention are crucial to improving outcomes. Ongoing monitoring for complications such as sepsis, abscess formation or organ failure is essential during recovery.

Clinical considerations

Effective communication is a vital part of caring for patients with peritonitis. Explain the condition clearly so that the patient and their family understand that peritonitis is a serious, potentially life-threatening inflammation of the abdominal lining requiring prompt medical attention and treatment.

Patients should be informed about the treatment plan, including rest, intravenous fluids, antibiotics and any necessary surgical procedures, and why these interventions are required. Preparing the patient for procedures is also important; explaining what to expect with nasogastric tubes, feeding tubes or surgical drains can reduce anxiety and help the patient understand how these devices support recovery and comfort.

Providing reassurance and emotional support is essential, encouraging patients to ask questions and become active participants in their care. Family involvement is also valuable, as relatives can help observe warning signs and support treatment adherence.

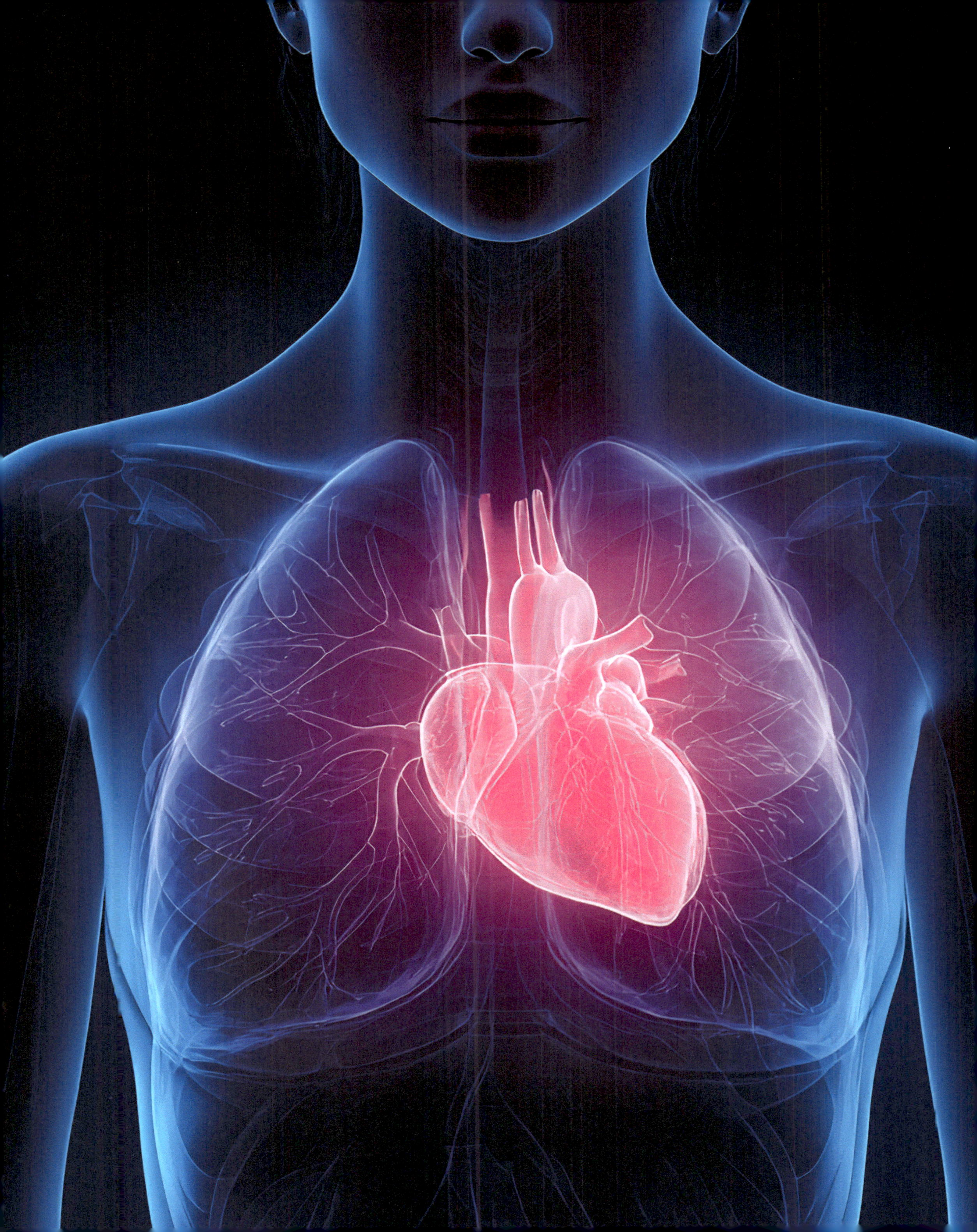

30 Crohn's disease

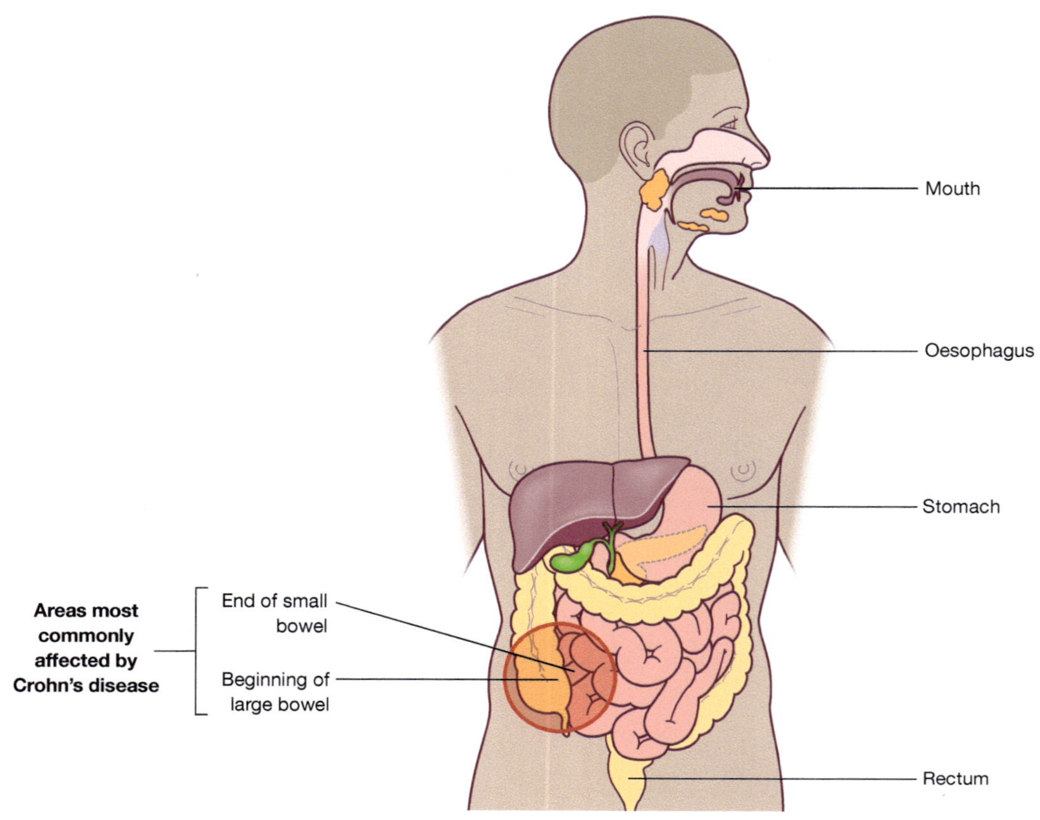

Figure 30.1 Areas affected by Crohn's disease.

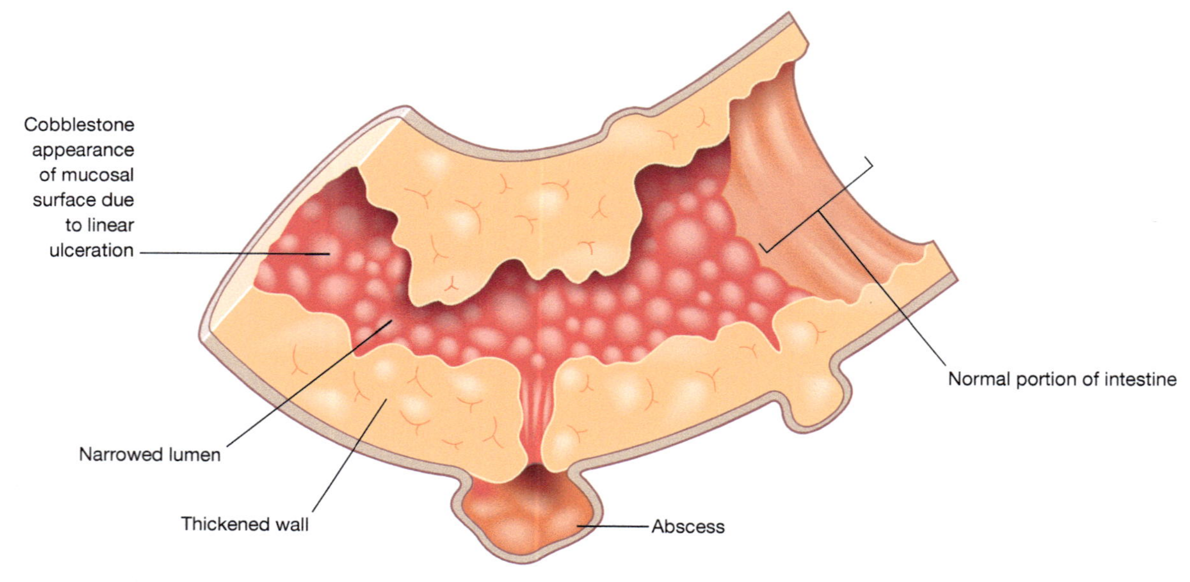

Figure 30.2 Cobblestone appearance of the colon.

Overview

Crohn's disease is a long-term inflammatory condition that affects the lining of the digestive tract. It can occur anywhere from the mouth to the anus, but it most commonly begins in the terminal part of the small intestine (the ileum) (see Figure 30.1). Unlike other gut conditions, Crohn's disease typically causes patchy inflammation, with some sections of the intestine inflamed and others remaining normal.

The gastrointestinal (GI) tract is a continuous tube starting at the mouth and ending at the anus. Food passes down the oesophagus into the stomach, where it is broken down by acids and enzymes, and then enters the small intestine, which has three sections: the duodenum, jejunum, and ileum. The small intestine is primarily responsible for digestion and absorption of nutrients into the bloodstream. From the ileum, the digestive contents pass into the large intestine (colon and rectum), where water is absorbed and the remaining material is stored as faeces, which are eventually expelled via the anus.

In Crohn's disease, inflammation can cause thickening of the intestinal wall, ulceration and the formation of fistulas or strictures (narrowed sections of bowel). This can lead to abdominal pain, diarrhoea, fatigue and unintentional weight loss. Patients may also experience blood or mucus in the stool. Chronic inflammation can sometimes lead to complications, including intestinal obstruction, malnutrition or increased risk of colorectal cancer.

Although the exact cause of Crohn's disease is unknown, it is thought to involve a combination of genetic, immune and environmental factors. There is no cure, but treatments such as anti-inflammatory medications, immunosuppressants, biologic therapies, and sometimes surgery can help control symptoms, reduce inflammation, and prevent complications.

Understanding the anatomy and function of the GI tract may help those who provide care and support to people to appreciate why Crohn's disease can affect digestion, nutrient absorption and overall health and well-being, and why careful monitoring and treatment are essential.

Pathophysiology

Crohn's disease is a chronic inflammatory condition of the GI tract, characterised by patchy, discontinuous inflammation. These affected segments are known as skip lesions; they are separated by normal-appearing bowel.

The inflammation in Crohn's disease is transmural, involving the entire thickness of the bowel wall, from the mucosa to the muscular layers. This deep inflammation contributes to the development of ulcers, fissures and a characteristic cobblestone appearance of the mucosa (Figure 30.2). Transmural involvement also predisposes patients to complications such as strictures, where the bowel narrows; fistulas, abnormal connections forming between the bowel and other structures; and abscesses, localised collections of pus.

The inflammatory process interferes with normal digestion and absorption, particularly when the jejunum or ileum is affected. Nutrients such as carbohydrates, proteins, fats, vitamins and folate may be inadequately absorbed. Involvement of the terminal ileum can impair vitamin B_{12} and bile salt absorption, while chronic ulceration can result in protein loss and slow GI bleeding, contributing to anaemia.

The exact cause of Crohn's disease is unknown, but it is believed to arise from a combination of genetic susceptibility, abnormal immune responses and environmental triggers. Dysregulated immune activity leads to chronic inflammation, tissue injury and impaired healing, driving the relapsing and progressive nature of the disease.

Risk factors

Crohn's disease arises from a combination of genetic, environmental and immune factors. A family history significantly increases risk, suggesting a hereditary component. Genetic mutations can predispose individuals to abnormal immune responses in the gut. Smoking is a well-established environmental risk factor associated with more severe disease and higher relapse rates. Other contributors include highly processed diets, low fibre intake and gut microbiome imbalances (this occurs when the normal balance of beneficial and harmful microorganisms is disrupted), which may trigger inappropriate immune activation. Certain medications, such as non-steroidal anti-inflammatory drugs, may exacerbate inflammation. Crohn's can develop at any age, but typically presents in adolescence or early adulthood.

Signs and symptoms

The symptoms of Crohn's disease vary depending on which part of the digestive tract is affected. Common symptoms include diarrhoea, abdominal pain, fatigue, weight loss, fever, malaise and anaemia. Stools are often liquid or semi-formed and may contain blood or mucus, especially if the colon is involved. The disease typically follows a relapsing-remitting pattern, with long periods of mild or no symptoms interrupted by flare-ups, when symptoms become more severe. Additional features can include loss of appetite, nausea, and, in children, delayed growth or development. Some patients also experience extra-intestinal manifestations, such as joint pain, skin rashes or eye inflammation.

Management

Diet and nutrition

Eating a balanced diet is important for overall health and supporting recovery. Some patients may be sensitive to certain foods that can trigger flare-ups, such as high-fat, very fibrous or spicy foods. Identifying and avoiding these foods, with guidance from a dietitian, can help manage symptoms. During acute flare-ups, a liquid or soft diet may reduce bowel irritation while providing essential nutrients. In severe cases, enteral nutrition via feeding tubes or parenteral nutrition via intravenous infusion may be necessary to maintain adequate nutrition.

Medication

Crohn's disease is treated with a range of medications depending on disease activity. Corticosteroids are effective for short-term flare control but are not used long-term due to side effects such as weight gain, osteoporosis and diabetes. Immunosuppressants (azathioprine, mercaptopurine and methotrexate) help reduce immune-mediated inflammation. Antibiotics may be used to prevent or treat infections. For moderate to severe or steroid-refractory disease, biologic therapies such as anti-TNF agents (infliximab and adalimumab) or other targeted treatments are used to control inflammation and induce remission.

Surgery

Approximately 70–80% of people with Crohn's disease require surgery at some point. Surgery is reserved for cases where medication cannot control symptoms or when complications arise, such as strictures, fistulas or abscesses. The inflamed bowel segment is removed, and the remaining intestine is reconnected (bowel resection with anastomosis). Surgery can provide long-term remission, but disease recurrence is common, so ongoing medical therapy is usually required.

Complications

Certain complications of Crohn's disease are common consequences of chronic inflammation and may even be the first presentation in some patients. Intestinal obstruction frequently develops due to repeated inflammation, scarring and fibrosis, resulting in bowel strictures.

Perforation of the bowel is rare but can lead to generalised peritonitis. Chronic inflammation, particularly in the colon, increases colorectal cancer risk; long-standing disease raises risk by approximately 5–6 times compared with the general population.

Other complications include abscesses and fistulas, a direct consequence of transmural inflammation, which allow abnormal connections or pus-filled cavities to form between the bowel and other organs or the skin.

> ### Clinical considerations
>
> Patients with Crohn's disease may experience frequent diarrhoea, urgency, incontinence or abdominal distension, which can be distressing. Maintaining dignity is essential and includes providing private toileting, sensitive communication and ensuring the patient does not feel hurried or judged. During examinations or procedures, explain what is happening, obtain consent and maintain privacy. Acknowledge the emotional impact of unpredictable symptoms on social life, work and travel.

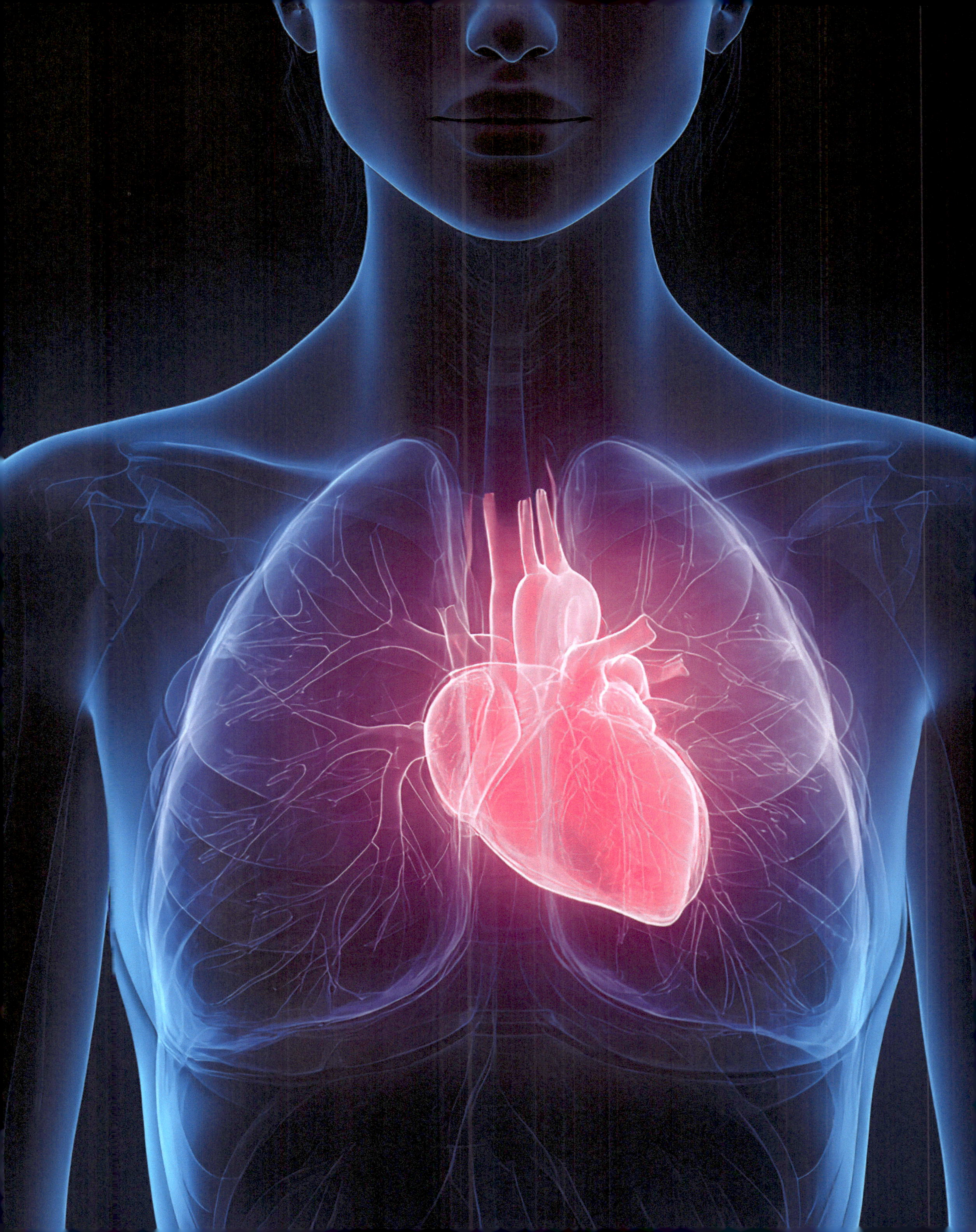

31 Peptic ulcer

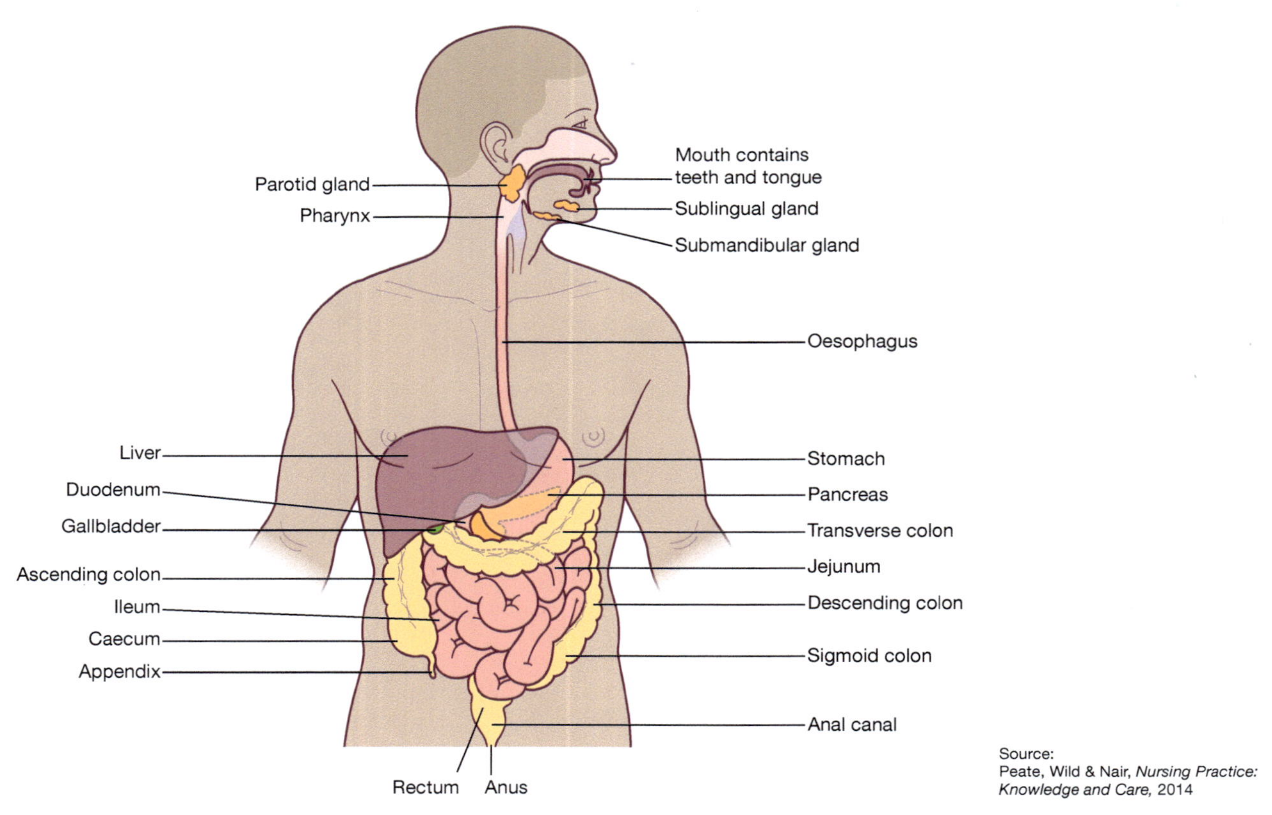

Figure 31.1 Digestive system.

Source:
Peate, Wild & Nair, *Nursing Practice: Knowledge and Care*, 2014

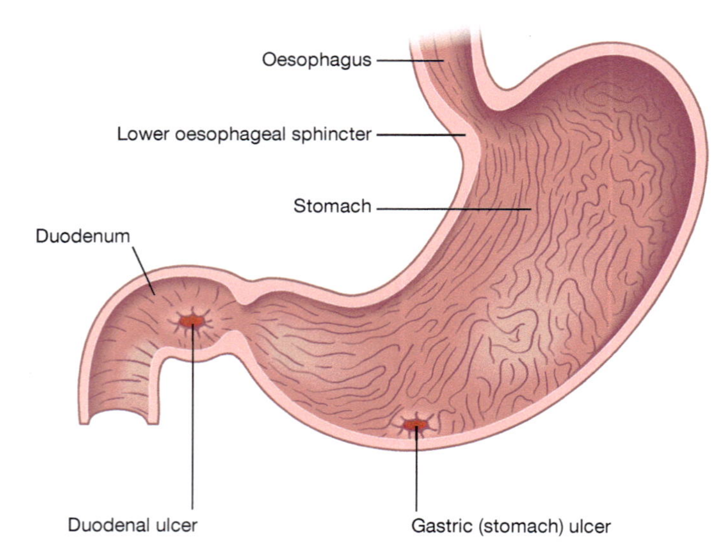

Figure 31.2 Peptic (gastric) ulcer.

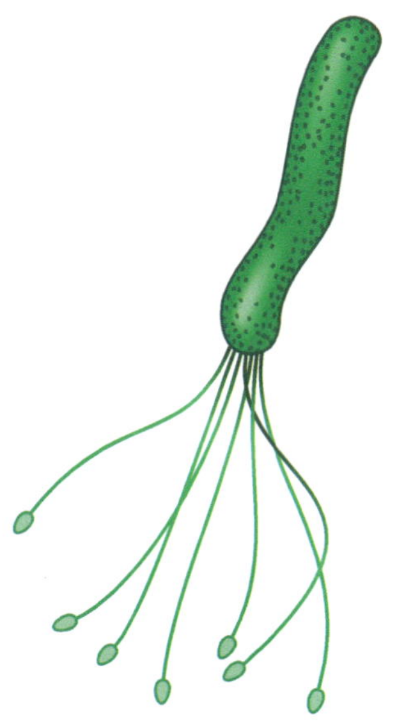

Figure 31.3 Diagram of a *H. Pylori*.

Overview of anatomy and physiology

Food passes down the oesophagus (gullet) into the stomach (Figure 31.1). The stomach makes acid, which is not essential but helps to digest food. After being mixed in the stomach, food passes into the duodenum (the first part of the small intestine). In the duodenum and the rest of the small intestine, food mixes with enzymes (chemicals). The enzymes come from the pancreas and from cells lining the intestine. The enzymes break down (digest) the food, which is absorbed into the body.

The stomach may be divided into seven major sections. The cardia is a 1–2 cm segment distal to the oesophagogastric junction. The fundus refers to the superior portion of the stomach that lies above an imaginary horizontal plane that passes through the oesophagogastric junction. The antrum is the smaller distal quarter to a third of the stomach. The narrow 1–2 cm channel that connects the stomach and duodenum is known as the pylorus. The lesser curve refers to the medial shorter border of the stomach, whereas the opposite surface is the greater curve.

Pathophysiology

Ulcers are caused when there is an imbalance between the digestive juices produced by the stomach and the various factors that protect the lining of the stomach. Symptoms of ulcers may include bleeding. On rare occasions, an ulcer may completely erode the stomach wall.

Mucus lines the digestive tract and acts as a barrier against the acidic gastric secretions. Too little mucus production coupled with too much acid production will leave the digestive tract vulnerable to acid erosion and ulceration. Erosion of the mucosal lining may result in the formation of a fistula. The fistula would allow the acidic gastric contents to leak out into the peritoneum, resulting in peritonitis. Stress, caffeine, cigarette smoking and alcohol consumption increase acid production. Medications such as non-steroidal anti-inflammatory drugs (NSAIDs) and aspirin inhibit prostaglandins, which protect the mucosal lining.

Causes

A peptic ulcer is a break or erosion in the mucosal lining of the stomach or duodenum (Figure 31.2). The main cause is *Helicobacter pylori* infection, which releases enzymes and toxins that weaken the protective mucous layer, allowing stomach acid to damage the tissue. The body responds with an inflammatory reaction, which further contributes to mucosal erosion and ulcer formation (Figure 31.3). NSAID use is another common cause, as these drugs reduce mucosal protection.

Rare causes include gastrin-secreting tumours (Zollinger–Ellison syndrome), which increase acid production. Smoking and a family history of peptic ulcer are recognised risk factors. Stress and caffeine may worsen symptoms but do not directly cause ulcers.

Understanding this pathophysiology is important because it informs treatment strategies, including eradication of *H. pylori*, acid suppression therapy and avoidance of NSAIDs and other aggravating factors.

Signs and symptoms

Some patients with a peptic ulcer may have no symptoms, particularly if the ulcer is small. When symptoms occur, they commonly include epigastric pain, heartburn, bloating, belching and reduced appetite. The pain is usually described as burning or gnawing and may sometimes radiate to the back.

The timing of the pain can vary: it often occurs 1–2 hours after meals in gastric ulcers and may improve or worsen depending on food intake. In duodenal ulcers, pain may appear several hours after eating or at night. Symptoms may come and go over days or weeks, reflecting periods of ulcer activity and relative remission.

Management

Management of peptic ulcer disease aims to heal the ulcer, prevent complications and reduce the risk of recurrence. Once a peptic ulcer is diagnosed, those offering people care and support should help patients identify modifiable lifestyle factors that may worsen symptoms or delay healing. These modifiable lifestyle factors include smoking, heavy alcohol consumption and excessive caffeine intake. While stress does not directly cause ulcers, it can exacerbate symptoms. Patients should be supported in implementing practical strategies to reduce these risks, such as smoking cessation, limiting alcohol and moderating caffeine intake.

Most duodenal and many gastric ulcers are caused by *H. pylori* infection. Eradicating this bacterium is essential, as failure to do so significantly increases the risk of ulcer recurrence once acid-suppressing therapy is stopped. Standard treatment involves triple therapy, which combines two antibiotics and a proton pump inhibitor (PPI). The PPI reduces gastric acid, allowing the antibiotics to work more effectively and promoting ulcer healing. Therapy typically lasts 7–14 days depending on local protocols.

In addition to *H. pylori* eradication, acid suppression alone may be used when *H. pylori* is absent or when NSAID-induced ulcers are suspected. PPIs are preferred over histamine H2 receptor antagonists due to greater efficacy. Patients should be advised about commitment to the full course of therapy, as incomplete treatment reduces effectiveness and increases the risk of antibiotic resistance.

Follow-up care includes monitoring for symptom resolution, managing complications such as bleeding or perforation, and advising on long-term prevention strategies. Those patients who are taking NSAIDs may need alternative pain management or protective medications, such as PPIs. Education should emphasise symptom recognition, when to seek urgent care, and the importance of regular medical review.

By combining lifestyle modification, *H. pylori* eradication, acid suppression and patient education, healthcare professionals can promote healing, reduce recurrence and improve quality of life for individuals with peptic ulcer disease.

Medication

A 4–8 week course of medication that greatly reduces stomach acid is usually recommended to allow ulcers to heal. The most commonly used drugs are PPIs, which act on the stomach lining (parietal cells) to reduce acid production. Examples include esomeprazole, lansoprazole, omeprazole, pantoprazole and rabeprazole, available under various brand names.

Sometimes another class of medicines, called H2 blockers (H2 receptor antagonists), is used. These reduce acid through a different mechanism and include cimetidine, famotidine and nizatidine.

By greatly reducing stomach acid, these medications allow the ulcer to heal and relieve symptoms such as pain and heartburn.

Diet

Patients with a peptic ulcer should receive advice to help manage symptoms. Eating small, regular meals can reduce discomfort, but patients should follow patterns that suit them. Spicy foods do not cause ulcers but may worsen symptoms in some individuals. Alcohol, caffeine and NSAIDs should be moderated, as these can delay healing or aggravate symptoms. Advice should be tailored to the patient, supporting nutrition while minimising discomfort.

Clinical considerations

Endoscopy is usually recommended for patients who present with alarm features, such as unexplained weight loss, persistent vomiting, gastrointestinal bleeding or new dyspepsia in individuals over 55 years. The procedure allows direct visualisation of the ulcer, assessment of its size and severity, and the opportunity to take biopsies for *H. pylori* testing or to exclude malignancy. Patients are advised to fast for 6–8 hours before the procedure, and acid-suppressing medications may need temporary adjustment. Sedation is often offered to increase comfort, and healthcare professionals should explain the process clearly to reduce anxiety. Endoscopy results are used to guide treatment decisions.

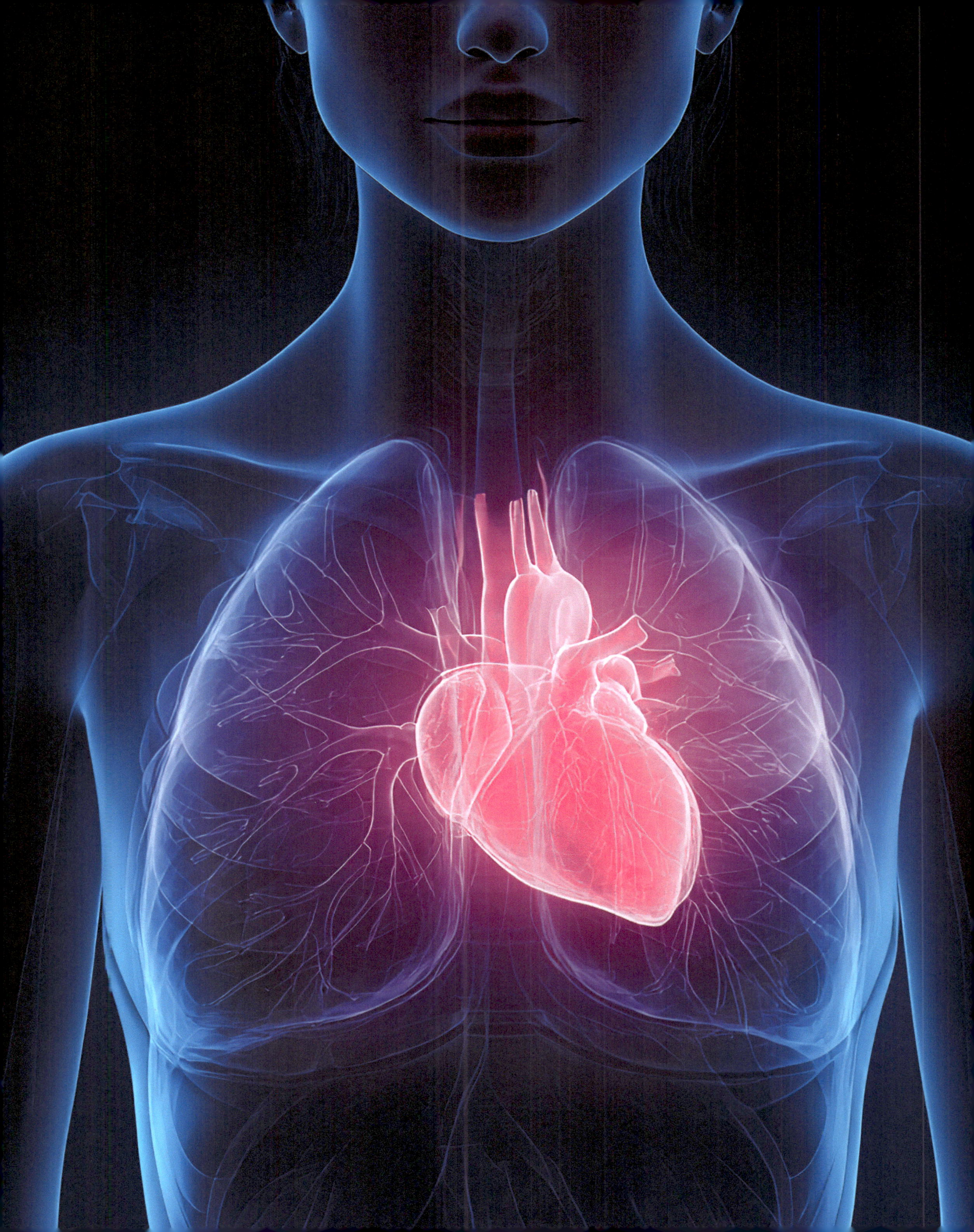

32 Ulcerative colitis

Figure 32.1 Diagram of the colon affected by ulcerative colitis.

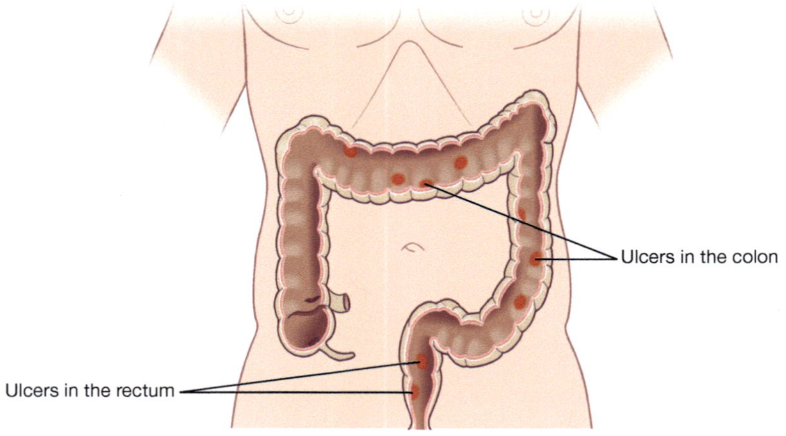

Figure 32.2 Common types of inflammatory bowel disease.

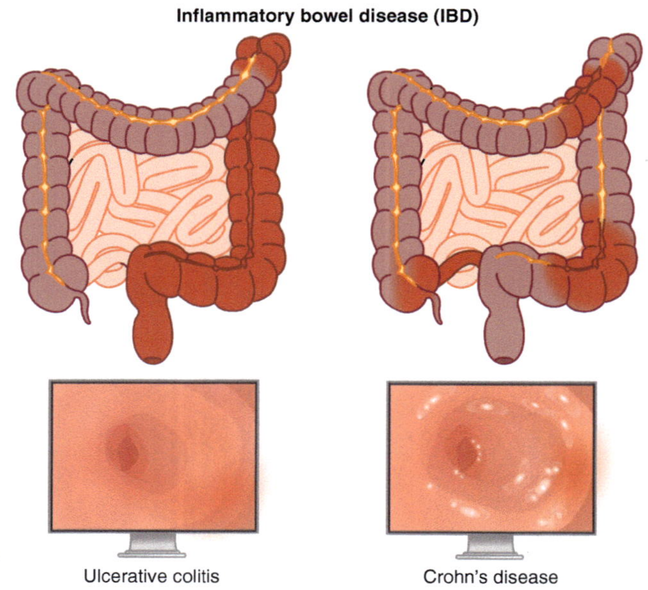

Source:
Peate et al. 2014/with
permission of John Wiley & Sons

Figure 32.3 Diagram showing colonoscopy procedure.

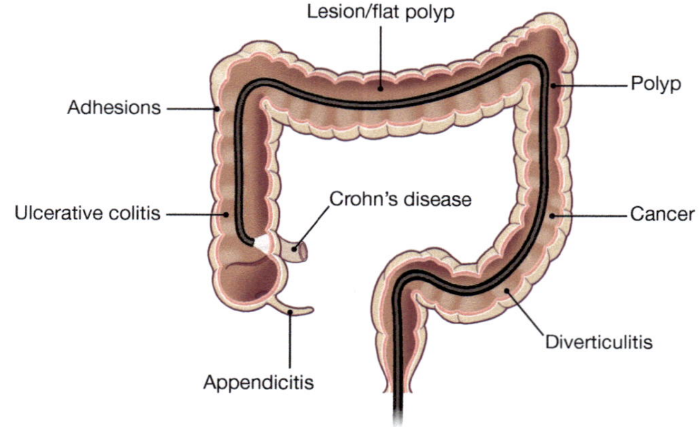

Overview

Ulcerative colitis is a disease where inflammation develops in the colon and the rectum (the large intestine) (Figure 32.1). Ulcerative colitis is one of the two main inflammatory bowel diseases; the other is Crohn's disease (see Chapter 31 of this book) (see Figure 32.2). Sometimes, ulcerative colitis only affects the rectum; when this occurs, this is called proctitis and is a less severe condition.

Ulcerative colitis occurs worldwide, but it is most common in North America and Northern Europe, particularly among people of Ashkenazi Jewish descent. Historically, it has been less common in Eastern Europe, Asia, South America and among people of African descent. For reasons that are not fully understood, the incidence of ulcerative colitis has been increasing in low- and middle-income countries in recent years.

Pathophysiology

Ulcerative colitis results from an abnormal immune response in genetically susceptible individuals, where the immune system reacts inappropriately to normal gut microbiota (these are a diverse community of microorganisms, including bacteria, viruses, fungi and other microbes, that naturally inhabit the gastrointestinal tract, primarily the intestines) and environmental triggers.

Genetic factors contribute significantly to susceptibility. Individuals with a first-degree relative affected by ulcerative colitis have an increased risk. Specific genes and those regulating epithelial barrier function and immune responses influence the disease's development. However, genetics alone is insufficient; environmental factors such as diet, infections and microbiome alterations also play a key role.

Inflammation in ulcerative colitis causes mucosal damage, leading to ulcer formation. These ulcers appear as small, red craters on the colonic lining and result in bleeding, oedema and mucosal destruction. The resulting symptoms include abdominal cramping, urgency and frequent defaecation, sometimes exceeding 10 bowel movements per day. Chronic blood loss may lead to iron deficiency anaemia.

Over time, repeated inflammation can cause pseudopolyps (benign, scar-like mucosal projections), mucosal remodelling and thickening of the colonic wall. Although ulcerative colitis is generally limited to the mucosa and submucosa, in severe or prolonged disease, it can lead to complications such as dehydration, electrolyte imbalance and malnutrition.

Ulcerative colitis is a multifactorial disease resulting from the interplay of genetic susceptibility, immune dysregulation and environmental factors. Understanding its pathophysiology helps explain both the clinical manifestations and potential complications and forms the basis for targeted therapeutic approaches.

Diagnosis

Ulcerative colitis is usually diagnosed through a combination of clinical assessment, endoscopic evaluation, histological examination and laboratory investigations, including non-invasive biomarkers. Endoscopy remains the cornerstone of diagnosis, typically undertaken using a sigmoidoscope or colonoscope (see Figure 32.3). During the procedure, the colonic mucosa is assessed for continuous inflammation, ulceration, erythema, loss of vascular pattern and pseudopolyps. Biopsies are obtained from multiple sites to confirm histology, exclude alternative diagnoses and assess inflammatory severity. Endoscopy also determines disease extent, classifying ulcerative colitis as proctitis, left-sided or extensive.

Laboratory investigations support diagnosis and disease monitoring. Blood tests can detect anaemia and elevated inflammatory markers, including C-reactive protein (CRP). Non-invasive faecal biomarkers, such as faecal calprotectin and lactoferrin, help distinguish ulcerative colitis from functional bowel disorders, assess disease activity and detect subclinical inflammation. Stool cultures and pathogen testing are performed to exclude infections that can mimic ulcerative colitis or trigger flares.

Cross-sectional imaging with CT or MRI enterography is recommended in complicated or severe disease to assess colonic extent, wall thickness or extra-luminal complications. Collectively, these investigations can enable clinicians to confirm diagnosis, quantify disease activity, determine extent and guide individualised management, including medical therapy, endoscopic surveillance and long-term follow-up.

Signs and symptoms

The symptoms of ulcerative colitis vary according to the extent of colonic involvement and the severity of inflammation. Commonly reported features include abdominal pain, diarrhoea containing blood and mucus, anaemia, weight loss and loss of appetite. Systemic symptoms such as malaise, fatigue and pyrexia are also common, and some individuals develop extra-intestinal manifestations affecting the joints, skin or eyes.

The severity of ulcerative colitis is typically classified as mild, moderate or severe, based on stool frequency, systemic symptoms and laboratory findings. In mild disease, patients usually experience fewer than four stools per day, with small amounts of blood and little or no systemic disturbance. Moderate disease is associated with four to six stools daily, more pronounced bleeding and mild systemic upset, including low-grade fever or fatigue. Severe disease, sometimes referred to as acute severe ulcerative colitis, presents with six or more bloody stools per day, pyrexia, tachycardia and anaemia, accompanied by significant elevation in inflammatory markers.

Clinically, a patient with severe disease may appear acutely unwell, pale, pyrexial and dehydrated, with tachycardia and hypotension indicating systemic inflammatory response and fluid depletion. Accurate assessment of disease activity is essential to guide treatment, determine hospital admission and prevent complications such as perforation or toxic megacolon (this is an acute dilatation and paralysis of the large intestine, accompanied by systemic toxicity).

Management

Those people who are living with ulcerative colitis often require holistic support that addresses both physical and psychological needs. Chronic symptoms such as diarrhoea, abdominal pain and urgency can be distressing and socially limiting, sometimes leading to anxiety, depression or isolation. Providing psychological support and access to counselling can help patients cope with the emotional impact of a long-term condition. Encouraging patients to express their concerns and connecting them with support groups or patient organisations, such as Crohn's & Colitis UK, can reduce isolation and improve self-management.

Adequate hydration and nutrition are essential, particularly during active disease flares when diarrhoea increases fluid and electrolyte loss. Water remains the preferred fluid; however, oral rehydration solutions may be beneficial if dehydration is significant. Patients should be advised to limit caffeine, alcohol and carbonated drinks, which may exacerbate symptoms. A balanced, individualised diet is recommended, and keeping a food and symptom diary can help identify triggers and tolerable foods.

Regular monitoring of fluid balance and electrolytes, especially sodium and potassium, is important in acute illness. Ongoing communication with the gastroenterology team, practice nurse or dietitian ensures timely support when symptoms worsen. Empowering patients with education about medication, nutrition and lifestyle adjustments promotes self-efficacy and helps maintain quality of life.

Clinical considerations

Living with ulcerative colitis can significantly affect psychological and social well-being. Chronic symptoms may lead to anxiety, depression and social isolation. Patients may feel embarrassed, reluctant to engage in social activities or concerned about burdening others.

Healthcare professionals should provide psychological support and counselling and encourage patients to express concerns about the disease, treatment and lifestyle impact. Connection with peer support groups or patient organisations can reduce isolation and provide practical guidance.

Addressing both emotional and practical challenges enhances confidence, coping and quality of life for those living with ulcerative colitis.

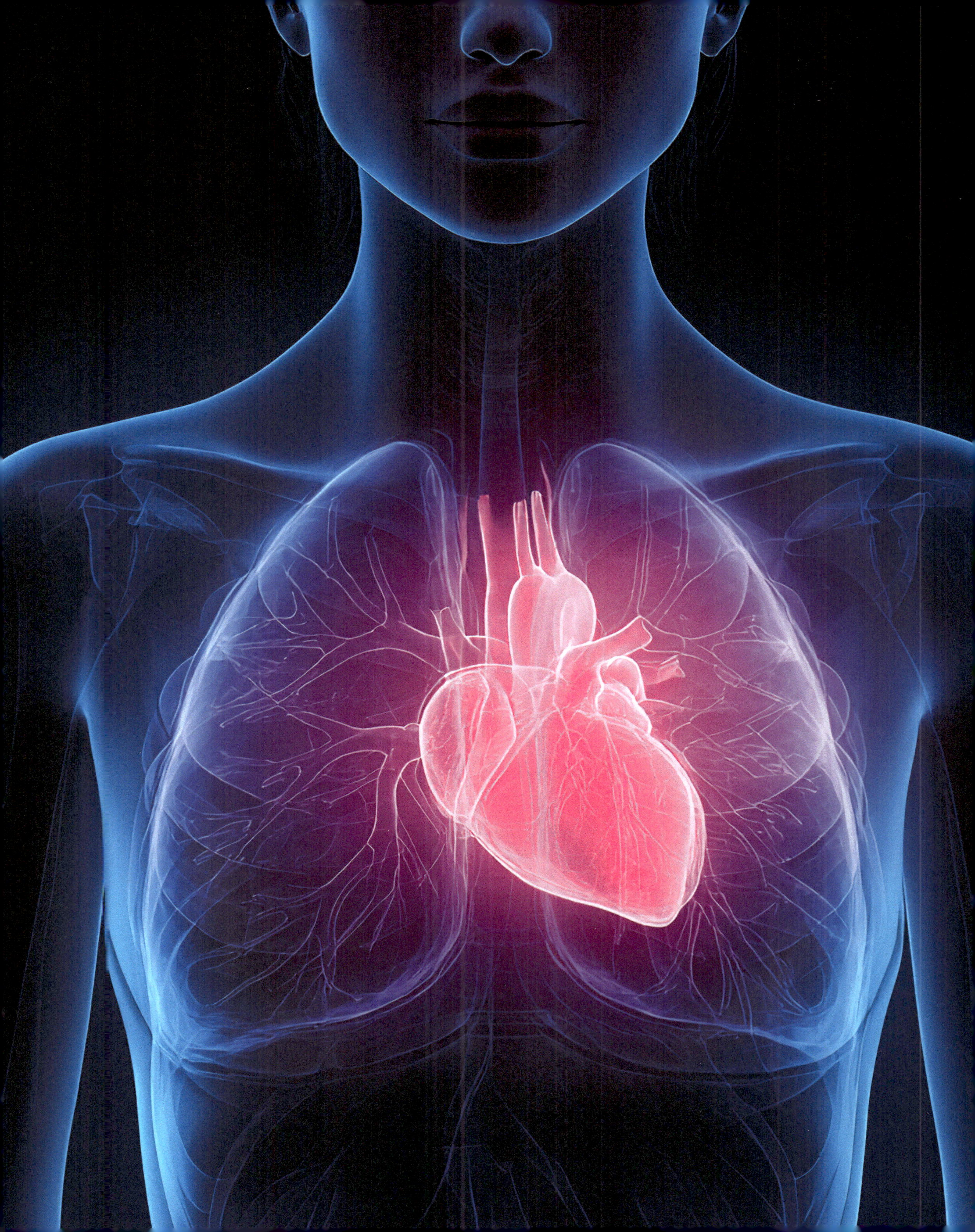

33 Bowel cancer

Figure 33.1 The large bowel (colon).

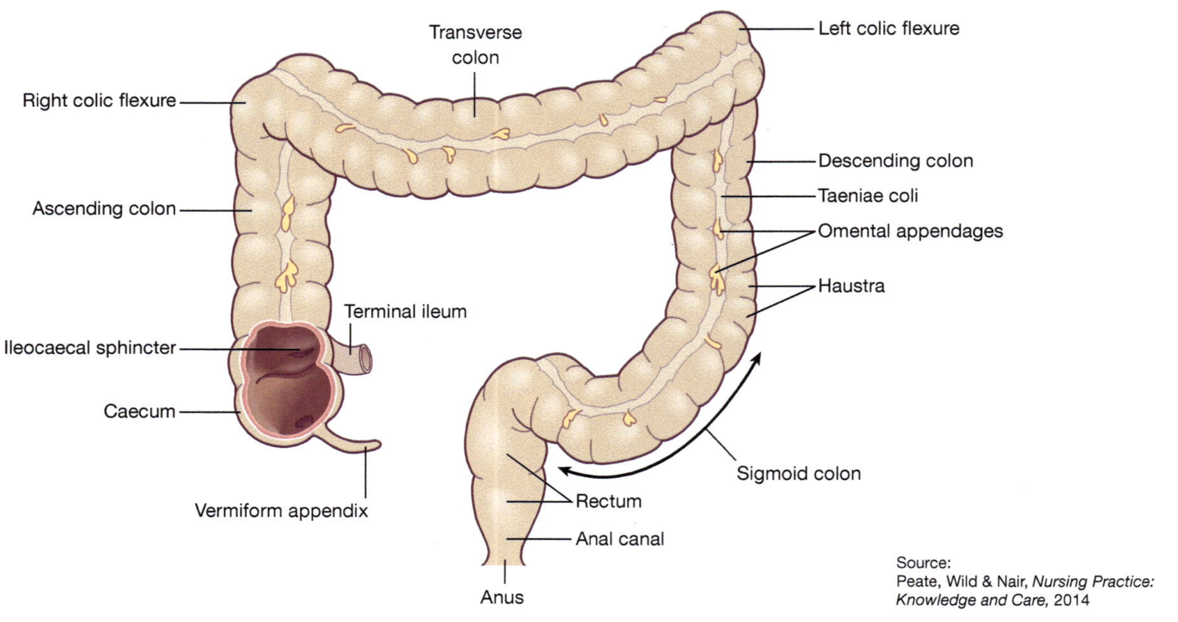

Source:
Peate, Wild & Nair, *Nursing Practice: Knowledge and Care*, 2014

Figure 33.2 Spread of cancer cells into the bloodstream and lymphatic system.

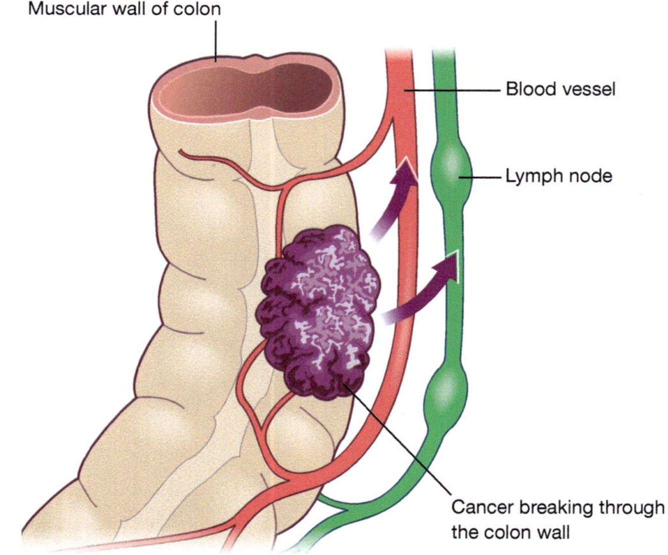

Overview

Bowel cancer (also known as colorectal cancer) affects the lower part of the digestive system, the large bowel and the rectum. It affects men and women equally and is the third most common type of cancer in men and the second most common in women. One in twenty people in the UK will develop bowel cancer in their lifetime.

The colon and rectum are parts of the gastrointestinal tract. The gastrointestinal tract commences at the mouth and terminates at the anus. When food or drink is consumed, it moves down the oesophagus and into the stomach. There, the stomach mixes and breaks down the food before passing it into the small intestine.

The small intestine (also called the small bowel) is around 6–7 m long; it is here where food is digested and absorbed. Undigested food, water and waste products are then passed into the large intestine (the large bowel). The main part of the large intestine is called the colon, which is about 1.5 m long. This is divided into four sections: the ascending, transverse, descending and sigmoid colon (Figure 33.1). Some water and salts are absorbed into the body from the colon. The colon leads into the rectum (back passage), which is about 15 cm long. The rectum stores faeces (stools) before they are passed out via the anus.

Pathophysiology

Cancer

Cancer is a disease of the body's cells. The human body is made up of billions of cells, which come in many different types. Cancer can arise from any cell type, leading to a wide variety of cancers. What all cancers have in common is that the cells are abnormal and they proliferate uncontrollably.

A malignant tumour is a mass of cancerous cells that continues to grow and divide. These tumours can invade nearby tissues and organs, causing damage. Cancer cells can also spread (metastasise) to other parts of the body. This occurs when cells break away from the primary tumour; they then travel through the bloodstream or lymphatic system and establish secondary tumours in new locations. These secondary tumours can then grow, invade surrounding tissues and potentially spread further.

The severity, responsiveness to treatment and prognosis of cancer vary depending on the type of cancer and the stage at diagnosis. Early detection often improves outcomes.

Bowel cancer

Bowel cancer is a cancer of the colon or rectum. The risk of developing this cancer increases with age. Bowel cancer can commence in any part of the colon or rectum, but it most frequently arises in the lower descending colon, the sigmoid colon or the rectum. Nearly all colorectal cancers are adenocarcinomas, which usually originate from adenomatous polyps, small growths found on the inner lining of the bowel.

Bowel cancer generally develops when a polyp becomes cancerous over time. In some cases, it can begin from a single abnormal cell in the bowel lining. Rare types of bowel cancer may arise from other cells in the colon or rectal wall, such as carcinoid tumours, lymphomas or sarcomas.

As cancer cells multiply, they form a tumour that can invade deeper layers of the colon or rectal wall. Some cells may enter the lymphatic system or bloodstream, allowing the cancer to metastasise to nearby lymph nodes or distant organs, most commonly the liver and lungs (see Figure 33.2). The risk of progression and prognosis will depend on the tumour's type, its location and stage at diagnosis, highlighting the importance of screening and early detection.

Signs and symptoms

In the early stages, colorectal cancer is often asymptomatic, particularly when the tumour is small. Symptoms generally develop as the cancer grows and vary depending on its location within the colon or rectum. Common clinical features include rectal bleeding, the presence of mucus in the stool, abdominal discomfort or pain, tenesmus (the sensation of incomplete bowel evacuation) and alterations in bowel habits, such as diarrhoea, constipation or a change in stool calibre.

Tumours in different regions of the colon may produce distinct patterns of symptoms. For example, cancers in the right colon often present with anaemia due to chronic blood loss, whereas those in the left colon or rectum are more likely to cause changes in stool consistency or obstruction.

As the tumour enlarges, it may cause a mechanical obstruction of the bowel, resulting in severe abdominal pain, distension, nausea and vomiting. Obstruction is a serious complication that often requires urgent medical intervention.

Early detection of colorectal cancer, either through screening programmes or timely investigation of warning symptoms, significantly improves prognosis. Recognising subtle changes in bowel habits, unexplained bleeding or other gastrointestinal symptoms is critical for the prompt diagnosis and effective management of colorectal cancer.

Management

The primary treatment for colorectal cancer remains surgical resection of the tumour, adjacent colon or rectum and regional lymph nodes. The extent of resection is determined by tumour location, lymphatic drainage and involvement of surrounding tissues. For most tumours of the ascending, transverse, descending and sigmoid colon, the affected segment is removed, and continuity of the bowel is restored through anastomosis. Whenever feasible, the anal sphincter is preserved to avoid the need for a permanent colostomy.

Rectal tumours often require more extensive procedures. An abdominoperineal resection involves the removal of the sigmoid colon, rectum and anus through combined abdominal and perineal incisions, resulting in a permanent colostomy. In selected patients with low-lying rectal tumours, sphincter-sparing procedures may be possible, depending on tumour size and the distance from the anal verge.

Adjuvant therapies play an important role, particularly for rectal cancer. Radiotherapy is rarely used for colon tumours, but it is frequently administered for rectal cancer to improve local control. It is often combined with chemotherapy, which increases the radiosensitivity of tumour cells. Additionally, systemic chemotherapy may be administered independently to treat micrometastatic disease and reduce the risk of recurrence.

Treatment plans are individualised according to tumour stage, location, histology and patient factors, with the goals of curative resection, minimising recurrence, preserving function and optimising survival.

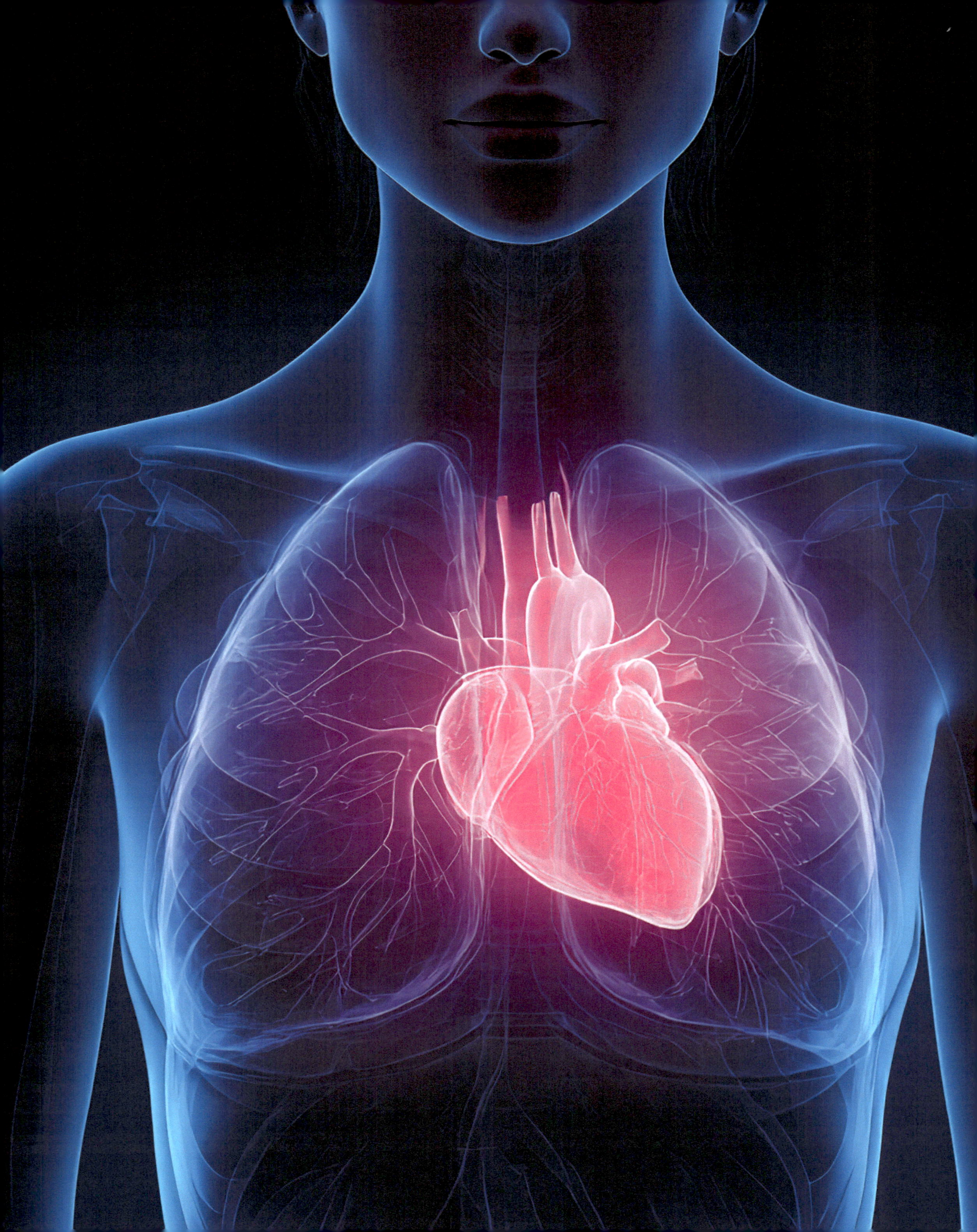

The hepatobiliary system

Chapters

34 Hepatitis

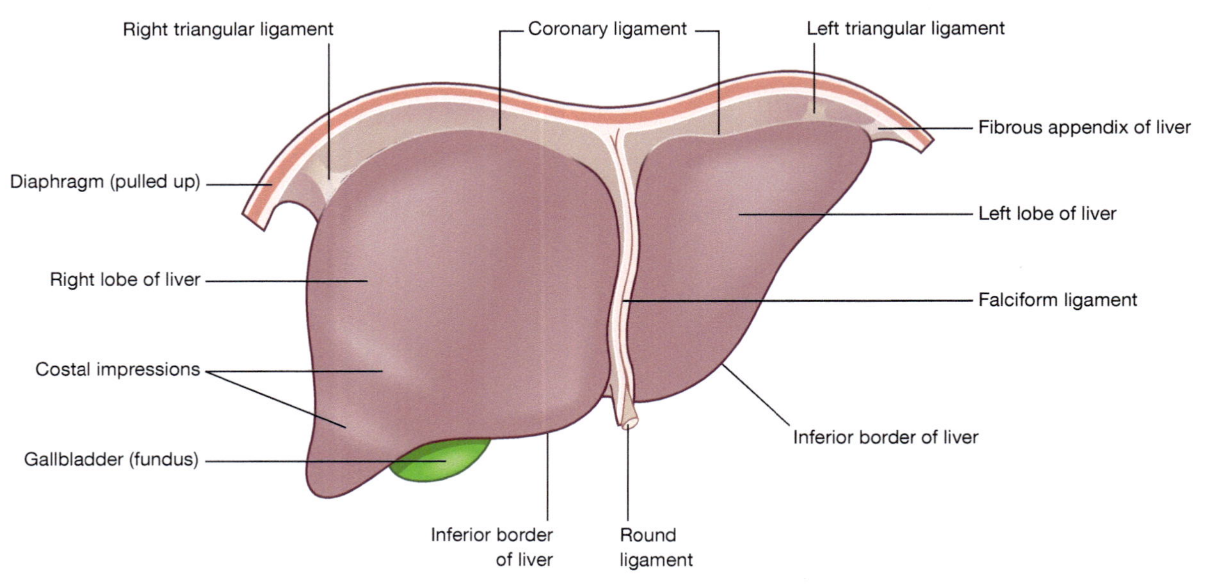

Figure 34.1 The liver

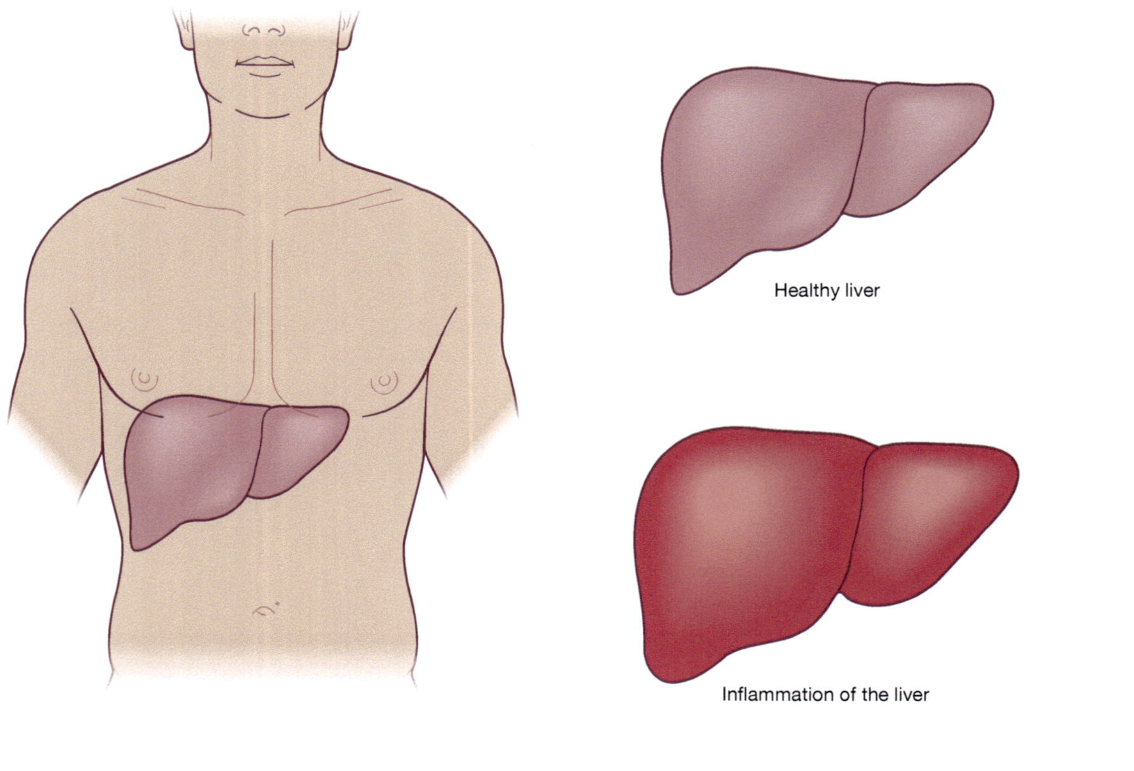

Figure 34.2 Normal and inflamed liver

Overview of anatomy and physiology

The liver is a large, solid organ; it is located on the right side of the abdomen. It weighs approximately 1.44–1.66 kg, has a reddish-brown colour, and has a firm, rubbery texture. The rib cage provides it with protection.

Anatomically, the liver is divided into two main lobes: the right and the left (Figure 34.1). Situated beneath the liver are the gallbladder, portions of the pancreas and sections of the intestines. These organs work closely together to support digestion, absorption and the processing of nutrients.

The liver's primary function is to filter blood from the digestive tract before it circulates to the rest of the body. It is also responsible for the detoxification of harmful substances and the metabolism of medications. During this process, the liver produces bile, which is released into the intestines to aid digestion. In addition, the liver synthesises vital proteins, including those necessary for blood clotting and other physiological functions, such as thermogenesis.

Blood supply to the liver is dual: the hepatic portal vein and the hepatic arteries. The hepatic portal vein provides about 75% of the liver's blood, carrying nutrient-rich blood from the gastrointestinal tract and associated organs, such as the stomach, intestines and pancreas, as well as blood from the spleen, so it can be processed and filtered by the liver. The hepatic arteries provide the remaining arterial blood. Both sources deliver oxygen, with roughly half of the liver's oxygen requirements met by each. Blood passes through specialised capillaries called sinusoids before collecting in the central vein of each lobule. These central veins merge to form the hepatic veins, which carry blood away from the liver and back into systemic circulation.

Pathophysiology

Hepatitis refers to inflammation of the liver (Figure 34.2). It can occur as a result of a viral infection or because the liver has been exposed to harmful substances such as alcohol, drugs or toxins.

Hepatitis A

Hepatitis A is an inflammation of the liver caused by the hepatitis A virus (HAV). It is transmitted primarily through the faecal–oral route, typically via ingestion of food or water contaminated with the faeces of an infected person. This mode of transmission is closely associated with poor sanitation and hygiene practices. In high-income countries, hepatitis A is less common due to improved sanitation and widespread vaccination. However, it can still occur, particularly among individuals who travel to areas with higher endemicity or engage in certain high-risk behaviours.

The infection is usually acute and self-limiting, with symptoms such as pyrexia, fatigue, loss of appetite, nausea, abdominal discomfort, dark urine and jaundice. Most individuals recover fully within a few weeks to months. There is no specific antiviral treatment for hepatitis A; management focuses on supportive care to relieve symptoms and ensure adequate hydration and nutrition. In rare cases, the infection can lead to severe liver failure, which may be fatal.

Vaccination is the most effective way to prevent hepatitis A.

Hepatitis B

Hepatitis B is caused by the hepatitis B virus (HBV), present in blood and certain body fluids, including semen and vaginal secretions, which can be transmitted through unprotected sexual contact, sharing needles or other injecting equipment, and from an infected mother to her baby during childbirth. Rarely, transmission can occur through close household contact or exposure to contaminated blood products.

Most adults who become infected with HBV can clear the virus and recover fully within a few months, often experiencing only mild symptoms. However, a small proportion of adults develop chronic hepatitis B, which can lead to serious long-term liver complications, including cirrhosis and hepatocellular carcinoma (liver cancer).

Acute hepatitis B may cause symptoms such as fatigue, fever, loss of appetite, nausea, abdominal discomfort, dark urine and jaundice. For many adults, once the infection is cleared, there is no lasting liver damage. There is no specific antiviral treatment for acute hepatitis B; management is supportive, including symptom relief, hydration and monitoring liver function.

Prevention is highly effective through vaccination.

Hepatitis C

Hepatitis C is caused by the hepatitis C virus (HCV), primarily present in blood. The virus is predominantly transmitted through blood-to-blood contact, such as sharing needles or medical equipment, and through contaminated blood transfusions. Although HCV can also be present in other bodily fluids such as saliva, semen and vaginal fluids, transmission via these routes is extremely rare.

Many individuals with hepatitis C experience no noticeable symptoms, or they may have mild, flu-like symptoms, leading to the infection often going undiagnosed. Approximately 15–25% of people will spontaneously clear the virus within 6 months. In the remaining 75–85%, the virus persists, leading to chronic hepatitis C. Chronic infection can increase the risk of long-term liver complications, including cirrhosis and hepatocellular carcinoma.

Signs and symptoms

The symptoms of acute hepatitis can vary widely between individuals. Some patients remain asymptomatic. Commonly reported symptoms include general malaise, loss of appetite, myalgia and arthralgia, jaundice (yellowing of the skin, sclerae and mucous membranes), dark urine and pale-coloured stools.

Management

Those who provide care play a key role in preventing the transmission of hepatitis. Emphasis should be placed on personal hygiene, including hand washing after using the toilet and before food preparation. For those who inject drugs, discuss the risks of sharing needles or other equipment. Those who are sexually active should be encouraged to follow safer sexual practices.

Patients with acute or chronic hepatitis are usually managed in community settings, with hospitalisation rarely required. Care provision focuses on preventing the transmission of infection and supporting the person.

Fatigue and weakness are common in acute hepatitis. While strict bed rest is rarely necessary, ensuring adequate rest periods and limiting strenuous activities may help recovery. Many patients may be unable to resume normal activities for 4 weeks or longer.

Patients with acute or chronic hepatitis are usually treated in community settings; rarely is hospitalisation required. Nursing care focuses on preventing the spread of the infection to others and promoting the client's comfort and ability to provide self-care. An important goal when caring for patients with acute viral hepatitis is preventing the spread of the infection.

Fatigue and possible weakness are common in acute hepatitis. Many patients with acute hepatitis may be unable to resume normal activity for 4 weeks or more.

Clinical considerations

Prevention of transmission relies on good personal hygiene, particularly thorough hand washing after using the toilet and before handling food. Patients should be advised to avoid sharing needles or any personal items that may be contaminated with blood. Safe sexual practices help reduce the risk of infection. Vaccination against hepatitis A and B should be offered where indicated. Information giving is key, ensuring patients understand how hepatitis is transmitted and the measures they can take to prevent spreading the infection to others.

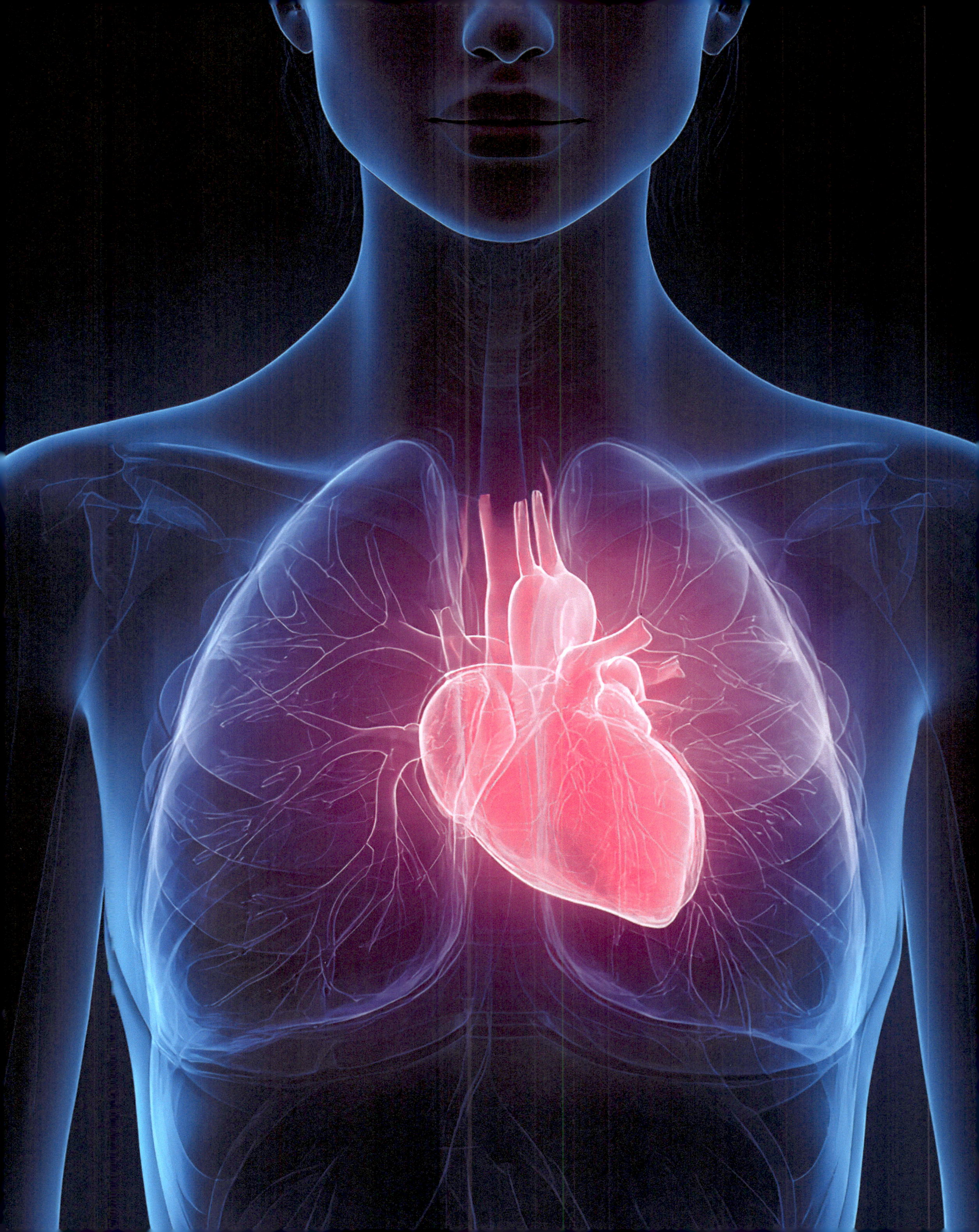

35 Cholecystitis

Figure 35.1 The gall bladder and its ducts, and location of the sphincter of Oddi.

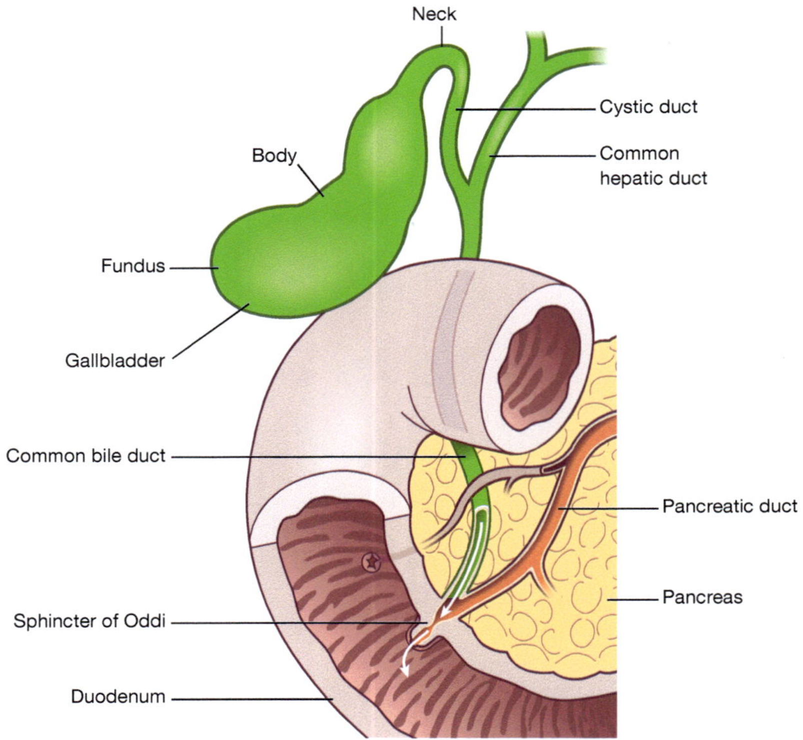

Figure 35.2 Gallstones in the gall bladder and the ducts.

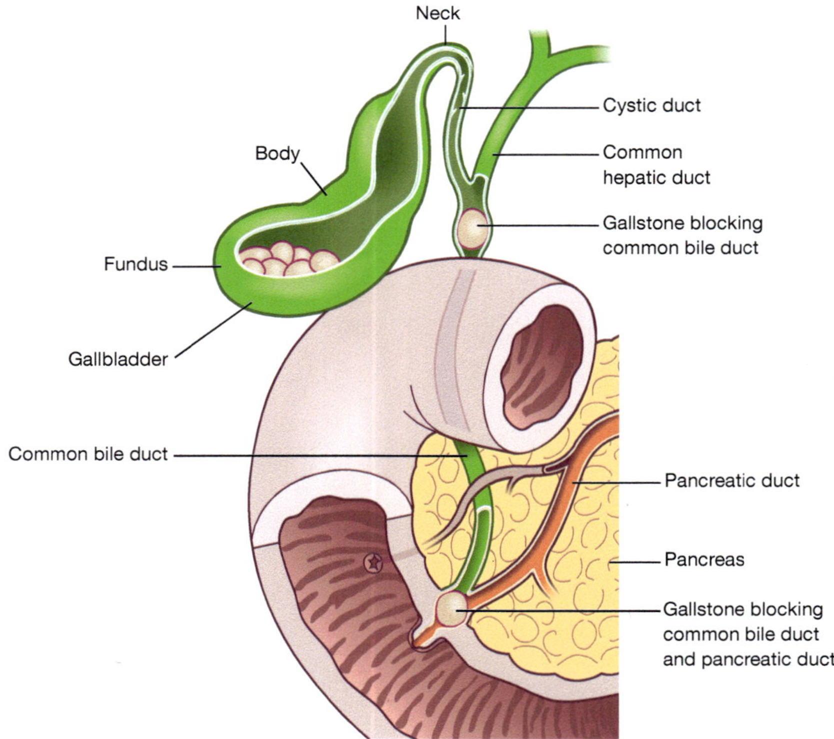

Overview of anatomy and physiology

The gallbladder is a hollow muscular sac; it is located just beneath the liver. It measures approximately 8 cm in length and 4 cm in diameter when it is fully distended. The gallbladder is divided into three regions: fundus, body and neck (Figure 35.1).

Bile production is the liver's primary digestive function. Bile is a greenish, watery solution containing bile salts, cholesterol, bilirubin, electrolytes, water and phospholipids, which are essential for emulsifying fats and promoting their absorption. The liver produces approximately 700–1200 mL of bile daily. When bile is not required for digestion, the sphincter of Oddi (Figure 35.1) located at the duodenal entry point remains closed, causing bile to back up through the cystic duct into the gallbladder for storage.

The gallbladder concentrates and stores bile. When fat-containing food enters the duodenum, cholecystokinin (CCK), a hormone, stimulates the gallbladder to contract and bile is released through the cystic duct, which joins the hepatic duct to form the common bile duct, allowing bile to enter the duodenum.

Pathophysiology

Cholecystitis is inflammation of the gallbladder; it is most often caused by obstruction of the cystic duct by gallstones (Figure 35.2). An acute obstruction leads to bile accumulation; there is increased intraluminal pressure, along with inflammation, which can progress to necrosis or infection if this is severe. Chronic cholecystitis develops from repeated acute episodes or persistent irritation, resulting in fibrosis, wall thickening and impaired gallbladder motility.

Gallstones (cholelithiasis) are small concretions, usually composed primarily of cholesterol (around 80%), with the remainder containing bile pigments and calcium salts. Stone formation involves three main factors: abnormal bile composition, biliary stasis and gallbladder inflammation. Supersaturation of bile with cholesterol, associated with obesity, high-calorie diets, rapid weight loss and certain medications, allows cholesterol to precipitate and form stones.

Genetic predisposition also plays a role; variants in genes regulating cholesterol metabolism and bile acid transport can increase the risk of gallstone formation. Hormonal influences, particularly elevated oestrogen and progesterone (e.g. during pregnancy), can reduce bile flow and gallbladder contractility, contributing to stone formation. Inflammation promotes water and bile salt reabsorption, which concentrates bile further and increases lithiasis risk.

Overall, cholecystitis results from a combination of mechanical obstruction, biochemical bile changes, genetic susceptibility, hormonal effects and inflammation, which together compromise gallbladder function and can lead to pain, infection or complications such as empyema or perforation.

Diagnosis

Patients often provide a history of sudden-onset, severe right upper quadrant abdominal pain, sometimes radiating to the right shoulder or back. Pain frequently occurs after a fatty meal. Associated symptoms may include nausea, vomiting, anorexia and fever. A history of recurrent biliary colic due to gallstones suggests chronic cholecystitis. Risk factors include female sex, obesity, rapid weight loss, pregnancy and oestrogen therapy.

Examination may reveal tenderness in the right upper quadrant, sometimes with guarding. A positive Murphy's sign, pain on inspiration while pressing under the right costal margin, is highly suggestive of gallbladder inflammation. Pyrexia may indicate acute inflammation or infection. Jaundice may be present if bile duct obstruction occurs.

Blood tests support the diagnosis. White blood cell count is often elevated, indicating inflammation or infection. Liver function tests may show raised bilirubin, alkaline phosphatase and alanine aminotransferase, particularly if obstruction is present.

Ultrasound is the first-line imaging modality, as it is painless and can detect gallstones, gallbladder wall thickening and pericholecystic fluid. If the diagnosis is uncertain, CT or HIDA scans may be used.

Diagnosis is made by correlating clinical history, physical findings, laboratory results and imaging, allowing timely management to prevent complications.

Management

Those patients with acute gallbladder disorders may experience severe pain, nausea and vomiting, and in rare cases, complications can lead to shock. Initial management includes hospital admission, pain control with appropriate analgesia and keeping the patient nil by mouth if surgery is anticipated. Intravenous fluids should be administered to prevent dehydration, and vital signs should be monitored regularly, with attention to signs of shock or systemic infection. Laboratory tests, including urea, electrolytes and renal function, should be monitored, and ongoing assessment is needed until the patient stabilises.

Surgery

Cholecystectomy can be performed either laparoscopically (keyhole surgery) or via an open approach. Laparoscopic cholecystectomy is the preferred method for most gallbladder disorders, as it requires only small abdominal incisions, resulting in minimal scarring, lower postoperative pain and a faster recovery. Patients typically experience a shorter hospital stay, quicker return to normal diet and daily activities, and overall improved postoperative outcomes.

Open cholecystectomy may be necessary in cases of complicated anatomy, where there is severe inflammation, dense adhesions or intraoperative difficulties. Occasionally, a laparoscopic procedure may need to be converted to an open approach to ensure patient safety. Contemporary perioperative care often follows Enhanced Recovery After Surgery protocols, which optimise pain control, early mobilisation and nutritional support, further improving recovery and reducing complications.

Alternative treatment

Extracorporeal Shock Wave Lithotripsy: In this approach, high-energy shock waves are used to break up gallstones, allowing fragments to pass through the gastrointestinal tract. This is rarely used today, and it is only suitable for selected patients with few small stones.

Oral dissolution therapy: Small cholesterol stones may be dissolved slowly using ursodeoxycholic acid (UDCA), used mainly in those patients who are unfit for surgery. UDCA may also be used prophylactically in high-risk individuals.

Contact dissolution therapy: A chemical solvent may be introduced directly into the gallbladder. The intention is to dissolve stones, but this is rarely used due to technical complexity and potential toxicity.

Dietary considerations: After cholecystectomy, a low-fat diet is not required. Avoiding foods very high in fat and cholesterol may help prevent stone formation in patients who still have their gallbladder.

Clinical considerations

Effective management of cholecystitis begins with prompt pain control, often using NSAIDs or opioids as prescribed, to relieve severe right upper quadrant discomfort. Patients may experience nausea and vomiting, so keeping them nil by mouth and providing antiemetic medication is important. Intravenous fluids should be administered to maintain hydration, and vital signs should be monitored regularly to detect any signs of shock or systemic infection. Laboratory tests, including white blood cell count and liver function tests, along with imaging such as ultrasound, help guide diagnosis and ongoing management. Ensuring patient comfort through careful positioning and support can also reduce pain and anxiety, contributing to overall recovery.

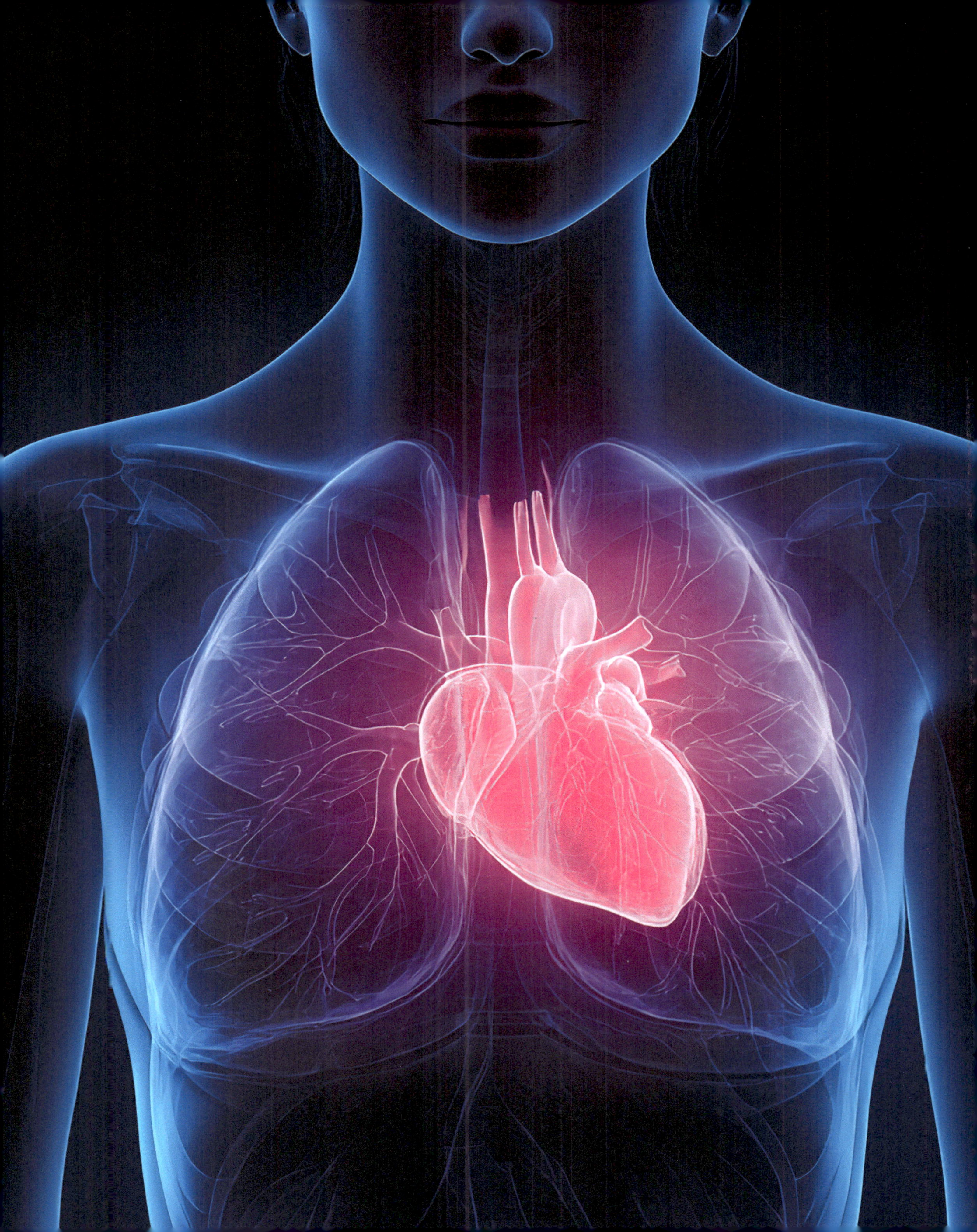

36 Pancreatitis

Figure 36.1 The pancreas.

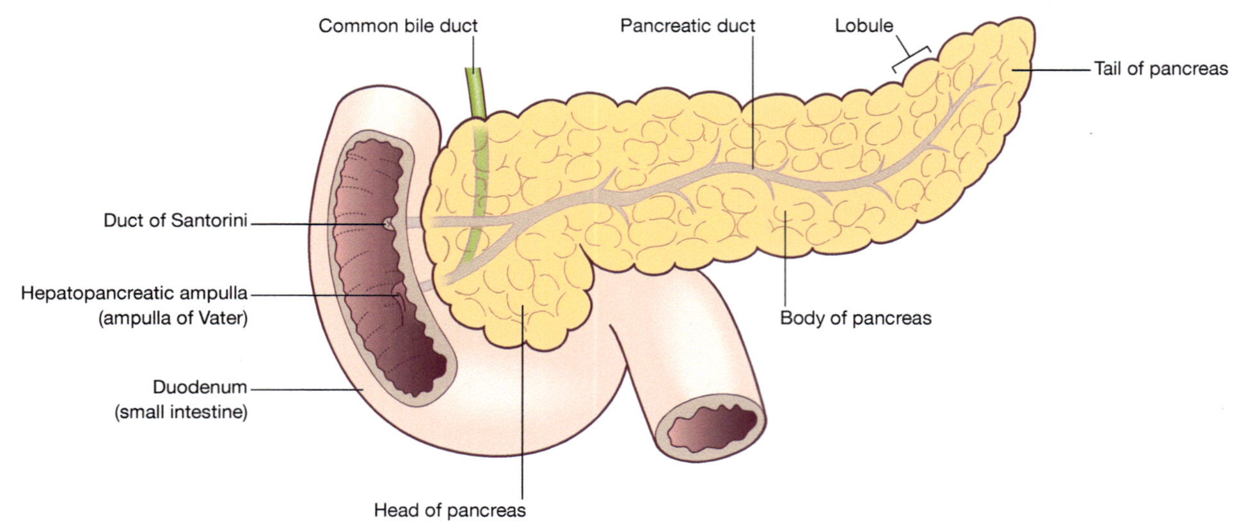

Figure 36.2 An inflamed pancreas due to gallstone blocking the duct.

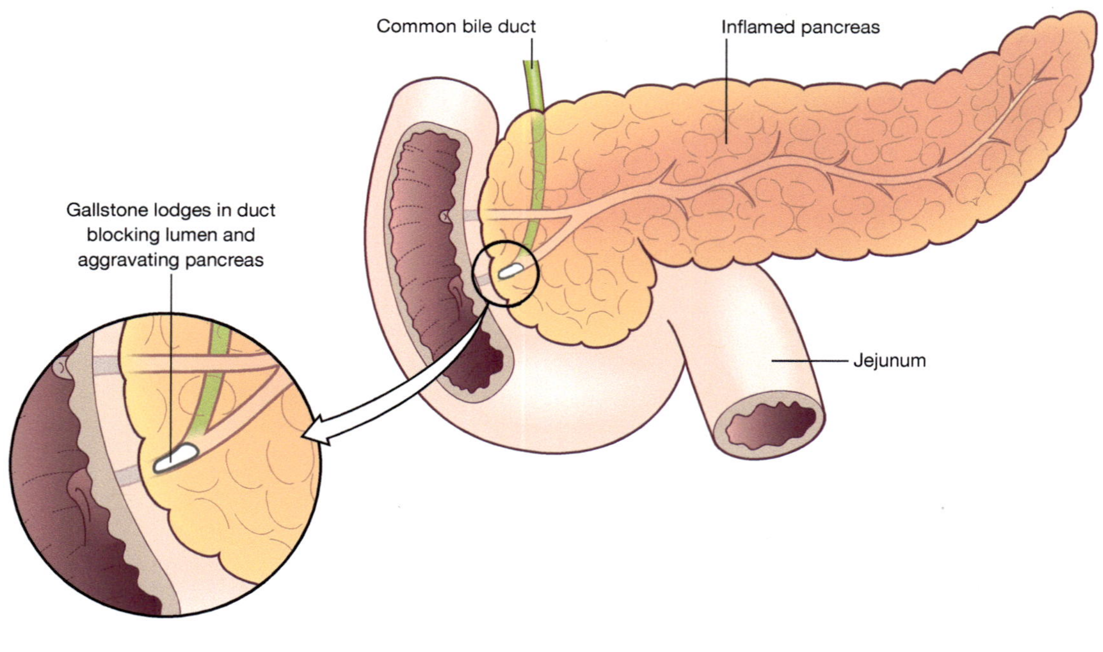

Overview of anatomy and physiology

The pancreas is located in the upper part of the abdomen, across the back of the body, behind the stomach and in front of the spine. It lies approximately at the level of the first and second lumbar vertebrae, and it extends horizontally from the curve of the duodenum on the right side to the spleen on the left. The pancreas measures about 15 cm in length; it is elongated and tapering in shape. The broad, rounded part next to the duodenum is called the head of the pancreas. The central section is known as the body, and the narrow tapering end is referred to as the tail (Figure 36.1).

The pancreas performs two vital functions: producing digestive enzymes to aid food breakdown and secreting hormones that regulate metabolism. Enzymes are specialised chemicals that speed up bodily reactions, while hormones act as messengers carried in the bloodstream to influence distant cells and tissues.

Pancreatic secretions pass through small ducts that merge into the main pancreatic duct. This duct joins the bile duct, which carries bile from the liver and gallbladder, before both open into the duodenum, where the pancreatic juices help digest food.

Pathophysiology

Acute pancreatitis

In acute pancreatitis, inflammation of the pancreas develops rapidly, usually over several days. The condition may resolve completely without lasting damage, although in severe cases it can cause extensive tissue injury and result in systemic complications.

Under normal conditions, pancreatic enzymes are produced in an inactive form and will only become activated once they have reached the duodenum. In acute pancreatitis, these enzymes become prematurely activated within the pancreas itself, which leads to autodigestion of pancreatic tissue. This triggers inflammation, oedema and varying degrees of necrosis. The release of inflammatory mediators can extend beyond the pancreas, resulting in systemic inflammation and organ failure in severe cases. Common causes include:

Gallstones: The most frequent cause in the UK. A gallstone may lodge in the common bile duct or at the ampulla of Vater, obstructing the outflow of pancreatic enzymes (see Figure 36.2). The resulting increase in ductal pressure and enzyme activation initiates inflammation.

Alcohol: Another major cause. Alcohol is thought to increase the permeability of pancreatic ducts and stimulate enzyme secretion, leading to premature activation and inflammation. Symptoms often develop within 6–12 hours after heavy alcohol intake, though in some individuals, pancreatitis may occur even after small amounts due to heightened pancreatic sensitivity.

Autoimmune pancreatitis: Occurs when the body's immune system attacks pancreatic tissue; often associated with other autoimmune disorders such as Sjögren's syndrome (a chronic autoimmune disorder) or primary biliary cholangitis.

Chronic pancreatitis

Chronic pancreatitis is characterised by persistent inflammation of the pancreas, which occurs over months to years. Unlike acute pancreatitis, the inflammation is usually less intense, but repeated or ongoing injury leads to progressive fibrosis, glandular atrophy and loss of both exocrine and endocrine function. The replacement of normal pancreatic tissue with scar tissue impairs enzyme production, resulting in malabsorption and nutritional deficiencies, and can eventually affect insulin production, leading to diabetes. Mechanisms and causes include:

Alcohol: The most common cause (around 70% of cases). Chronic alcohol intake leads to repeated episodes of low-grade inflammation, oxidative stress, and toxic effects on pancreatic cells, gradually causing fibrosis and ductal strictures. Men aged 40–50 years are most frequently affected, often after decades of heavy drinking.

Genetic factors: Rare hereditary conditions, such as mutations associated with cystic fibrosis or other gene defects, can predispose individuals to chronic pancreatic injury.

Autoimmune: The immune system attacks the pancreas, leading to inflammation, fibrosis and functional loss. This can be associated with other autoimmune disorders, such as Sjögren's syndrome or primary biliary cholangitis.

Over time, these processes lead to structural damage, chronic pain and pancreatic insufficiency, which are hallmarks of the disease.

Signs and symptoms

The pain that is often associated with chronic pancreatitis typically occurs in the epigastrium or left upper abdomen, and this may radiate to the back. Some individuals will experience persistent mild to moderate abdominal discomfort between acute exacerbations. This pattern is particularly common in people who continue to consume alcohol after diagnosis.

Over time, chronic inflammation can lead to exocrine pancreatic insufficiency, resulting in malabsorption, steatorrhoea (fatty, pale, bulky and foul-smelling stools), weight loss and nutrient deficiencies. These symptoms usually develop many years after the initial onset of pain. Additional features can include nausea, vomiting, anorexia and jaundice (especially if there is biliary obstruction). Endocrine dysfunction may also occur, with diabetes developing in over half of patients with long-standing chronic pancreatitis.

Management

Treatment of acute pancreatitis is primarily supportive, and a detailed assessment of needs is needed so as to respond in a patient-centred holistic manner. Pain is controlled with the use of analgesics (opioids and non-opioid analgesia such as paracetamol or non-steroidal anti-inflammatories); antiemetics may be required, and intravenous fluids are given to maintain hydration and perfusion.

Oral intake may be temporarily withheld in severe acute pancreatitis, but early enteral nutrition is preferred once nausea and abdominal pain allow, as this supports gut function and reduces complications. Antibiotics are only indicated if infected pancreatic necrosis or another infection occurs. Once the patient can tolerate oral intake, a low-fat diet may be recommended, and alcohol should be avoided.

In chronic pancreatitis, lifelong pancreatic enzyme replacement may be required. Proton pump inhibitors may be prescribed to optimise enzyme function. Patients should avoid alcohol, and nutritional support should address malabsorption and deficiencies as needed.

Clinical considerations

Patients with acute pancreatitis require regular monitoring of vital signs, fluid balance, pain and laboratory tests. Oxygen saturation should be checked; note that pulse oximetry may be less accurate in darker-pigmented skin; clinical assessment of perfusion and respiration is essential. Imaging may be needed to identify complications such as gallstones or pancreatic necrosis. Observe for signs of systemic involvement, including hypotension, tachycardia, respiratory distress, jaundice or infection. Nutrition is assessed, alongside patient support on alcohol avoidance and dietary recommendations.

37 Liver cancer

Figure 37.1   The liver segments

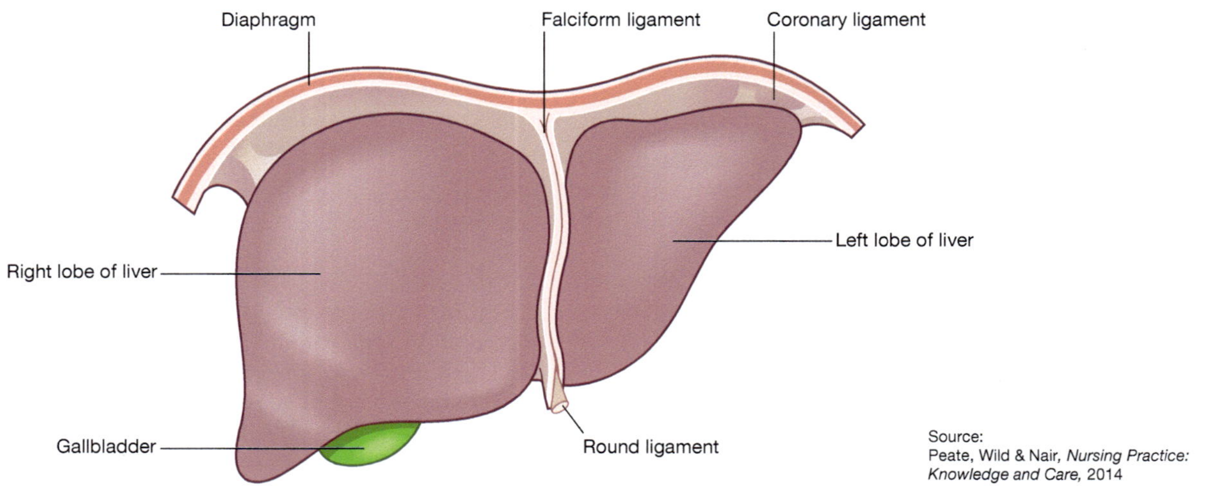

Source:
Peate, Wild & Nair, *Nursing Practice: Knowledge and Care,* 2014

Figure 37.2   Cirrhosis of the liver

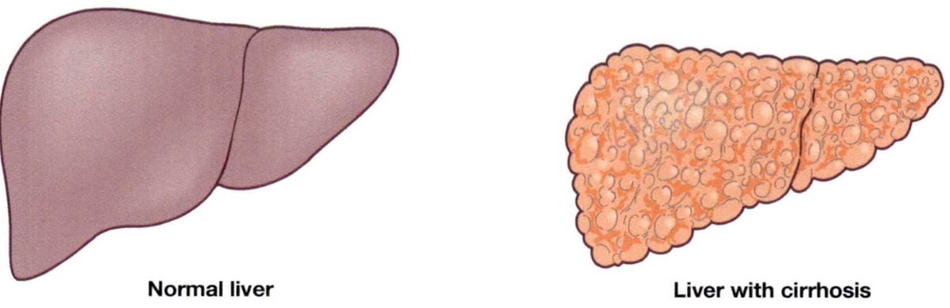

Figure 37.3   Drainage of ascites from the abdomen

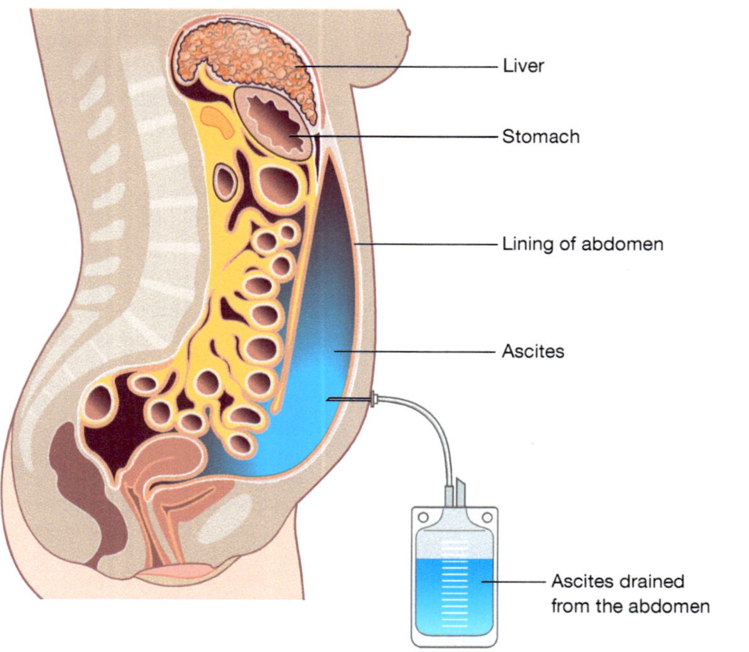

Overview of anatomy and physiology

The liver is the second-largest organ in the body after the skin. It lies mainly below the right lung, protected by the lower ribs, and extends partially across the midline into the left upper quadrant. The liver is divided into two main lobes, the right (largest) and left, as well as two smaller lobes: the caudate and quadrate. Functionally, it is further divided into eight segments based on vascular supply (see Figure 37.1).

The liver is one of the most complex organs in the body; it performs over 500 functions. Its key roles include producing bile to aid fat digestion, synthesising proteins (including clotting factors), metabolising nutrients, as well as the detoxification of harmful substances.

Pathophysiology

Primary liver cancer, though historically uncommon in the UK, has been increasing in incidence, partly due to rising rates of chronic liver disease and viral hepatitis. Globally, it is the sixth most common cancer, with the highest prevalence in Eastern Asia.

Approximately 80–90% of primary hepatic malignancies are hepatocellular carcinomas (HCC), arising from hepatocytes, while the remainder are cholangiocarcinomas, which originate in the bile duct epithelium. Most cases develop in the context of chronic liver injury from alcoholic cirrhosis, hepatitis B or C infection or, increasingly, non-alcoholic fatty liver disease (NAFLD).

Tumours may be localised to one area, form multiple nodules, or diffusely infiltrate the liver surface. As they grow, they disrupt hepatic architecture and vascular flow, leading to biliary obstruction, jaundice, portal hypertension and metabolic disturbances such as hypoalbuminaemia, hypoglycaemia and coagulopathy. Some tumours also produce biologically active substances, resulting in paraneoplastic syndromes such as polycythaemia, hypoglycaemia or hypercalcaemia. Primary liver cancers typically grow rapidly and metastasise early, often to the lungs or regional lymph nodes.

Secondary, or metastatic, liver cancer refers to the spread of malignant cells to the liver from a primary tumour located elsewhere. It is far more common than primary liver cancer, reflecting the liver's role as a major filter for blood. The most frequent primary sites include the colon, pancreas, stomach, lung and breast, although almost any cancer can metastasise to the liver.

Risk factors

The risk of developing HCC increases with age, with approximately 70% of cases occurring in people over 65 years. Liver cirrhosis, characterised by widespread scarring and distortion of hepatic architecture, is a major risk factor for HCC. Cirrhosis may result from chronic viral hepatitis (hepatitis B or C), long-term heavy alcohol consumption, NAFLD associated with obesity or rarer inherited conditions such as haemochromatosis (see Figure 37.2). Primary biliary cholangitis, formerly known as primary biliary cirrhosis, is another cause of chronic liver injury that can predispose to HCC. Although cirrhosis substantially increases the likelihood of HCC, only a proportion of individuals with cirrhosis develop liver cancer each year, with the precise risk depending on the underlying cause and severity of liver disease.

Chronic hepatitis B or C infection not only contributes to cirrhosis but also has direct carcinogenic effects on hepatocytes, further increasing HCC risk. Patients with viral hepatitis are advised to avoid alcohol, as excessive intake compounds liver damage and accelerates carcinogenesis. Smoking is an independent risk factor for HCC and has a synergistic effect in individuals who also consume alcohol or have viral hepatitis.

Additional risk factors include metabolic syndrome, diabetes and obesity, which are increasingly important in the UK due to rising rates of NAFLD. The combination of these factors – chronic liver injury, metabolic stress and environmental exposures – leads to hepatocyte damage, genomic instability and the eventual development of malignant tumours. Preventative strategies focus on viral hepatitis vaccination and treatment, lifestyle modification and surveillance in high-risk populations.

Signs and symptoms

Jaundice may develop if the liver is unable to function properly due to cancer or an underlying condition such as cirrhosis. It can also result from obstruction of the bile ducts by a tumour, which causes bile to back up into the bloodstream. Clinically, jaundice presents as yellowing of the skin and the sclerae (whites of the eyes) and can cause intense itching (pruritus). Other signs include dark urine and steatorrhoea.

In some cases, fluid may accumulate in the abdomen and legs, leading to ascites (see Figure 37.3). Additional symptoms can include loss of appetite, unintentional weight loss, nausea, vomiting and fever. These features often reflect both impaired liver function and the systemic effects of malignancy.

Management

Patients with liver cancer should avoid alcohol and any substances that could further damage the liver. Pain management is a priority, and both patients and their families often benefit from emotional, practical and symptom management support. Not all liver cancers are curable; discussions about treatment options, prognosis and care goals should be conducted sensitively, allowing the patient and family to express concerns, fears or frustrations. In the early stages, patients may remain independent, but as the disease progresses, they will require increasing assistance. Referral to a specialist cancer or palliative care team is recommended to support symptom control, psychosocial needs and advance care planning.

Surgery

Surgical resection is a potentially curative treatment for primary liver cancer; however, only a minority of patients are eligible for this approach due to tumour size, location or underlying liver disease such as cirrhosis. Removal of a liver lobe, known as a lobectomy or hemi-hepatectomy, may be performed if sufficient healthy liver remains, as the liver has the capacity to regenerate.

Liver transplantation is another curative option for selected patients, particularly those with small, unresectable tumours confined to the liver and no evidence of extrahepatic disease. Tumours that are too large, multiple beyond established criteria or spread outside the liver make transplantation unsuitable, as residual cancer cells elsewhere would remain and the surgery would not be curative.

Chemotherapy

Transarterial chemoembolisation (TACE) is a locoregional therapy (treatment that is delivered directly to a specific area or region of the body, rather than affecting the whole body systemically) in which chemotherapy is delivered directly into the artery supplying a liver tumour, followed by embolisation of the tumour-feeding vessels. TACE is primarily used for patients who are not candidates for surgical resection or as a bridging therapy before liver transplantation. It may be combined with other treatments, such as radiofrequency ablation or surgery, to improve outcomes.

Clinical considerations

Liver transplantation can be curative for hepatocellular carcinoma confined to the liver and unsuitable for resection. Preoperative assessment includes evaluation of liver function, comorbidities and infection risk. Post-transplant, patients require lifelong immunosuppression and regular monitoring for graft function, cancer recurrence and complications. Support for nutrition, rehabilitation and psychosocial needs is important. Transplant is not suitable for patients with extrahepatic spread or uncontrolled disease.

The urinary system

Chapters

38 Renal failure

Figure 38.1 Renal system.

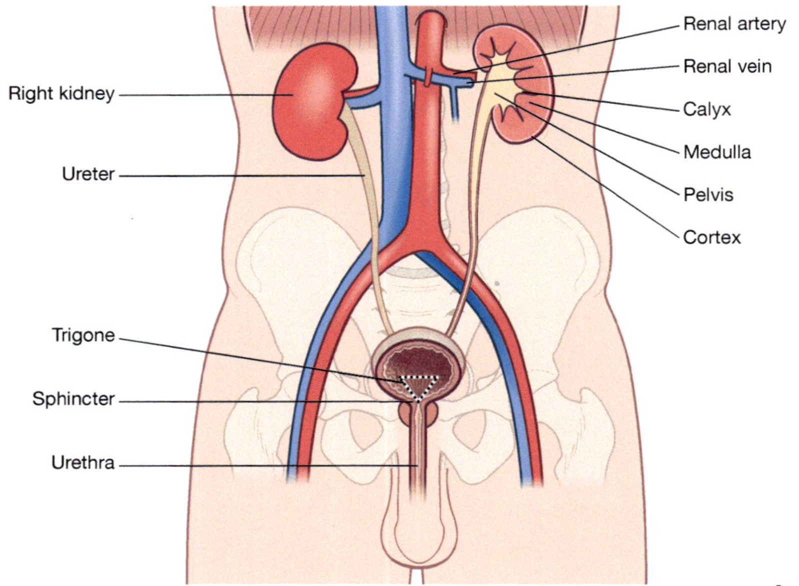

Source:
Peate, Wild & Nair, *Nursing Practice: Knowledge and Care,* 2014

Figure 38.2 The structures of a nephron.

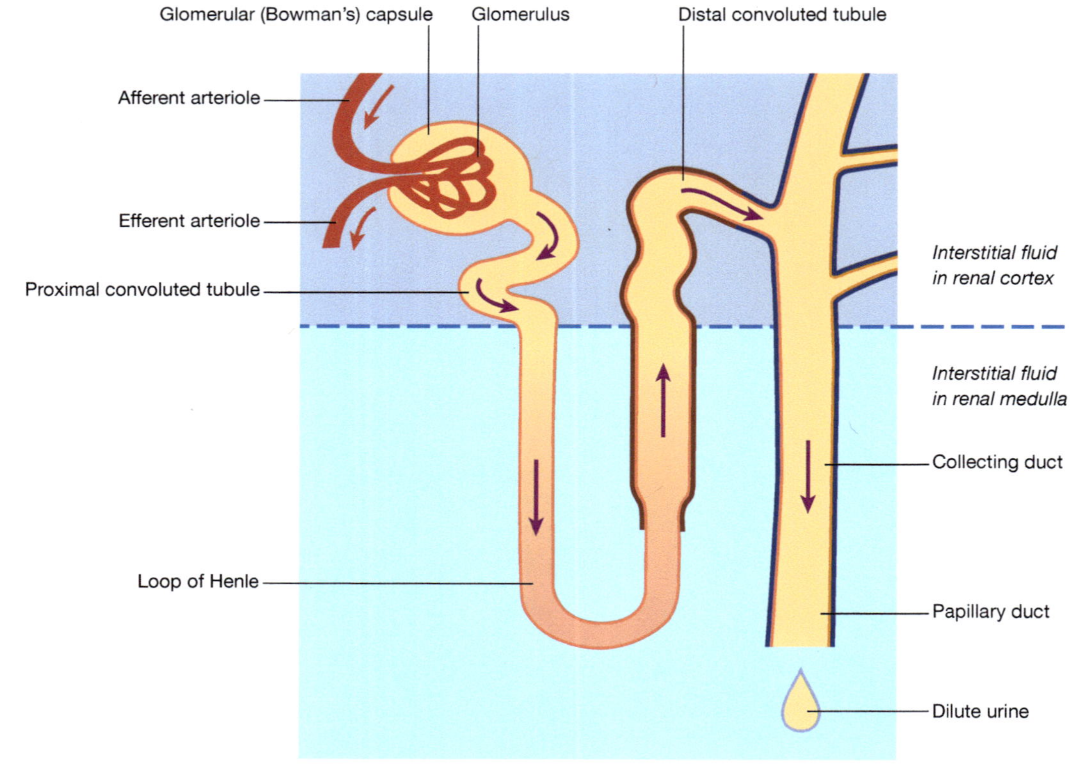

Source: Peate I & Nair M *Fundamentals of Anatomy and Physiology for Student Nurses (2011)*

Overview of anatomy and physiology

The body normally contains two kidneys, positioned within the abdominal cavity at a slightly oblique angle on either side of the vertebral column, spanning the levels of the twelfth thoracic vertebra to the third lumbar vertebra. Each kidney measures approximately 10–12 cm in length, 5–7 cm in width and 3–4 cm in thickness. They are bean-shaped, with a convex outer surface and a concave inner surface. At the centre of the concave border lies an indentation called the renal hilum, which serves as the entry and exit point for the ureter, renal artery, renal vein, lymphatic vessels and nerves (Figure 38.1).

The nephron is the kidney's structural and functional unit. Each nephron operates independently, producing a very small amount of urine. It can be divided into distinct regions: the Bowman's capsule, glomerulus, proximal convoluted tubule, loop of Henle, distal convoluted tubule and collecting ducts (Figure 38.2).

Blood supply

The kidneys receive their blood supply directly from the aorta via the renal arteries, and blood is returned to the inferior vena cava through the renal veins. They receive approximately 20% of the cardiac output. The paired renal arteries arise at the level of L2 and enter each kidney through the renal hilum, the passageway into the organ. At the hilum, the renal vein lies anteriorly, the renal artery lies posterior to the vein, and the renal pelvis lies most posteriorly. The renal veins carry blood from the kidneys back to the inferior vena cava, with the left renal vein being longer than the right as it crosses the midline to reach the inferior vena cava.

Functions

The kidneys perform several vital functions, including the filtration and excretion of metabolic waste products such as urea, creatinine and ammonium; the regulation of electrolytes, fluid, and acid–base balance; and the stimulation of red blood cell production. They also help regulate blood pressure through the renin–angiotensin–aldosterone system, controlling water reabsorption and maintaining intravascular volume. Additionally, the kidneys reabsorb essential nutrients such as glucose and amino acids, and they have important hormonal functions, including the production of erythropoietin, the activation of vitamin D to calcitriol and the regulation of calcium and phosphate metabolism.

Pathophysiology

Acute kidney injury

Acute kidney injury (AKI) is an abrupt decline in renal function, resulting in the kidney's inability to maintain fluid, electrolyte and acid–base balance. It is primarily detected and monitored by serial serum creatinine measurements, which rise acutely, while urine output typically decreases. Although the glomerular filtration rate (GFR) declines, estimates such as eGFR (estimated GFR) may be unreliable in the acute setting due to the lag in creatinine rise.

Aetiology

Prerenal

Prerenal causes arise from conditions that reduce renal perfusion without direct damage to the kidney tissue. These include volume depletion resulting from haemorrhage, severe vomiting or diarrhoea, burns or excessive diuretic use. Cardiac failure, cirrhosis, nephrotic syndrome and systemic hypotension can also reduce effective circulating volume and lead to prerenal AKI. In addition, renal hypoperfusion may occur due to the effects of non-steroidal anti-inflammatory drugs or selective cyclooxygenase-2 (COX-2) inhibitors, which impair prostaglandin-mediated vasodilation of the afferent arteriole. Angiotensin-converting enzyme inhibitors and angiotensin II receptor antagonists (AIIRAs or ARBs) can also contribute by reducing efferent arteriolar tone. Other causes include abdominal aortic aneurysm, renal artery stenosis or occlusion, and hepatorenal syndrome.

Intrarenal

Intrarenal causes involve direct injury to the kidney parenchyma, affecting the glomeruli, tubules, interstitium or renal vasculature. Glomerular diseases such as glomerulonephritis, thrombosis or haemolytic uraemic syndrome can impair filtration. Tubular injury, most commonly in the form of acute tubular necrosis, may result from prolonged ischaemia or exposure to nephrotoxins such as aminoglycoside antibiotics, radiocontrast media or myoglobin in rhabdomyolysis. Vascular causes include vasculitis, polyarteritis nodosa, thrombotic microangiopathy, cholesterol emboli, renal artery stenosis, renal vein thrombosis, malignant hypertension and eclampsia.

Postrenal

Postrenal causes result from obstruction to urinary outflow at any level of the urinary tract. Common examples include renal or ureteric calculi, prostatic hypertrophy or malignancy, retroperitoneal fibrosis, bladder tumours, pelvic malignancy, urethral strictures and papillary necrosis. Obstruction increases hydrostatic pressure within the urinary tract, impairing glomerular filtration and, if prolonged, causing irreversible damage to renal tissue.

Chronic kidney disease

Chronic kidney disease (CKD) results from irreversible damage to nephrons, leading to a gradual loss of kidney function. It is classified into five stages of increasing severity. In the early stages, as some nephrons are lost, the remaining healthy nephrons compensate by increasing their filtration (hyperfiltration) and sometimes hypertrophying. Over time, this adaptive process can damage the remaining nephrons, causing a progressive decline in kidney function, which may continue even after the initial injury has resolved.

Signs and symptoms

Symptoms and signs of renal failure vary depending on the stage of the disease. In the early stages, kidney disease may be asymptomatic; the person may feel well. As kidney function declines, the kidneys fail to filter waste properly, leading to the accumulation of nitrogenous wastes in the blood, a condition called azotaemia. When renal failure causes noticeable clinical effects, it is termed uraemia.

Symptoms may include fatigue, weakness, loss of appetite, nausea, vomiting, diarrhoea, weight loss and difficulty urinating. Swelling of the legs, ankles, feet, face or hands and shortness of breath due to fluid in the lungs are also common. Changes in urine, such as haematuria, may be noticed.

Signs observed on examination or through investigations can include pitting oedema, pulmonary oedema and hypertension. Pale skin from anaemia may be present, and in severe uraemia, neurological signs such as confusion, lethargy or even seizures may occur. Laboratory findings often reveal elevated urea and creatinine, electrolyte imbalances (e.g., hyperkalaemia), metabolic acidosis and abnormal urinalysis showing proteinuria or haematuria.

Management

The management of renal failure depends on whether it is AKI or CKD. A thorough assessment, including vital signs, weight, fluid intake and output, medical history, and understanding of the disease, is essential. Nutrition is carefully managed: in AKI, protein intake may be moderately restricted to reduce nitrogenous waste, while carbohydrates are increased to provide calories and spare protein. In CKD, prolonged protein restriction is avoided to prevent malnutrition, and once dialysis begins, a high-protein diet is recommended. Water and sodium intake are regulated to maintain fluid balance.

Medications are used to treat underlying causes and control complications. These include antihypertensives, diuretics for fluid overload, erythropoiesis-stimulating agents for anaemia, phosphate binders and vitamin D analogues for bone-mineral disorders, and sodium bicarbonate for metabolic acidosis. Nephrotoxic drugs should be avoided or adjusted.

Renal replacement therapy (RRT), including haemodialysis, peritoneal dialysis or continuous RRT, is required when the kidneys cannot maintain fluid, electrolyte and waste balance. RRT removes nitrogenous wastes, corrects electrolyte imbalances, removes excess fluid and maintains acid–base balance. In CKD, long-term planning for dialysis or kidney transplantation is essential.

Clinical considerations

Renal replacement therapy is initiated when the kidneys are unable to maintain normal fluid, electrolyte and waste balance, typically in cases of severe acute kidney injury or end-stage chronic kidney disease. The main types of RRT include haemodialysis, where blood is filtered through a machine to remove waste and excess fluid; peritoneal dialysis, which uses the peritoneal membrane as a natural filter; and continuous renal replacement therapy, used for critically ill or haemodynamically unstable patients in intensive care settings.

Care focuses on close monitoring of vital signs, weight and fluid balance, as well as assessment of the vascular access or peritoneal catheter site for signs of infection or complications. The overall goal of renal replacement therapy is to maintain homeostasis until kidney function recovers in acute kidney injury or to sustain life in chronic kidney disease, where renal recovery is unlikely.

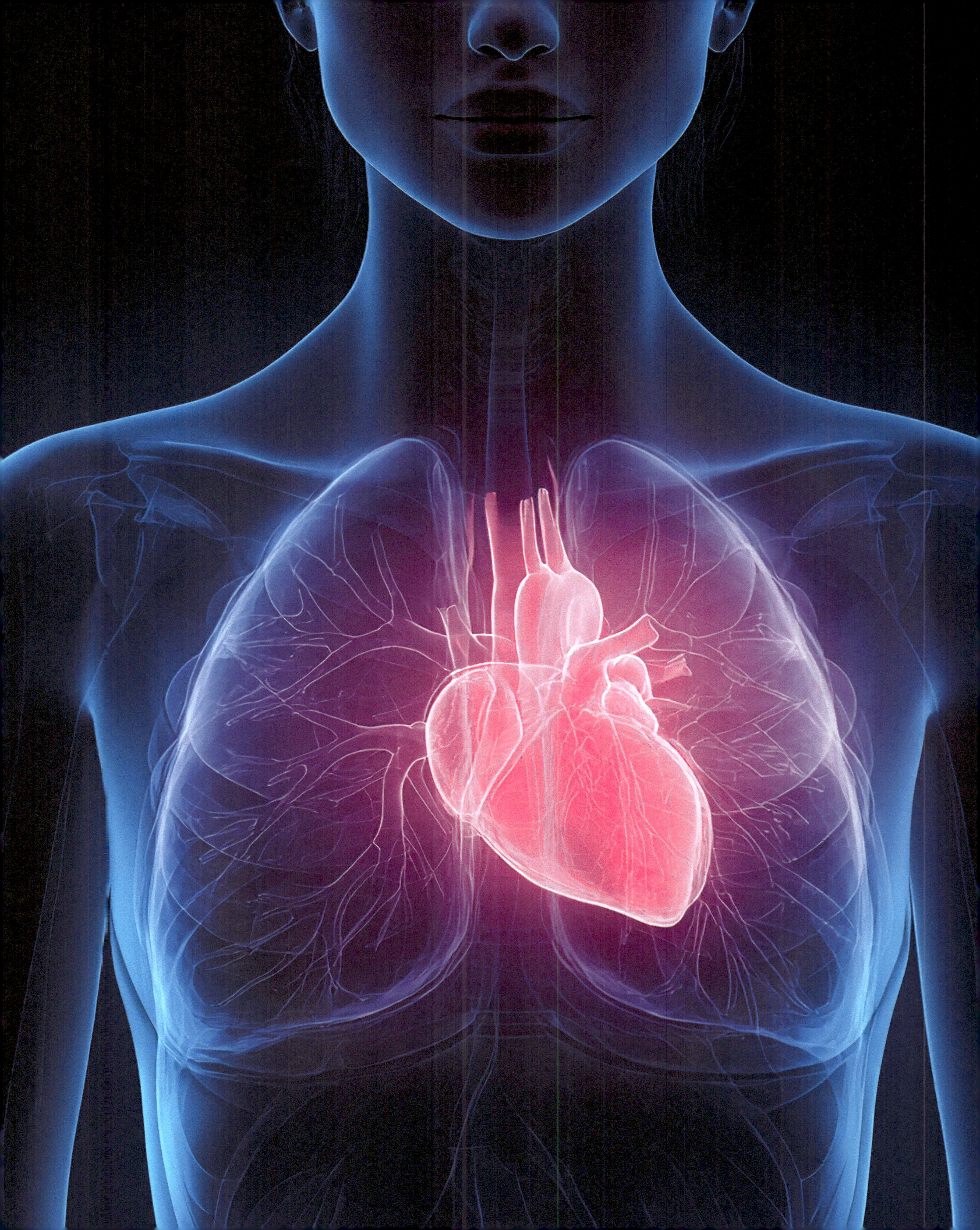

39 Pyelonephritis

Figure 39.1 Anatomy of the kidney.

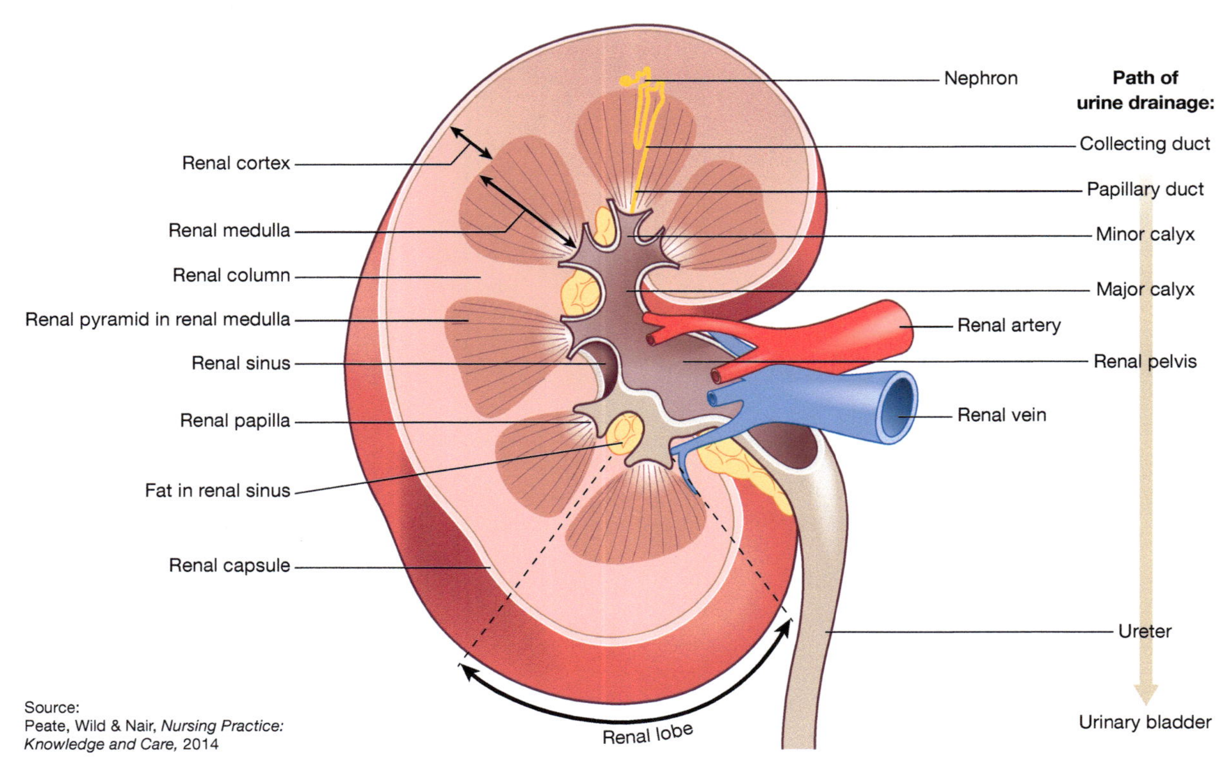

Source:
Peate, Wild & Nair, *Nursing Practice:
Knowledge and Care,* 2014

Figure 39.2 A kidney affected by chronic pyelonephritis.

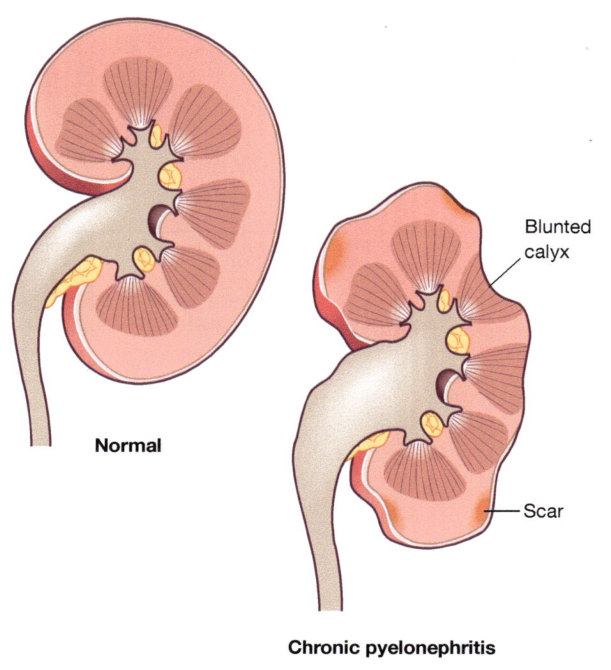

Figure 39.3 Causes of hydronephrosis.

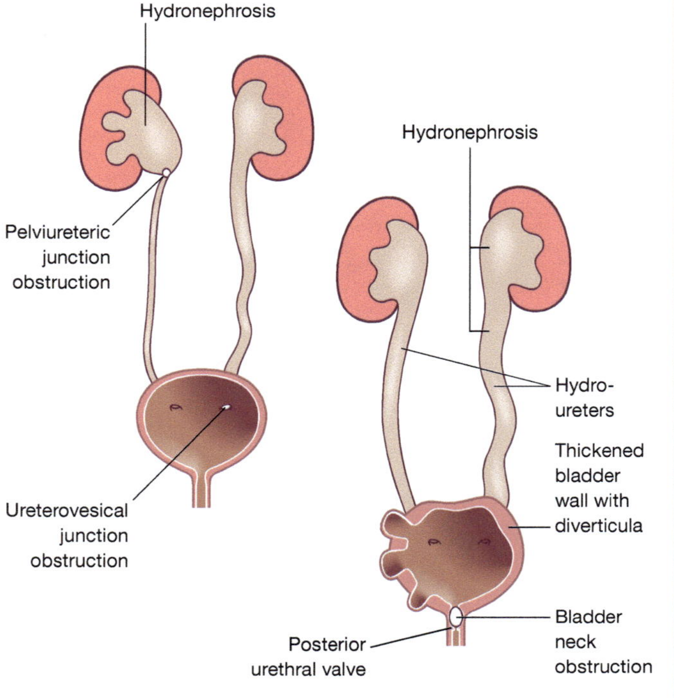

Overview

The kidneys, located on either side of the upper posterior abdomen, filter the blood to remove waste products and excess water, producing urine.

The urine drains from the kidneys through narrow muscular tubes called ureters, one from each kidney, which transport it to the urinary bladder. Blood enters the kidneys through the renal arteries and passes into millions of tiny filtering units called nephrons. Each nephron removes waste products, excess salts and water from the blood to produce urine. This is the filtering process. The bladder acts as a temporary storage organ for urine. When the bladder becomes full, urine is expelled from the body through the urethra during the process of micturition (passing urine); see Figure 39.1. Pyelonephritis is a bacterial infection of the renal pelvis and kidney tissue. It is a type of upper urinary tract infection (UTI) that typically arises when bacteria ascend from the bladder (as in cystitis) up the ureters to the kidneys.

Causes of pyelonephritis

Most cases of pyelonephritis arise as a complication of a lower UTI, usually cystitis. Bacteria that commonly inhabit the gastrointestinal tract, particularly *Escherichia coli*, can enter the urinary tract via the urethra and colonise the bladder. If the infection is not effectively treated, bacteria may ascend the ureters to infect the kidneys, resulting in pyelonephritis. The risk of this ascending infection is increased by factors such as urinary tract obstruction, vesicoureteric reflux (a condition in which urine flows backward from the bladder into one or both ureters and sometimes up to the kidneys, instead of flowing normally from the kidneys to ureters to bladder to urethra), indwelling urinary catheters or underlying conditions including diabetes mellitus and immunosuppression. Prompt recognition and management are essential to prevent complications such as renal scarring or sepsis.

Pathophysiology

Pyelonephritis is an inflammatory condition affecting the renal parenchyma (the functional tissue of the kidney) and pelvis, most commonly caused by bacterial infection. It can be classified as acute or chronic. Acute pyelonephritis usually results from an ascending bacterial infection originating in the lower urinary tract, often caused by *E. coli*. The bacteria trigger an inflammatory response in the kidney, leading to symptoms such as fever, flank pain and pyuria. Chronic pyelonephritis typically arises from recurrent or persistent bacterial infections, often associated with structural abnormalities such as vesicoureteric reflux or urinary tract obstruction, and can result in renal scarring and long-term impairment of kidney function.

Acute pyelonephritis

Acute pyelonephritis usually results from a bacterial infection that ascends from the lower urinary tract to the kidney. Conditions such as asymptomatic bacteriuria or cystitis can precede the development of acute pyelonephritis. Risk factors include pregnancy, which predisposes due to physiological ureteral dilation and slowed peristalsis, urinary tract obstruction and congenital urinary tract malformations. Additional contributing factors include urinary tract trauma, scarring, calculi (stones), structural kidney disorders such as polycystic or hypertensive kidney disease, and chronic systemic diseases such as diabetes mellitus.

Vesicoureteral reflux is a common risk factor resulting in bladder outflow obstruction.

Infection typically spreads from the renal pelvis to the renal cortex, affecting the pelvis, calyces and medulla. Infected renal tissue shows white blood cell infiltration, inflammation, and oedema, and localised cortical abscesses may develop. *E. coli* is responsible for approximately 85% of acute cases. Other organisms, including *Proteus* and *Klebsiella*, which normally inhabit the intestinal tract, are also common causes.

Chronic pyelonephritis

Chronic pyelonephritis is characterised by long-standing inflammation and scarring of the renal tubules and interstitial tissue (see Figure 39.2). It is a common cause of chronic kidney disease. The condition may develop following recurrent UTIs, vesicoureteral reflux or urinary tract obstruction. Structural or vascular abnormalities, such as severe hypertension, may also contribute to kidney damage over time.

Affected kidneys are typically smaller (contracted) with coarse surface scarring. If both kidneys are involved, asymmetry may be observed. Histological examination shows blunting and deformation of the calyces, along with coarse corticomedullary scarring, often most pronounced in the upper and lower poles in reflux-associated cases. In obstruction-related chronic pyelonephritis, features of hydronephrosis may also be present due to prolonged urinary stasis (see Figure 39.3).

Investigations and diagnosis

The diagnosis of UTI is primarily based on clinical history and urinalysis. A history of previous UTIs is important, particularly in patients with recurrent infections. Urine culture is indicated in high-risk patients (e.g. those who are pregnant, immunosuppressed or who have failed to respond to initial antibiotic therapy). In men with symptoms suggestive of a UTI, urine culture should always be performed, regardless of urinalysis results.

Imaging of the urinary tract may be warranted to identify underlying structural abnormalities, obstruction or renal stones. Ultrasound of the kidneys and bladder is recommended in cases of complicated pyelonephritis, recurrent infection or when anatomical abnormalities are suspected. This helps guide management and prevent further renal damage.

Signs and symptoms

Patients with UTI may present with dysuria, urinary urgency, frequency, nocturia and haematuria. Systemic features such as pyrexia, tachycardia, shaking chills, flank pain and malaise are more common in acute pyelonephritis. In chronic pyelonephritis, symptoms may be mild, intermittent or absent, allowing the disease to progress gradually and potentially result in renal scarring or chronic kidney disease.

Urinalysis often reveals cloudy, malodorous urine with positive dipstick results for blood, protein, leukocytes and nitrites. A midstream urine (MSU) specimen should be sent for microscopy and culture, although bacteriuria may not always correlate with symptoms. If a urinary catheter is in place, a catheter specimen is acceptable. Microscopy typically shows pyuria (the presence of pus in the urine).

Blood cultures should be obtained if there is suspicion of systemic infection. They are positive in approximately 12–20% of patients with acute pyelonephritis and can help guide targeted antimicrobial therapy.

Management

The primary objective in managing UTIs is to identify the cause and provide appropriate treatment. Patients should receive reassurance, health information and psychological support. Those with acute pyelonephritis should be encouraged to rest as needed, maintain adequate hydration, and be monitored for systemic signs such as fever, tachycardia and malaise, which may indicate worsening infection.

Antibiotic therapy for acute pyelonephritis can be prescribed for 7–14 days. In severe cases, treatment is started intravenously in hospital and changed to oral antibiotics once the patient stabilises. Mild cases in otherwise healthy adults may be managed entirely with oral therapy. Antibiotic choice should be guided by local resistance patterns and adjusted according to urine culture and sensitivity results. Blood pressure should be monitored and controlled to slow the progression of chronic kidney damage; ACE inhibitors are preferred when indicated.

In rare cases, pyelonephritis can lead to renal abscess formation, which is difficult to treat with antibiotics alone. Percutaneous drainage under imaging guidance, such as nephrostomy insertion, is typically required to manage the abscess.

Clinical considerations

Prompt antibiotic therapy is essential in pyelonephritis to prevent complications such as sepsis or renal damage. Treatment should begin as soon as infection is suspected, ideally after urine and blood cultures are taken. The initial antibiotic should cover *Escherichia coli* and other Gram-negative organisms, guided by local resistance patterns and refined once culture results are available.

Severe or complicated cases require intravenous antibiotics initially. Milder infections may be treated with oral antibiotics alone. Treatment duration is usually 7–14 days, depending on clinical response. Renal function should be monitored.

Patients are advised to complete the full course of antibiotics, maintain hydration and attend follow-up to ensure full recovery and prevent recurrence.

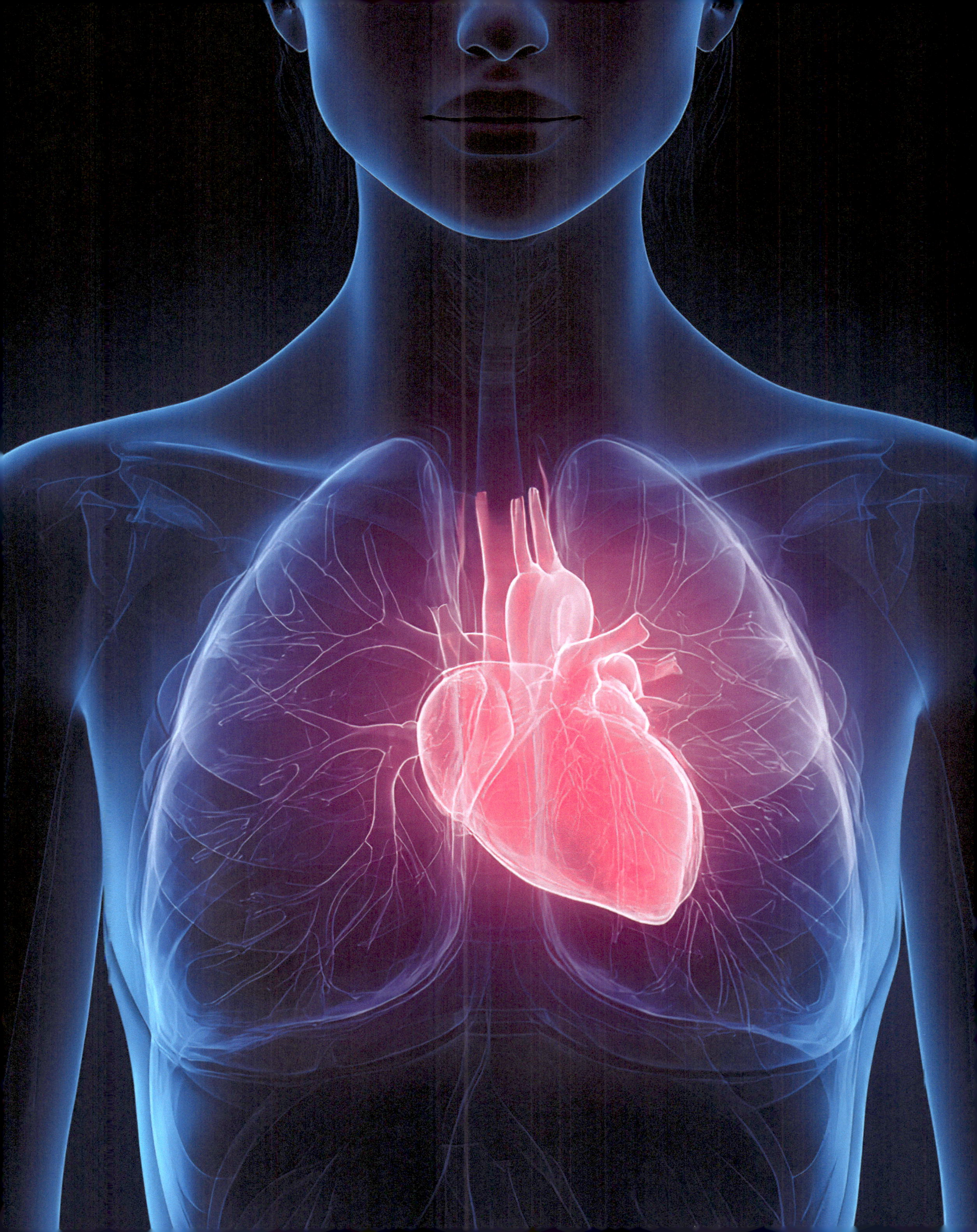

40 Renal calculi

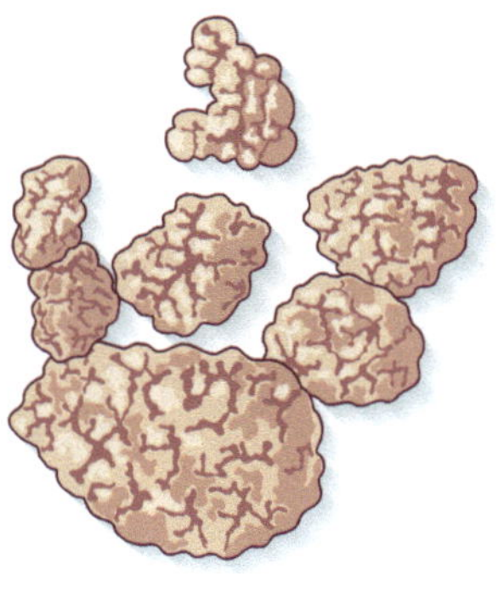

Figure 40.1 Calcium oxalate stones.

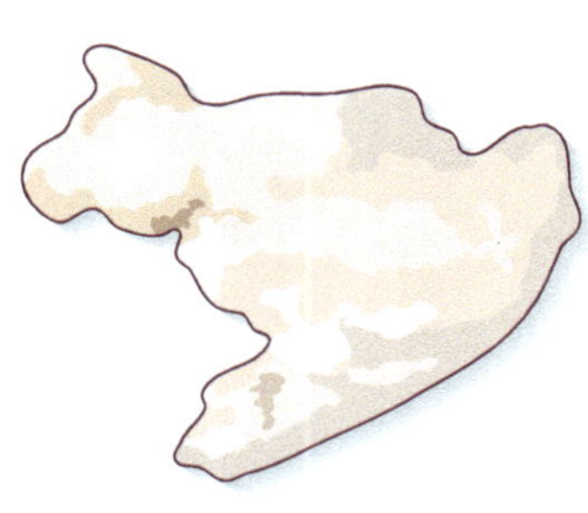

Figure 40.2 Struvite stone.

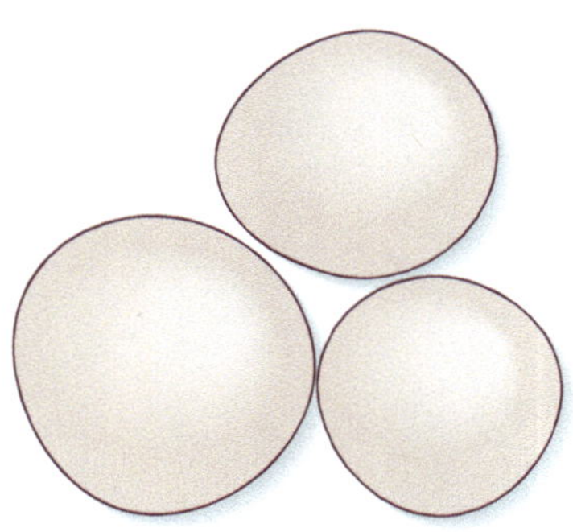

Figure 40.3 Uric acid stones.

Figure 40.4 Cystine stone in the bladder.

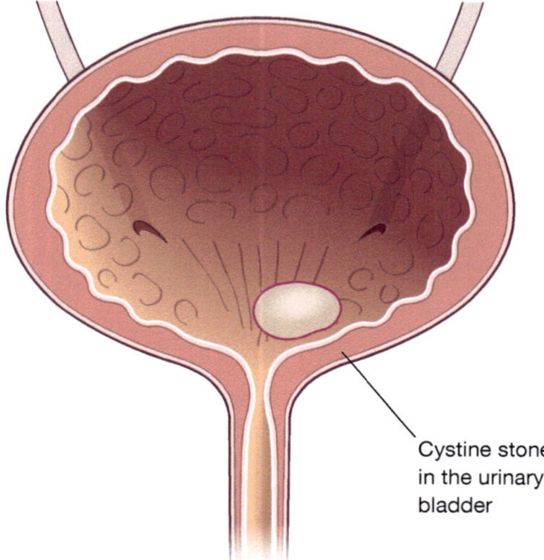

Figure 40.5 Shock waves to break kidney stones.

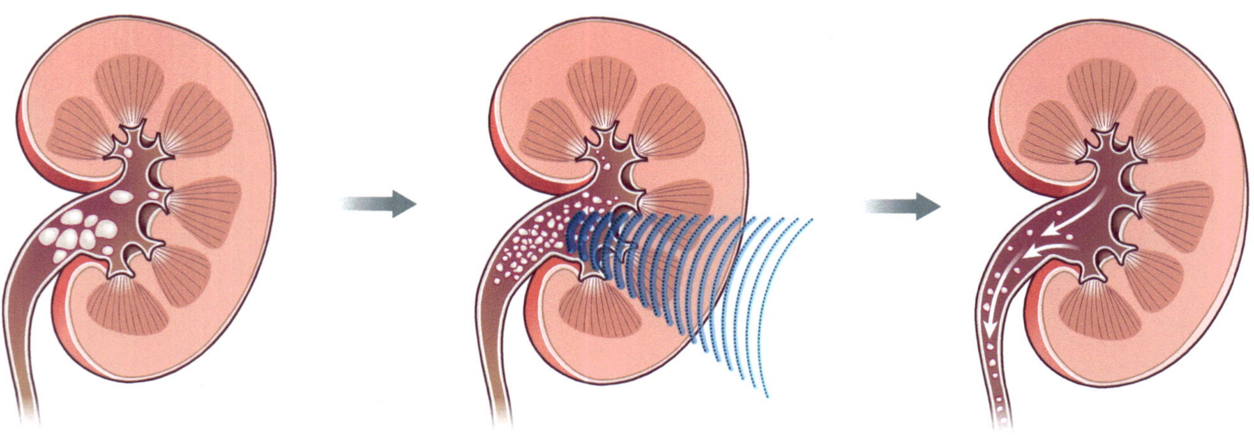

Overview

The kidneys normally maintain homeostasis by balancing water conservation with the excretion of poorly soluble substances, such as calcium salts. This balance is influenced by a number of factors, including diet, environmental temperature and physical activity. Protective substances present in the urine, such as pyrophosphate, citrate and glycoproteins, help inhibit the formation of renal stones by preventing crystal nucleation and aggregation.

Renal calculi, commonly known as kidney stones, are solid concretions (solid masses of mineral salts or other substances) or crystals that form in the kidneys from minerals and salts normally found in the urine. They form when the urine becomes supersaturated with salts and minerals, including calcium oxalate, struvite (magnesium ammonium phosphate), uric acid and cystine. Approximately 60–80% of stones contain calcium. Stones vary in size; they range from small gravel-like particles to large staghorn calculi. They may remain at their site of formation or migrate along the urinary tract, producing symptoms such as pain and/or haematuria.

Although most stones are idiopathic (there is no known cause), several risk factors have been identified. The greatest risk is a personal or family history of urinary calculi, which may reflect a genetic predisposition to high urinary mineral concentrations or a congenital deficiency of protective factors. Other contributors include dehydration, immobility, excess dietary intake of calcium, oxalate or protein, and medical conditions such as gout, hyperparathyroidism, urinary stasis or recurrent infections.

Pathophysiology

Three main factors contribute to renal stone formation (urolithiasis): supersaturation of urine, nucleation of crystals and a deficiency of inhibitory substances. When the concentration of an insoluble salt in the urine becomes very high (supersaturation), crystals may form. Normally, these crystals disperse and are excreted because the bonds between them are weak. However, a stable nucleus can develop, around which more crystals aggregate to form a stone. In most cases, kidney stones develop when crystals deposit and grow around a small framework of organic material in the urine, such as mucoproteins or glycoproteins, which act as a scaffold to promote stone formation. Only a small trigger, such as a high-salt meal or naturally concentrated urine overnight, may be sufficient to initiate crystallisation in supersaturated urine. Adequate hydration generally prevents stone growth. The acidity of the urine and the presence of natural inhibitors determine how easily crystals can form and grow into stones.

Most (75–80%) kidney stones are calcium stones (calcium oxalate and/or calcium phosphate), often associated with hypercalciuria. Uric acid stones develop when uric acid concentration is high, are more common in men, and may be linked to gout. Genetic factors contribute to both calcium and uric acid stones. Struvite stones occur in the setting of urinary tract infection with urease-producing bacteria (e.g. *Proteus*) and can grow into staghorn calculi that fill the renal pelvis and calyces. Cystine stones are rare and result from a genetic defect in cystine transport.

Calcium stones: Most kidney stones are calcium stones, usually in the form of calcium oxalate (Figure 40.1). Oxalate is a naturally occurring substance that is found in food; certain fruits, vegetables, nuts and chocolate are particularly rich in oxalate. The liver also produces oxalate. Factors that increase urinary calcium or oxalate include dietary intake, high doses of vitamin D, intestinal bypass surgery and metabolic disorders. Calcium stones may also occur as calcium phosphate.

Struvite stones: these stones form in response to urinary tract infections, which are often caused by urease-producing bacteria (Figure 40.2). Struvite stones can grow rapidly, becoming very large. They may cause few symptoms initially, often developing within the renal pelvis without causing significant urinary obstruction. They are commonly associated with recurrent urinary tract infections.

Uric acid stones: uric acid stones develop in individuals with low fluid intake, excessive fluid loss, high-protein diets or gout (Figure 40.3). Genetic factors may also increase the risk.

Cystine stones: these are rare stones that occur in people with the hereditary disorder cystinuria, which causes excessive excretion of certain amino acids in the urine (Figure 40.4).

Signs and symptoms

Kidney stones may not cause symptoms while they remain in the kidney. Symptoms typically occur when a stone moves within the kidney or passes into the ureter, the tube connecting the kidney to the bladder. Common signs include severe, colicky flank pain that may radiate to the groin, haematuria, dysuria, urinary urgency, cloudy or offensive-smelling urine and nausea or vomiting. Pyrexia and chills may occur if a urinary tract infection is present. The pain may change location or intensity as the stone moves through the urinary tract.

Management

The treatment of kidney stones depends on the type, size and the underlying cause. The majority of stones can be managed conservatively, with simple measures, and do not usually require invasive procedures.

Hydration: patients should generally be encouraged to maintain adequate hydration, aiming for 2–2.5 L of fluid daily, primarily water, to help flush the urinary system. Urine should be clear or nearly clear. However, fluid intake should be adjusted in patients with heart failure, kidney failure or other conditions requiring fluid restriction.

Analgesia: passing even a small stone may cause the patient significant discomfort. Mild to moderate pain can usually be managed with oral analgesics such as ibuprofen or paracetamol. Severe pain may require stronger medications, including intravenous opioids and antispasmodics, and may indicate the need for urgent imaging or intervention.

Antibiotics: if there is a urinary tract infection, appropriate antibiotic therapy should be prescribed.

Stones that cannot be managed conservatively because they are too large to pass spontaneously, if they cause persistent bleeding, obstruction, kidney damage or recurrent urinary tract infections, may require invasive treatment. Options include extracorporeal shock wave lithotripsy (ESWL), laser lithotripsy or percutaneous ultrasonic lithotripsy (Figure 40.5).

Clinical considerations

Management of kidney stones focuses on hydration, pain relief, infection control and monitoring for complications. Encourage adequate fluid intake, typically 2–2.5 L per day, unless contraindicated. Mild discomfort can often be managed with oral NSAIDs or paracetamol; severe pain may require opioids, intravenous analgesia or antispasmodics. Urinary tract infections should be treated promptly with appropriate antibiotics. Stones that are too large to pass spontaneously may require invasive interventions, including extracorporeal shock wave lithotripsy, laser lithotripsy or percutaneous procedures.

41 Bladder cancer

Figure 41.1 Urinary bladder.

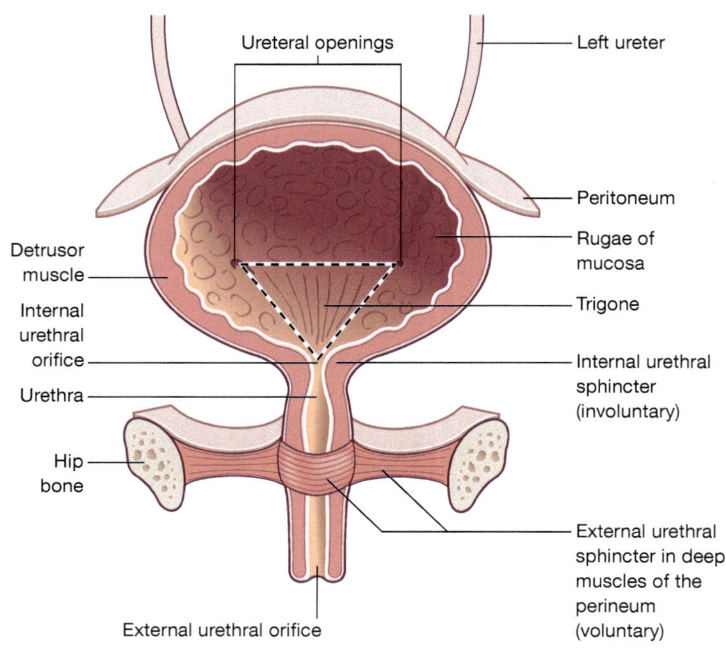

Source:
Peate et al. 2014/with permission of John Wiley & Sons

Figure 41.2 Male urethra.

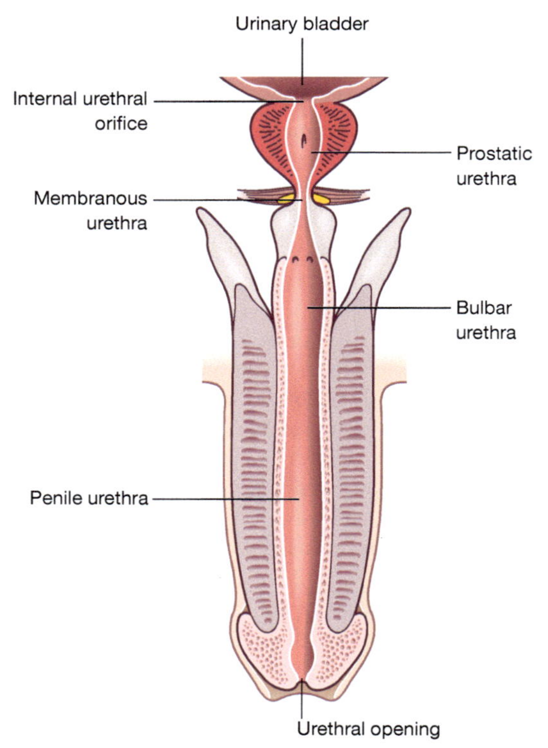

Figure 41.3 Female urethra.

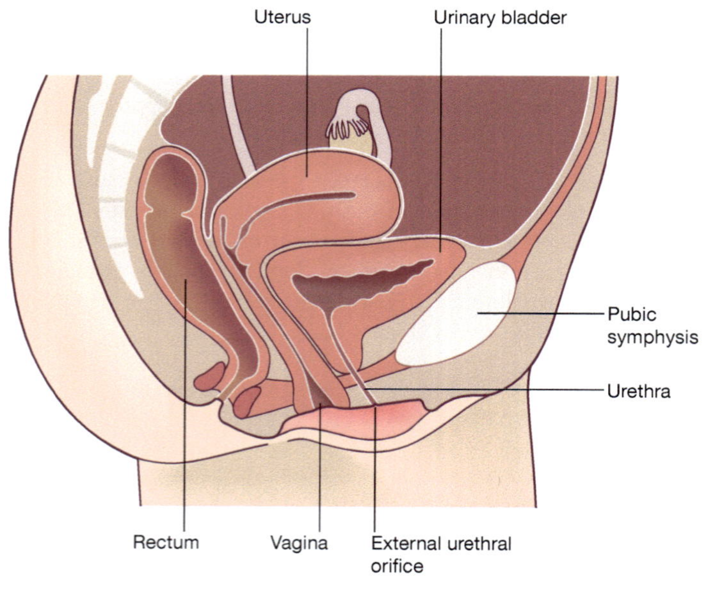

Source:
Peate et al. 2014/with permission of John Wiley & Sons

Figure 41.4 Staging of bladder cancer.

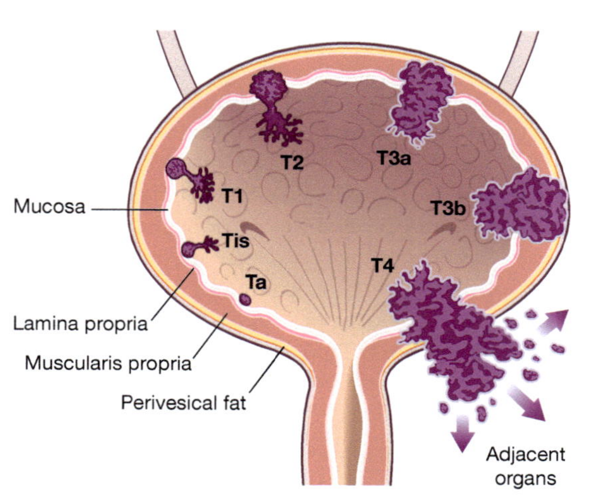

Source:
Peate et al. 2014/with permission of John Wiley & Sons

Overview

The urinary bladder is a muscular sac that is located in the pelvis, just above and behind the pubic bone. When the bladder is empty, it is roughly the size and shape of a pear, with its apex pointing forward and the neck tapering into the urethra.

Urine is produced in the kidneys, and it travels down two tubes, the ureters, to the bladder. The bladder stores urine, allowing urination to be both infrequent and voluntary. Its walls are made up of detrusor muscle, which stretches to accommodate increasing volumes of urine. In a healthy adult, the bladder can normally hold 400–600 mL of urine.

In the floor of the bladder is a small triangular area called the trigone. The trigone is formed by the two ureteral orifices and the internal urethral orifice. The area is very sensitive to expansion, and once stretched to a certain degree, the urinary bladder signals the brain of its need to empty. The signals become stronger as the bladder continues to fill. During urination, the bladder muscles contract, and two sphincters (valves) open to allow urine to flow out. Urine exits the bladder into the urethra, which carries urine out of the body.

The flow of urine through the urethra is controlled by the internal and external urethral sphincters. The internal sphincter is composed of smooth muscle; this relaxes involuntarily when the bladder reaches a threshold volume, and this contributes to the sensation of urgency. The external sphincter is made of skeletal muscle and is under voluntary control, allowing urine to be passed or withheld as needed (see Figure 41.1).

Urethra

The male urethra is a narrow fibromuscular tube that conducts urine from the bladder and semen from the ejaculatory ducts to the exterior. Although a single tube, it is divided into three anatomically distinct segments: prostatic, membranous and spongy (penile). The male urethra, as it passes through the penis, is longer than the female urethra, measuring approximately 20 cm in adults (Figure 41.2).

The female urethra is a shorter, narrower fibromuscular tube, approximately 3–5 cm in length (Figure 41.3), that conducts urine from the bladder to the exterior. It is embedded in the anterior vaginal wall and opens just above the vaginal opening. Because of its short length, the female urethra is more susceptible to ascending urinary tract infections, but it is solely a urinary conduit.

Pathophysiology

Bladder cancer most commonly arises from the urothelial cells that line the bladder, which are responsible for forming a protective barrier and allowing the bladder to stretch as it fills. The development of bladder cancer occurs when these cells undergo genetic and molecular changes, disrupting normal cell cycle regulation. Such changes lead to uncontrolled proliferation, evasion of programmed cell death (apoptosis) and abnormal tissue growth, forming a tumour. Superficial bladder tumours remain confined to the urothelial lining and often cause fewer symptoms, whereas invasive tumours penetrate the muscular wall of the bladder, increasing the risk of local tissue destruction, bleeding and obstruction (see Figure 41.4).

Cancer cells can also metastasise, spreading via the bloodstream or lymphatic system to distant organs such as the lungs, liver or bones, where they form secondary tumours. The likelihood of metastasis and tissue damage is higher in invasive tumours compared with superficial lesions.

Early detection of bladder cancer is crucial. Superficial tumours are usually more amenable to treatment, including surgical resection or intravesical therapy, and are associated with a better prognosis. In contrast, invasive or metastatic bladder cancer often requires more aggressive treatment and carries a poorer outlook. Understanding the cellular origins and mechanisms of tumour progression is essential for effective management and improved patient outcomes.

Signs and symptoms

The most common symptom of bladder cancer is haematuria, which may be visible (gross) or detected only on urinalysis (microscopic). Haematuria is often painless and intermittent, and while it can result from other conditions such as urinary tract infections or kidney stones, it is never considered normal and should always be evaluated promptly. Other possible symptoms include loss of appetite, unintentional weight loss, back or abdominal pain and painful urination (dysuria). Less commonly, patients may experience urinary frequency, urgency or recurrent infections. Early recognition of these signs is important for prompt diagnosis and improved outcomes.

Management

Treatment of bladder cancer depends on the location, size and stage of the tumour, including whether it has invaded the bladder wall or spread to other parts of the body.

Minimally invasive/bladder-preserving therapy

Transurethral resection of bladder tumour (TURBT) is the primary treatment for non-muscle-invasive bladder cancer. This procedure removes visible tumours from the bladder lining. TURBT is usually followed by intravesical therapy (medication instilled directly into the bladder via a catheter) with mitomycin C (a chemotherapy agent) or Bacillus Calmette–Guérin (BCG) immunotherapy, which helps destroy residual cancer cells and reduce the risk of recurrence.

Surgical management

Radical cystectomy is the standard treatment for muscle-invasive bladder cancer. It involves the removal of the bladder and, depending on sex, the adjacent reproductive organs. For tumours invading the bladder wall but not other organs, partial cystectomy or combined chemoradiotherapy may be considered for selected cases where the tumour invades the bladder wall but has not spread beyond it.

Radiotherapy and chemotherapy

Radiotherapy may be used before surgery to shrink tumours, as palliative therapy, or in combination with systemic chemotherapy to reduce relapse. Patients may experience hair loss, nausea, vomiting or mucositis; those caring for people should provide emotional support, listen actively and respond to concerns.

Clinical considerations

Supporting patients with bladder cancer requires a holistic, patient-centred approach. Information about the type and stage of cancer, treatment options and potential side effects is essential, along with guidance on follow-up and monitoring. Emotional support should be offered, allowing patients to express concerns and involving family or carers as appropriate. Symptom management, including pain, urinary discomfort, fatigue, nausea and post-surgical care, is vital. Care should be individualised, respecting patient preferences, comorbidities and psychosocial needs, and promoting shared decision-making throughout treatment.

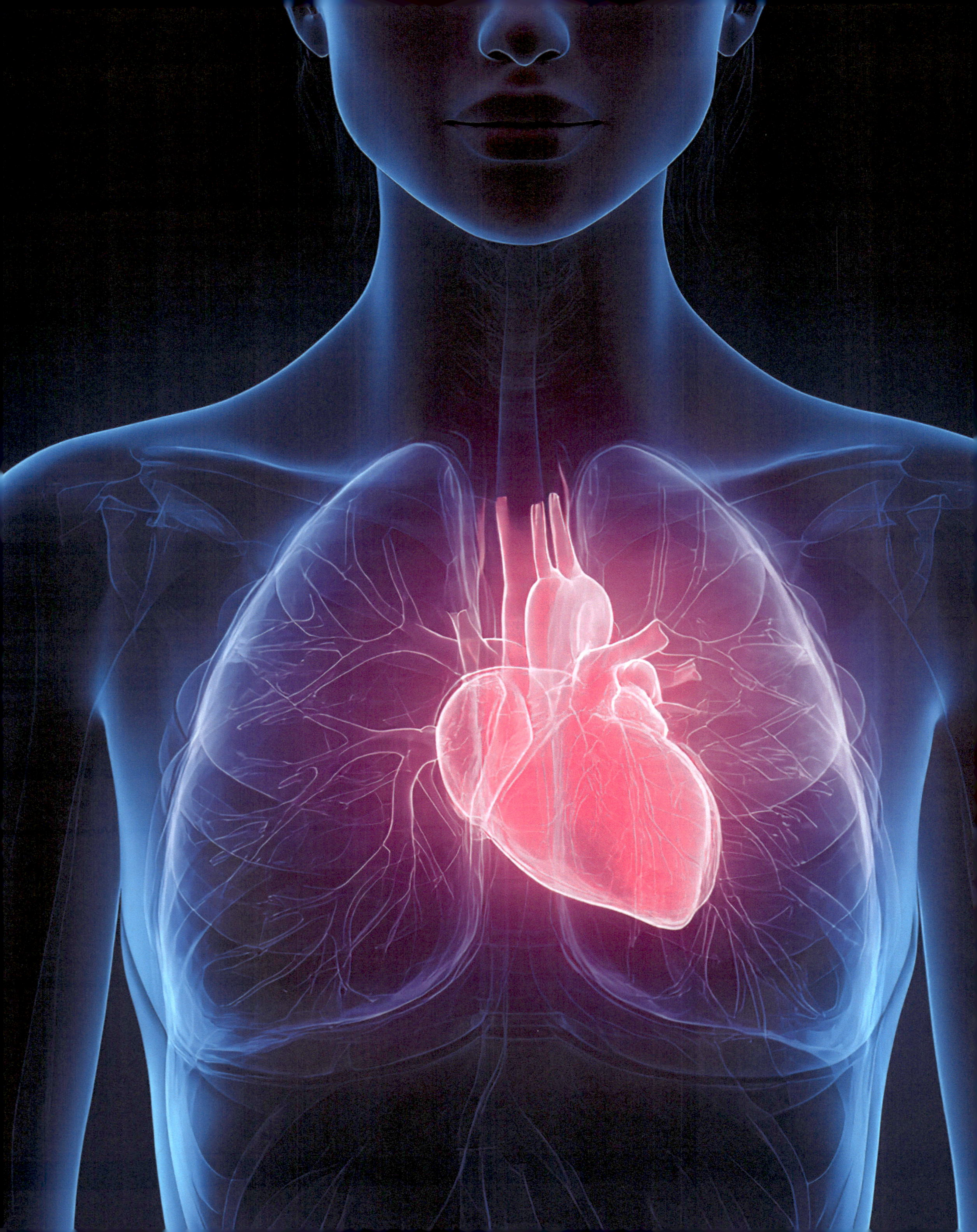

The male reproductive system

Chapters

42 Benign prostatic hyperplasia

Figure 42.1 The prostate gland is situated at the apex of the bladder, surrounding the proximal urethra.

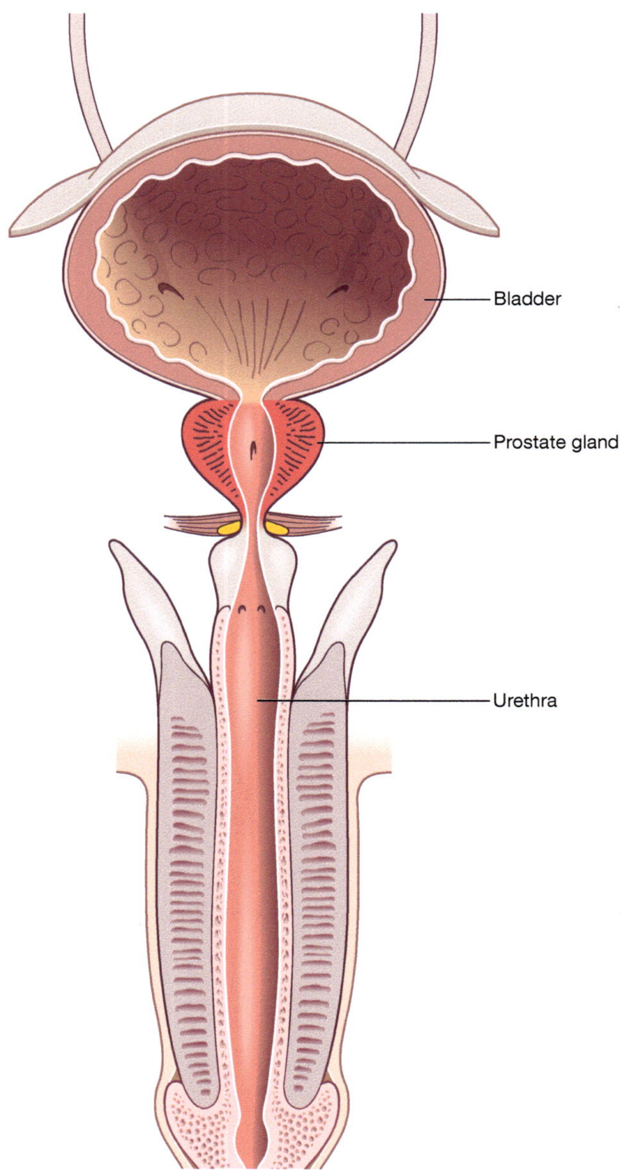

Box 42.1 Considerations for treatment.

- Treatment is normally only necessary if the symptoms are bothersome or complications are present
- Where the symptoms do not cause the man any difficulties the watchful waiting approach is advocated (provided that malignancy has been excluded) where treatment may not be required
- All treatment options have advantages and disadvantages

Overview

Benign prostatic hyperplasia

Benign prostatic hyperplasia (BPH), also known as benign prostatic enlargement (BPE), refers to a non-malignant increase in the size of the prostate gland. It is a common, but not inevitable, age-related condition and is considered a normal part of the ageing process in many men.

As the prostate gland enlarges, it can compress the urethra where it passes through the gland, leading to lower urinary tract symptoms (LUTS) such as difficulty starting urination, weak stream, incomplete bladder emptying and increased frequency, particularly at night (Figure 42.1).

BPH is the most common prostate disorder in men, typically occurring after the age of 50 years. It can significantly impact the quality of life. The condition is less common before age 45 years and tends to be more severe in men of African or Afro-Caribbean origin than in white men. Prostatic enlargement commonly occurs with advancing age due to benign prostatic hyperplasia.

Pathophysiology

The exact cause of BPH is not fully understood, but its development is closely linked to hormonal changes that are associated with ageing. Enlargement of the prostate is dependent on the androgen dihydrotestosterone (DHT), which is formed from testosterone by the enzyme 5-alpha reductase. DHT binds to androgen receptors within the nuclei of prostatic cells, which stimulates cellular growth and results in glandular and stromal hyperplasia (an increase in the number of cells). This process is influenced by an altered balance between oestrogens and androgens in ageing men.

The prostate contains numerous alpha-1 adrenergic receptors within its smooth muscle and capsule, as well as at the bladder neck. Stimulation of these receptors contributes to increased smooth muscle tone and dynamic obstruction of the bladder outlet, worsening LUTS.

Because the prostate is enclosed within a fibromuscular capsule and confined within the pelvis, enlargement often results in inward compression of the prostatic urethra. The bladder must generate greater pressure to overcome this resistance, leading to detrusor hypertrophy (an increase in cell size) and bladder wall trabeculation (where the bladder wall appears thickened, ridged or irregular). Over time, the bladder may become irritable and less efficient at emptying, resulting in increased residual urine and, in severe cases, acute or chronic urinary retention.

The fact that men without testosterone (e.g. those men with congenital or acquired hypogonadism) do not develop BPH highlights that androgen signalling is essential for prostate enlargement, and it provides a foundation for understanding both the pathophysiology and targeted treatments.

Signs and symptoms

BPH commonly causes LUTS due to compression of the urethra and obstruction of urine flow. Men may experience increased urinary frequency, particularly at night (nocturia), hesitancy or delay in initiating urination and a reduced force or weak urinary stream. Incomplete bladder emptying can lead to post-void dribbling, overflow incontinence and prolonged voiding time.

In advanced cases, severe urethral compression may cause acute urinary retention, where the man is unable to pass urine at all. Chronic urinary obstruction can increase the risk of urinary tract infections (UTIs) and, if untreated, may eventually lead to hydronephrosis and renal impairment.

Investigations

Assessment of men with suspected BPH begins with a detailed history and physical examination, including a digital rectal examination (DRE) to evaluate prostate size, consistency and nodularity.

Urinalysis should be performed to detect blood, leukocytes, bacteria, protein or glucose. If abnormalities are detected, a urine culture may be indicated to exclude UTI as a cause of irritative voiding symptoms.

Prostate-specific antigen (PSA) testing may be considered, though routine screening for prostate cancer remains controversial and should follow an informed discussion with the patient. Blood tests, including electrolytes, urea and creatinine, can help screen for chronic renal insufficiency, particularly in men with high post-void residual (PVR) volumes.

Imaging studies are recommended in selected cases. Ultrasound (abdominal, renal or transrectal) and intravenous urography can assess prostate and bladder size, evaluate hydronephrosis and measure PVR. Transrectal ultrasonography (TRUS) provides detailed measurements of prostate dimensions and volume and may guide TRUS-guided biopsy in men with elevated PSA. Imaging of the upper urinary tracts is indicated for patients with haematuria, a history of urolithiasis, elevated creatinine, high PVR or prior upper UTIs.

Management

Management of BPH depends on symptom severity, prostate size, patient comorbidities and treatment preferences. Both medical and surgical approaches are available (see Box 42.1).

Medical

Medical therapy is often the first-line treatment for men with moderate-to-severe LUTS. Alpha-1 adrenergic blockers relax the smooth muscle at the bladder neck and within the prostate, improving urine flow and reducing voiding symptoms. These drugs should be used with caution in those men who are prone to postural hypotension or syncope. 5-alpha-reductase inhibitors (5-ARIs), such as finasteride and dutasteride, block the conversion of testosterone to dihydrotestosterone, reducing prostate volume over time. They are particularly indicated in men with a prostate volume greater than 30 mL, elevated PSA (greater than 1.4 ng/mL), or a high risk of disease progression, although they may affect sexual function.

Surgery

Surgery is reserved for men with large prostates, significant LUTS unresponsive to medical therapy or complications such as acute urinary retention, failed voiding trials, recurrent gross haematuria, UTIs or renal impairment due to obstruction.

Open prostatectomy is indicated for very large prostates (greater than 75 g), in the presence of bladder stones or diverticula, or when patients are not suitable for transurethral surgery.

Transurethral resection of the prostate (TURP) remains the gold standard for surgical management of moderate-sized prostates. It is effective, avoids abdominal entry and provides durable symptom relief, although it carries risks such as bleeding, infection, urethral stricture or retrograde ejaculation.

Holmium laser enucleation of the prostate (HoLEP) is increasingly preferred for larger prostates, offering lower morbidity, shorter catheterisation times and durable outcomes. It is suitable for prostates of all sizes and is becoming a first-line surgical option where available.

Minimally invasive procedures are typically reserved for smaller prostates (less than 30 g) or patients unfit for more invasive surgery. These include:

- Transurethral incision of the prostate (TUIP) – a surgical incision at the bladder neck to relieve obstruction without tissue removal.
- Transurethral needle ablation (TUNA) – uses radiofrequency energy to ablate prostatic tissue and reduce obstruction.

Choice of surgical approach should be guided by prostate size, symptom severity, comorbidities and patient preference, with shared decision-making central to care planning.

Clinical considerations

Management of BPH depends on symptom severity, prostate size and patient preference. Medical therapy with alpha-1 blockers or 5-alpha-reductase inhibitors is first-line for moderate symptoms. Surgery is reserved for men with large prostates, persistent symptoms or complications such as urinary retention, recurrent infections, haematuria or renal impairment. Options include TURP, HoLEP, open prostatectomy or minimally invasive procedures (TUIP, TUNA) for smaller prostates or those unfit for major surgery. Ongoing care involves monitoring urinary function and providing education and support regarding treatment effects and lifestyle measures.

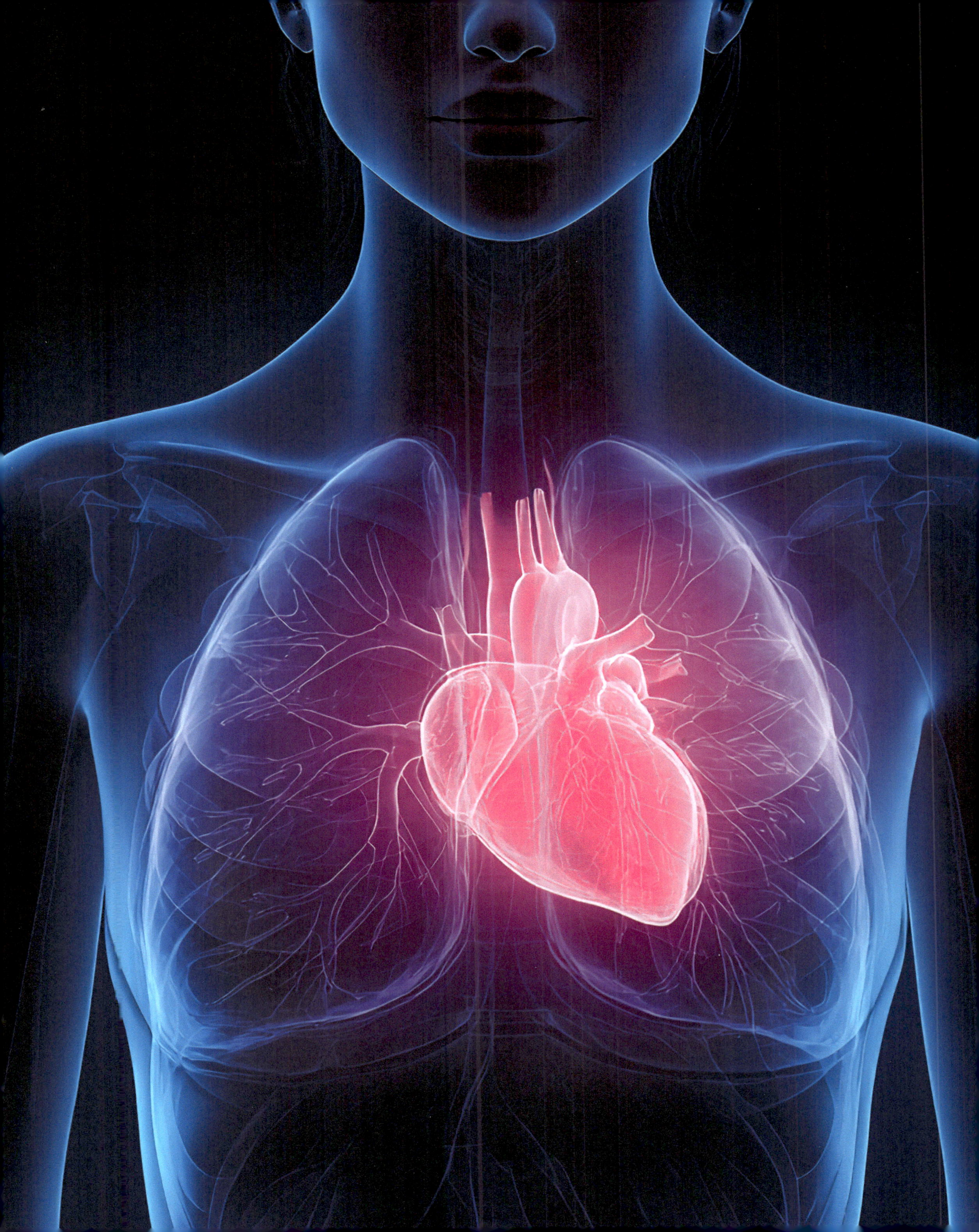

43 Testicular torsion

Figure 43.1 Comparison of a normal testicle and testicular torsion.

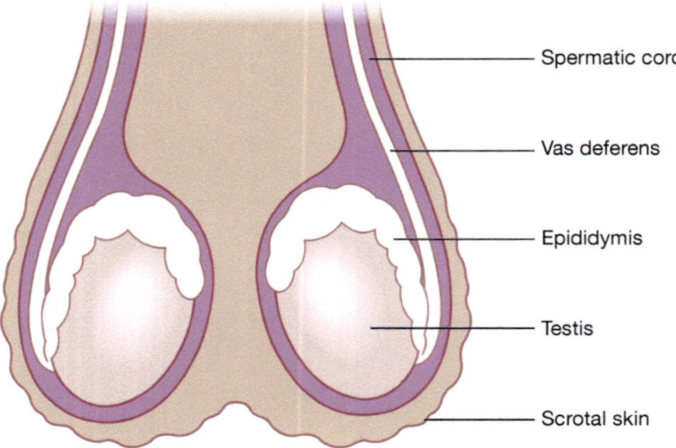

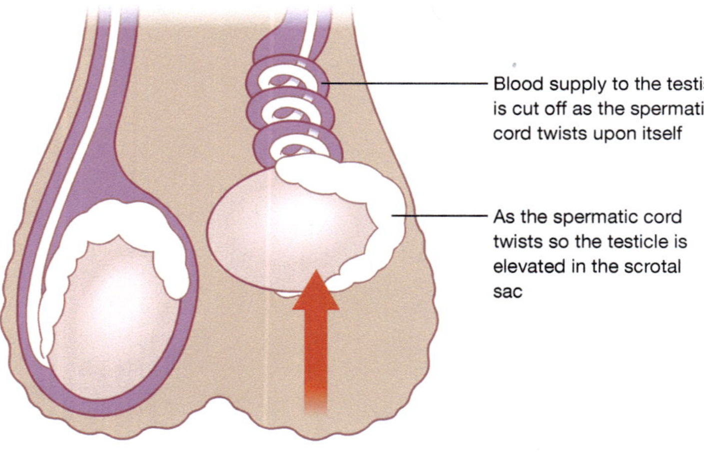

Testicular torsion

Testicular torsion refers to the abnormal twisting of the spermatic cord, usually resulting from rotation of the testis or the mesorchium, the fold of tissue that connects the testis to the epididymis (see Figure 43.1). This twisting compromises the arterial blood supply and venous drainage of the testis, leading to sudden, severe scrotal pain and swelling that are not relieved by rest or elevation.

The condition most commonly affects adolescents between the ages of 12 and 16 years but may occur at any age, including the neonatal period or even in utero. The onset is typically abrupt, and the affected testis may appear elevated and tender, often with an absent cremasteric reflex.

Testicular torsion is a urological emergency requiring immediate surgical intervention. Prompt detorsion and fixation of both testes (bilateral orchidopexy) within 4 to 6 hours of symptom onset are crucial to preserve testicular viability. Delayed treatment can result in testicular infarction, necessitating orchidectomy, which may affect future fertility and endocrine function. Prognosis is excellent with early recognition and timely surgical management.

Contents of the spermatic cord:

- Ductus deferens and associated vessels and nerves
- Testicular artery
- Pampiniform plexus (forming the testicular vein)
- Genital branch of the genitofemoral nerve.

Pathophysiology

Testicular torsion occurs when the testis rotates on its vascular pedicle causing twisting of the spermatic cord and compromising blood flow. The torsion may be spontaneous or triggered by minor trauma, physical exertion or sudden movements, and it is almost always unilateral. It can occur at any time, whether the patient is sitting, standing or even asleep. Prompt recognition is critical, as prolonged torsion can result in irreversible testicular damage.

The condition can be classified based on anatomical features and age. In neonates, the testis may not be fully fixed within the tunica vaginalis, creating increased mobility. This predisposes to extravaginal torsion, in which the testis and tunica vaginalis rotate together. This form is typically observed within the first 7–10 days of life and can occur in utero or shortly after birth.

In older children, adolescents and adults, intravaginal torsion is more common. Here, abnormal fixation of the testis to the tunica vaginalis allows it to rotate freely within the scrotum. A bell clapper deformity, a congenital anomaly in which the tunica vaginalis attaches high on the testis and allows a transverse orientation of the long axis, is a major predisposing factor. The testis can rotate between 90° and 180°, initially compromising venous outflow, leading to venous congestion, oedema and testicular swelling.

When torsion reaches 360° or more, arterial inflow is obstructed, causing ischaemia. In severe cases, torsion can exceed 720°, rapidly resulting in testicular infarction. The duration of torsion is equally critical: testicular salvage rates are highest when surgical detorsion occurs within 6–8 hours of symptom onset. After 12–24 hours, irreversible necrosis is likely, and orchidectomy may be required.

There is a recognised familial tendency, indicating a hereditary component, as first-degree relatives may be at increased risk. These congenital and structural factors are essential in understanding the pathophysiology and timing of torsion events.

The pathophysiological consequences include progressive tissue hypoxia, interstitial oedema and eventual cellular death. Persistent torsion also affects the spermatogenic epithelium, potentially impairing fertility even if the testis is salvaged. Pain arises from stretching of the spermatic cord, nerve ischaemia and oedematous swelling. The degree of torsion, speed of onset and underlying anatomical anomalies together determine the urgency of intervention and the likelihood of testicular recovery.

Signs and symptoms

Testicular torsion usually presents with sudden, severe unilateral scrotal pain, often radiating to the inguinal region or lower abdomen. The onset is typically acute and the pain is excruciating; gradual pain is uncommon. Pain may be accompanied by nausea, vomiting and general malaise, reflecting the severity of ischaemia; the patient is often reluctant to move. A history of intermittent scrotal pain may indicate previous episodes of partial torsion with spontaneous detorsion, which increases the risk of recurrent torsion and testicular loss. Prompt recognition and referral for surgical evaluation are essential in these cases.

On examination, the affected testis is usually swollen, tender and retracted superiorly, often lying in a horizontal position known as the 'bell clapper' position. The overlying scrotal skin may appear reddened and oedematous. The cremasteric reflex is typically absent on the affected side, which is a key diagnostic finding. In early torsion, the epididymis may be palpated in an abnormal anterior position, although progressive swelling can obscure this sign. Elevation of the testis toward the pubic symphysis exacerbates pain, distinguishing torsion from epididymitis, where pain may improve with lifting (negative Prehn's sign).

Pyrexia is uncommon early on but may develop if ischaemia persists for several hours. Urinary symptoms such as dysuria or frequency are generally absent, helping differentiate torsion from urinary tract infection or epididymo-orchitis.

Recognition of these classic features is time-critical, as testicular viability declines sharply after 6 hours of torsion. Immediate surgical intervention is required to restore perfusion and maximise the likelihood of testicular salvage, minimise ischaemic injury and preserve future fertility.

Investigations

Diagnosis of testicular torsion is primarily clinical, based on a thorough medical history and physical examination. Sudden, severe unilateral scrotal pain, a high-riding testis, horizontal lie, absent cremasteric reflex and scrotal swelling are key findings. When torsion is suspected, immediate surgical exploration is required; delaying surgery for laboratory tests or imaging risks permanent testicular loss. The principle is that a negative surgical exploration is far preferable to the loss of a viable testis.

No laboratory test is sufficiently sensitive or specific to confirm or exclude torsion. Routine blood tests, urinalysis or inflammatory markers may assist in evaluating alternative diagnoses (e.g. epididymitis), but they cannot reliably diagnose torsion.

Imaging is reserved for cases with low clinical suspicion or diagnostic uncertainty. Colour Doppler ultrasonography is the most valuable imaging modality, as it assesses intratesticular blood flow, helping to identify compromised perfusion. Nuclear scintigraphy can also detect perfusion deficits but is less commonly used in emergency settings due to limited availability and longer acquisition times.

In all cases where clinical suspicion is high, surgical exploration should not be delayed for imaging. Rapid intervention maximises the likelihood of testicular salvage and minimises ischaemic injury.

Management

If suspected, prompt intervention is essential to preserve testicular viability. Manual detorsion may be attempted as a temporary measure, but definitive treatment requires surgical exploration. Ideally, surgery should occur within 6 hours of symptom onset, as the likelihood of salvaging the testis decreases significantly after this window.

During surgery, the affected testis is detorsed and examined for viability. Orchiopexy is performed, anchoring the testis to the scrotal wall to prevent recurrence. The contralateral testis is usually fixed prophylactically, as anatomical predisposition may be bilateral.

If the testis is nonviable due to prolonged ischaemia or infarction, orchidectomy is necessary. Postoperative outcomes are significantly better with early intervention, highlighting the importance of rapid recognition and urgent surgical management.

Clinical considerations

Testicular torsion can compromise fertility if the affected testis undergoes infarction or requires orchidectomy. In cases where testicular salvage is uncertain or the patient presents late, discussion regarding sperm preservation may be appropriate. Sperm banking can be considered prior to surgery if feasible, particularly in adolescents or men with a solitary testis. Early urology referral is essential to assess the risks and options.

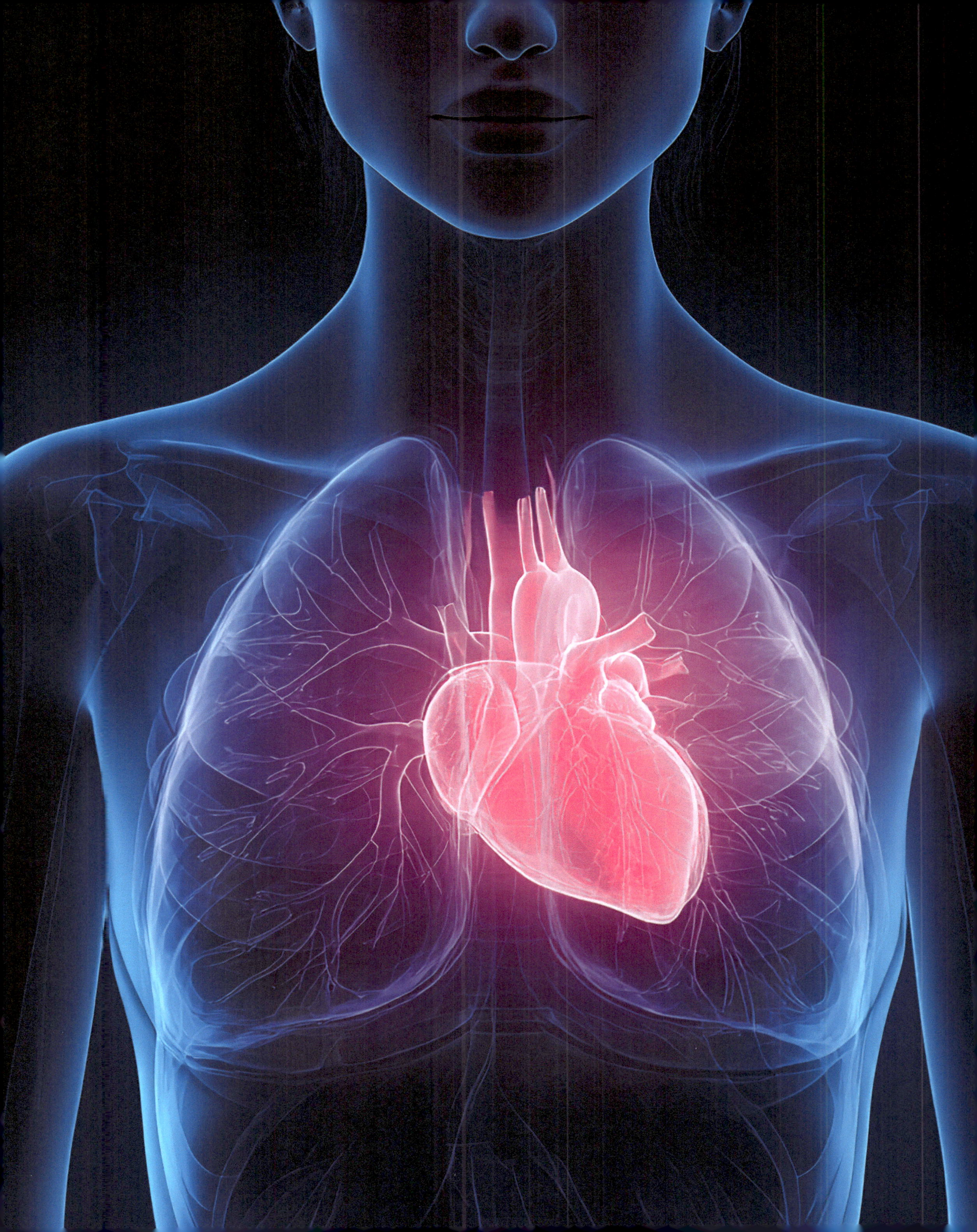

44 Erectile dysfunction

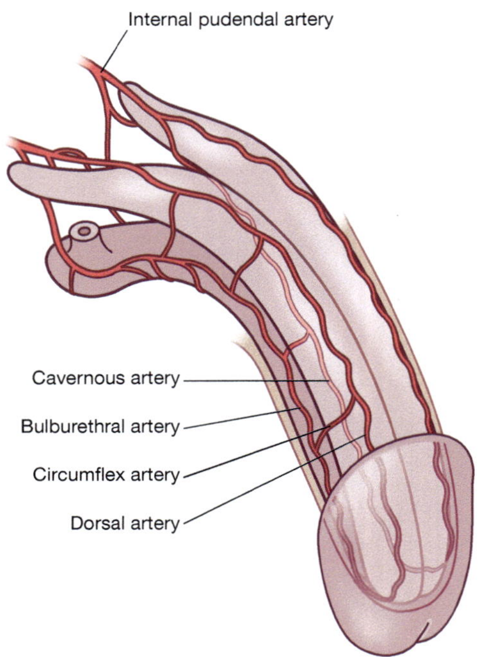

Figure 44.1 The arterial blood supply to the penis.

Figure 44.2 The normal erection process.

Table 44.1 Causes of erectile dysfunction.

Organic	Neurological	Hormonal
Vascular factors: • CVD • Atherosclerosis • Hypertension • Diabetes mellitus • Hyperlipidaemia • Smoking • Surgery or radiotherapy to pelvis or retroperitoneum • Trauma	• Central causes: – Parkinson's disease, stroke – multiple sclerosis – tumours – traumatic brain injury (causing hypothalamic-pituitary deficiency) – cerebrovascular disease – intervertebral disc disease – spinal cord disease or injury • Peripheral causes: – polyneuropathy – peripheral neuropathy – diabetes mellitus – alcoholism – uraemia – surgery (i.e. pelvis or retroperitoneum)	• Hypogonadism • Hyperprolactinaemia • Thyroid disease • Cushing's disease
Drugs • Antihypertensives • Beta-blockers • Diuretics • Antidepressants • Antipsychotics • Hormonal agents • Anticonvulsants • Antihistamines • Recreational drugs • H2 antagonists	**Anatomical** • Peyronie's disease • Micropenis and other penile anomalies	**Psychogenic** • Psychosexual factors: – disorders of sexual intimacy, lack of arousability – partner, performance or stress • Psychiatric illness: – generalised anxiety states – depression – psychosis

Overview

Erectile dysfunction

An understanding of penile anatomy is essential for the assessment and management of erectile dysfunction (ED). The common penile artery, a branch of the internal pudendal artery, divides into the dorsal, bulbourethral and cavernous arteries (Figure 44.1), which supply the tissues that are responsible for penile rigidity and tumescence.

Although ED is a benign condition, it can have a significant impact on the man's quality of life, as well as on his partner and family relationships. Prior to initiating treatment, a comprehensive assessment should be undertaken, including medical, sexual and psychosocial history, physical examination and appropriate investigations to identify underlying causes.

Pathophysiology

ED is the persistent inability to achieve or maintain an erection sufficient for satisfactory sexual performance. While ED was historically attributed primarily to psychological factors, it is now recognised that organic causes are predominant in most men, particularly vascular, neurological, hormonal or structural abnormalities. Awareness of these underlying mechanisms enables healthcare providers to engage men in open discussions about the impact of ED on quality of life.

Penile rigidity is governed by the contractile state of the corporal smooth muscle within the corpus cavernosum. The balance between contraction and relaxation is determined by central and peripheral neural inputs, as well as endothelium-derived factors. Contraction is mediated by agents including noradrenaline, endothelin-1, neuropeptide Y, prostanoids and angiotensin II, which maintain penile flaccidity by promoting smooth muscle tone.

Relaxation of the corporal smooth muscle, essential for erection, is primarily mediated via the nitric oxide (NO)–cyclic guanosine monophosphate (cGMP) pathway, along with other modulators such as acetylcholine, vasoactive intestinal polypeptide, pituitary adenylate cyclase-activating peptide, calcitonin gene-related peptide, adrenomedullin and adenosine. NO released from endothelial cells and nitrergic nerves activates guanylate cyclase, increasing cGMP levels and causing smooth muscle relaxation, resulting in penile engorgement and rigidity.

Structural abnormalities, impaired arterial inflow, venoocclusive dysfunction, hormonal deficiencies (e.g. low testosterone) and certain medications can disrupt this finely tuned system, leading to ED. Additionally, endothelial dysfunction, often associated with cardiovascular disease, diabetes or smoking, reduces NO availability, further impairing the erectile response.

Understanding the pathophysiology of ED highlights the interplay of vascular, neurological, hormonal and smooth muscle factors, providing a framework for tailored diagnostic assessment and management, including lifestyle modification, pharmacotherapy and, where indicated, device or surgical interventions.

Normal erectile process

Erections occur in response to tactile, olfactory and visual stimuli. Achieving and maintaining a full erection depends not only on penile structures but also on the integrity of peripheral nerves, vascular supply and biochemical events within the corpora cavernosa. The autonomic nervous system mediates erection, orgasm and tumescence (Figure 44.2).

Sexual stimulation triggers the release of neurotransmitters from cavernosal nerve endings and endothelial-derived relaxing factors, predominantly NO. This induces smooth muscle relaxation in penile arteries and arterioles, increasing blood flow, filling the sinusoids and producing penile expansion.

Detumescence occurs when neurotransmitter release ceases, second messengers such as cGMP are degraded by phosphodiesterase enzymes, and sympathetic nerve activity increases during ejaculation. Contraction of trabecular smooth muscle reopens venous channels, allowing blood to drain from the corpora, restoring flaccidity.

Signs and symptoms

Men with ED typically experience persistent difficulty in achieving or maintaining an erection sufficient for satisfactory sexual activity. This may present as a complete inability to attain an erection despite adequate sexual stimulation, or as a loss of rigidity during intercourse, making penetration difficult or impossible. Erections may be less firm than usual, or spontaneous erections, such as nocturnal or morning erections, may become infrequent or absent, often suggesting an underlying organic cause. In addition to the physical difficulties, men may experience a decreased sexual desire and the condition can lead to psychological consequences, including anxiety, frustration, low self-esteem and relationship stress. Erectile difficulties may occur intermittently or only in certain situations, which can indicate a predominantly psychogenic component. ED may also coexist with other systemic symptoms, such as those associated with cardiovascular disease, diabetes or hormonal disorders, which can provide important clues about the underlying aetiology. Some of the causes of ED are outlined in Table 44.1.

Investigations

The investigations required for ED depend on the information gathered during a detailed history and physical examination. Laboratory testing may be necessary. Tests help determine the patient's overall medical status, identify and characterise the type of dysfunction and guide whether further investigations are required. In making decisions about management or referral, the man's needs, expectations and priorities should always be discussed and incorporated into the plan.

Hormonal blood tests should be considered on a case-by-case basis, guided by the clinical presentation and may include testosterone, luteinising hormone, follicle-stimulating hormone and prolactin. Additional blood tests, such as haemoglobin, serum chemistry and lipid profile, can provide insight into contributing systemic conditions.

Vascular assessment of the penis can be undertaken using duplex ultrasonography to evaluate arterial inflow and venoocclusive function. Nocturnal penile tumescence testing helps differentiate organic from psychogenic causes: inadequate or absent nocturnal erections suggest organic dysfunction, while normal results point to a likely psychogenic aetiology. Men with traumatic vascular injuries may be considered for angiography if vascular reconstruction is a treatment option. Men with central nervous system disorders, peripheral neuropathy, diabetes or penile sensory deficits may benefit from targeted neurological evaluation.

Emerging diagnostic tools are expanding the options for detailed assessment. Dynamic contrast-enhanced MRI and high-resolution Doppler ultrasonography allow precise visualisation of penile perfusion and vascular integrity. Biomarkers of endothelial function and oxidative stress are being investigated as non-invasive indicators of early vascular dysfunction. While primarily in specialist or research settings, these tools may complement conventional assessments in complex or refractory cases.

Management

The goal of treatment is to help the patient achieve satisfactory sexual function while addressing underlying causes. A range of evidence-based options is available, and choice should be guided by physiological status, comorbidities and patient preference.

Pharmacotherapy

Phosphodiesterase type-5 inhibitors (PDE5 inhibitors) remain first-line therapy for ED, including sildenafil, tadalafil, vardenafil and avanafil. Effectiveness depends on intact neural and vascular pathways. For men with low libido and confirmed hypogonadism, testosterone replacement therapy may improve sexual function.

Intracavernosal and intraurethral therapy

For patients unresponsive to oral agents, intracavernosal injection of vasodilators, most commonly alprostadil, can be used. Intraurethral administration of alprostadil via a medicated urethral system for erection (MUSE) is another option.

Mechanical devices

Vacuum erection devices draw blood into the corpora cavernosa to induce an erection and are used with a constriction ring at the base of the penis to maintain rigidity.

Surgical interventions

Penile prosthesis implantation is reserved for men who do not respond to or cannot tolerate other therapies.

Psychosexual support

Sexual counselling is a vital component of management, addressing the psychological and relational aspects of ED.

Clinical considerations

PDE5 inhibitors (sildenafil, tadalafil and vardenafil) are contraindicated with nitrates or nicorandil due to the risk of severe hypotension. Caution is required in cardiovascular disease, severe hepatic or renal impairment, and conditions predisposing to priapism. Concomitant alpha-blockers may cause postural hypotension; start with the lowest effective dose. Take 30–60 minutes before sexual activity; sexual stimulation is required for effect. Common side effects include headache, flushing, dyspepsia and visual changes.

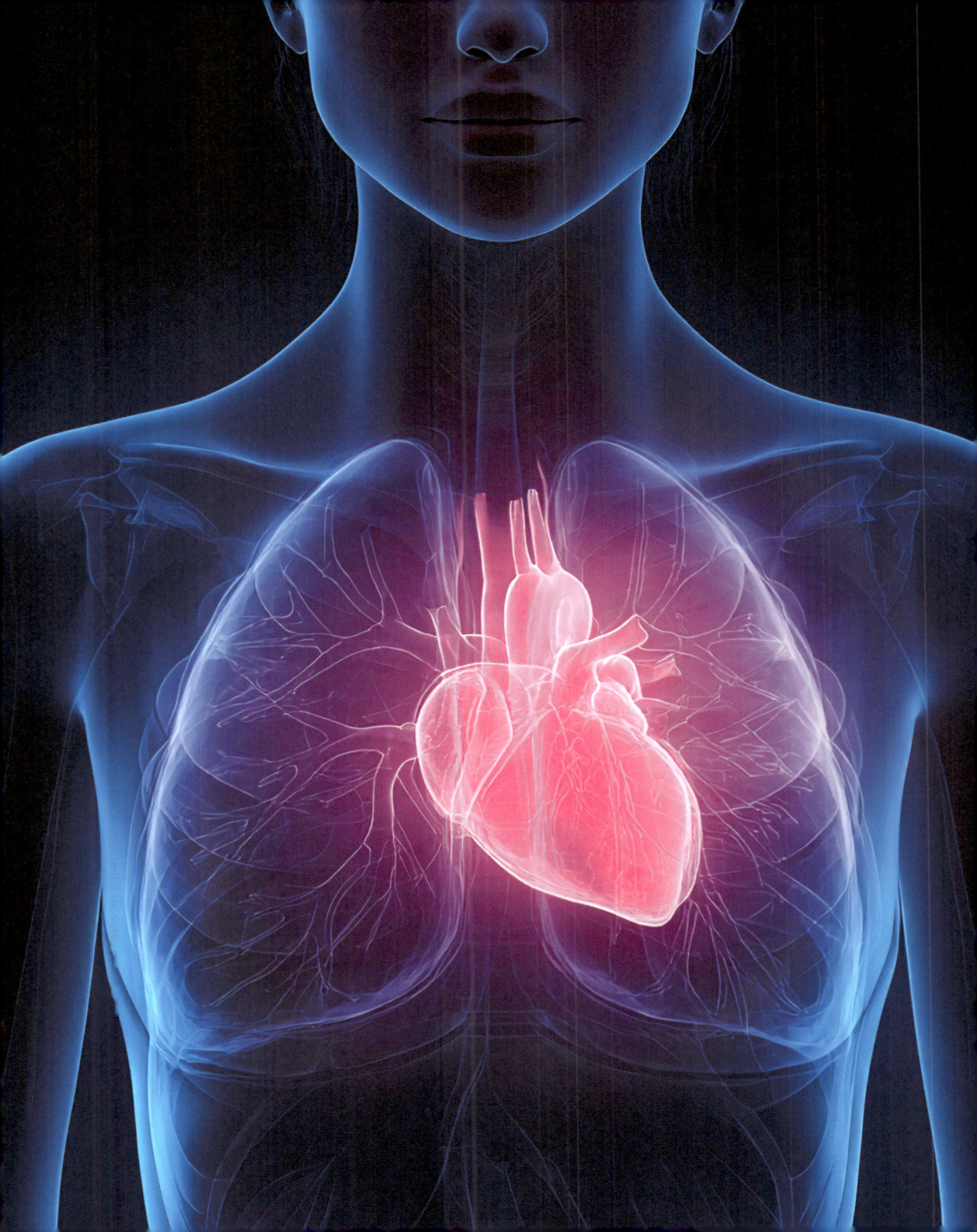

45 Prostate cancer

Figure 45.1   The zones of the prostate gland.

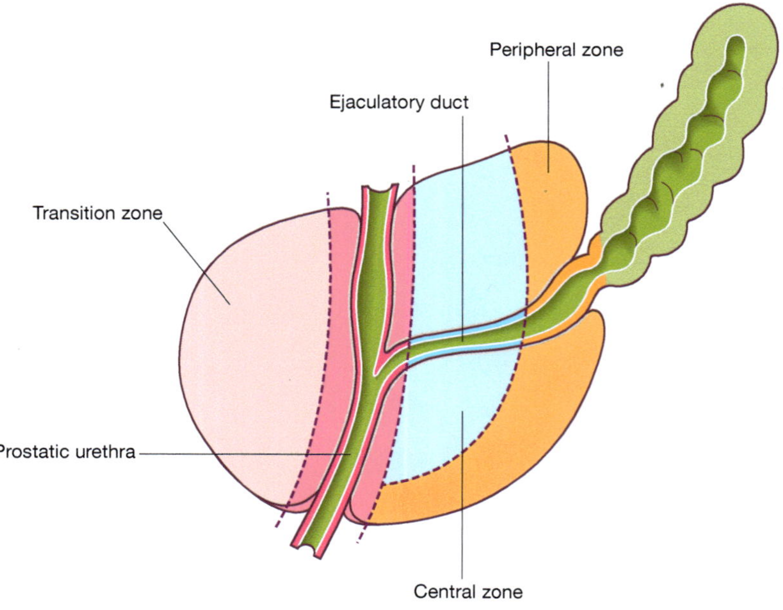

Box 45.1   Risk factors associated with prostate cancer.

- Ethnicity is an important risk factor, with a higher incidence in North America and Europe, particularly amongst black African or black Caribbean groups. Low rates are noted in China and Japan

- Risk increases 2–3 times if a first-degree relative is diagnosed at an early age. There is an increased risk with a family history of breast cancer. Possible responsible genes have been identified. Approximately 9% of all cases of prostate cancer have a genetic basis

- It has been suggested that diet may also be an important risk factor. Red meat and unsaturated fats increase risk, while vitamin E, selenium and lycopene (antioxidants) appear to have a protective effect

- Occupation: there is an increased risk with farming and exposure to radiation or cadmium

Box 45.2   Digital rectal examination.

Serial examinations over time are best. A nodule is suspicious for malignancy and requires evaluation. Findings such as asymmetry, difference in texture and bogginess are important clues and should be given consideration, along with the PSA level. Change in texture over time also suggests the need for a biopsy

DRE findings alone cannot accurately differentiate cysts or stones from cancer. The examiner should maintain a high degree of suspicion for non-cancerous disorders if the DRE results are abnormal. If cancer is detected, DRE findings form the basis of clinical staging of the primary tumour (tumour (T) stage in the tumour-node-metastases (TNM) staging system)

Box 45.3   PSA levels.

There is no one PSA reading considered normal. Levels vary from man to man and increase as the man ages. The following values are a rough guide:

- 3 ng/mL or less is considered to be in the normal range for a man under 60 years old

- 4 ng/mL or less is normal for a man aged 60–69

- 5 ng/mL or less is normal for men aged over 70

Prostate cancer

Most prostate cancers are adenocarcinomas, typically arising in the peripheral zone of the prostate gland (see Figure 45.1). While many prostate cancers are indolent and slow-growing, a subset can be clinically significant and aggressive, particularly in younger men. In the UK, prostate cancer is the second leading cause of cancer-related death in men, after lung cancer.

Pathophysiology

The exact cause of the disease remains unclear; both genetic and environmental factors contribute to risk. Mutations in genes are associated with increased susceptibility and are linked to more aggressive disease. Advancing age is a major risk factor, and life-long exposure to androgens influences prostate cell proliferation (see Box 45.1). Prostate cancers are typically androgen-dependent in the early stages but may progress to androgen-independent (castration-resistant) disease in advanced stages – early prostate cancers rely on male hormones to grow; advanced cancers can become resistant, and they can grow without them.

Tumour growth begins in the epithelial cells of the peripheral zone, where most prostate cancers arise. Cancer cells can invade locally, extend along the prostatic capsule and spread via lymphatic and haematogenous routes. The most common sites of metastasis are regional lymph nodes and bone, particularly the axial skeleton. Understanding these mechanisms is critical for risk stratification, treatment planning and prognostication.

Signs and symptoms

Symptoms

Prostate cancer often develops silently, and many cases are asymptomatic in the early stages. When symptoms do occur, they frequently overlap with those of benign prostatic conditions (see Chapter 42 of this book), making early detection based on symptoms alone unreliable. Common lower urinary tract symptoms such as urinary frequency, hesitancy, nocturia and a weak urinary stream are not specific to malignancy and do not in themselves increase the risk of prostate cancer.

As the disease progresses locally, patients may experience additional urinary symptoms, including a sensation of incomplete bladder emptying, urgency, urge incontinence and recurrent urinary tract infections. Locally invasive tumours can cause haematuria, dysuria, haematospermia, perineal or suprapubic pain and obstruction of the urinary tract, potentially leading to hydronephrosis, loin pain and renal impairment. Erectile dysfunction may also develop as a consequence of local tumour invasion or disruption of neurovascular structures.

Metastatic prostate cancer commonly involves the axial skeleton and regional lymph nodes. Patients may present with bone pain, sciatica or neurological symptoms resulting from spinal cord compression. Other systemic features can include fatigue, weight loss, anorexia and cachexia. Advanced disease may also manifest as obstructive nephropathy due to ureteric obstruction, lower-extremity lymphoedema or signs of venous thromboembolism.

On physical examination, a digital rectal examination (DRE) may reveal a hard, irregular or nodular prostate, asymmetry between lobes, induration, lack of mobility or palpable seminal vesicles (see Box 45.2). However, physical examination alone cannot reliably distinguish benign from malignant disease, and a biopsy is required to confirm the diagnosis. Determining whether the tumour is confined to the prostate or has extended beyond the capsule is crucial for treatment planning. Locally advanced disease may be indicated by obliteration of the lateral sulcus or involvement of the seminal vesicles. In patients with advanced or metastatic disease, examination may reveal cachexia, bony tenderness, overdistended bladder, lymphadenopathy or neurological deficits indicative of spinal cord involvement, highlighting the importance of a thorough systemic and neurological assessment.

Investigations

Screening for prostate cancer remains contentious. The main screening tools are prostate-specific antigen (PSA) testing and DRE. PSA testing detects elevated levels of PSA in the blood, while DRE allows assessment of gland texture, nodularity and asymmetry. Neither method alone can reliably confirm malignancy, and abnormal findings typically prompt further investigation (see Box 45.3).

In contemporary practice, men with raised PSA or abnormal DRE findings are increasingly evaluated with multiparametric MRI (mpMRI) before biopsy. mpMRI combines anatomical and functional imaging sequences; mpMRI combines several imaging techniques to detect and characterise cancer. T2-weighted imaging (T2WI) provides detailed anatomy, showing the size, shape and location of lesions. Diffusion-weighted imaging (DWI) highlights areas of restricted water movement, helping identify densely packed, potentially aggressive tumour cells. Dynamic contrast-enhanced imaging (DCE-MRI) uses a contrast agent to show abnormal blood flow patterns, which are often seen in cancerous tissue. Together, these sequences improve detection of clinically significant prostate cancer, guide targeted biopsies and assist in staging and treatment planning.

Transrectal ultrasound (TRUS) remains important for guiding prostate biopsies but is not recommended as a population screening tool due to a high false-positive rate. Biopsies, either systematic needle or template-guided, provide histological confirmation and grading of the tumour.

Further investigations focus on staging and risk stratification. MpMRI also assesses extraprostatic extension, seminal vesicle involvement and local tumour spread, aiding treatment planning. Imaging for metastatic disease may include bone scans to detect skeletal metastases and CT or PET/CT to assess lymph node or visceral involvement. Abdominal ultrasound may be used to evaluate urinary tract obstruction.

Management

Management is guided by staging and risk stratification, which assess the extent of disease locally, regionally and at distant sites. Investigations such as mpMRI, bone scan, CT or PET/CT, along with biopsy results, provide information on tumour size, extraprostatic extension, lymph node involvement and metastases. Accurate staging assists in selecting the most appropriate treatment, ranging from active surveillance for low-risk disease to surgery, radiotherapy or systemic therapies for locally advanced or metastatic cancer.

Low-risk localised prostate cancer

In men with small, well-differentiated (low-risk) prostate cancer, active surveillance is recommended, comprising regular PSA testing and clinical review, interval mpMRI and selective repeat biopsy to detect progression, with definitive treatment offered only if there is evidence of tumour growth or increased aggressiveness, an approach that lets many men avoid or delay the side effects of surgery or radiotherapy.

High-risk localised prostate cancer

High-risk localised prostate cancer is defined by adverse clinical, biochemical or histological factors. Management should be individualised after discussion at an MDT and shared decision-making with the patient, taking into account stage, comorbidity and life expectancy. Curative-intent options often combine local and systemic treatments: radical prostatectomy (with pelvic lymph node dissection) or external beam radiotherapy with long-term androgen deprivation therapy (ADT) are commonly used. Brachytherapy may be added to external beam radiotherapy. ADT can be delivered medically or surgically (orchidectomy). Less widely adopted or investigational approaches used selectively or in clinical trials include high-intensity focused ultrasound (HIFU) and cryotherapy (usually for focal therapy or salvage). Chemotherapy (e.g. docetaxel) and novel systemic agents are generally reserved for metastatic disease or selected high-risk patients within multimodal regimens or trials. Palliative care should be integrated when the disease is incurable or symptoms require optimisation.

Clinical considerations

PSA, a protein used as a biomarker for prostate disease, elevated levels are not specific to cancer. Benign prostatic hyperplasia, prostatitis, urinary retention and recent prostate manipulation (e.g. DRE, catheterisation, biopsy or ejaculation within 48 hours) can all transiently raise PSA. Results should be interpreted in the clinical context and confirmed with repeat testing if elevated.

Age-specific PSA reference ranges may improve accuracy. Inform men about the benefits and limitations of PSA testing, including the risk of false positives, overdiagnosis and anxiety.

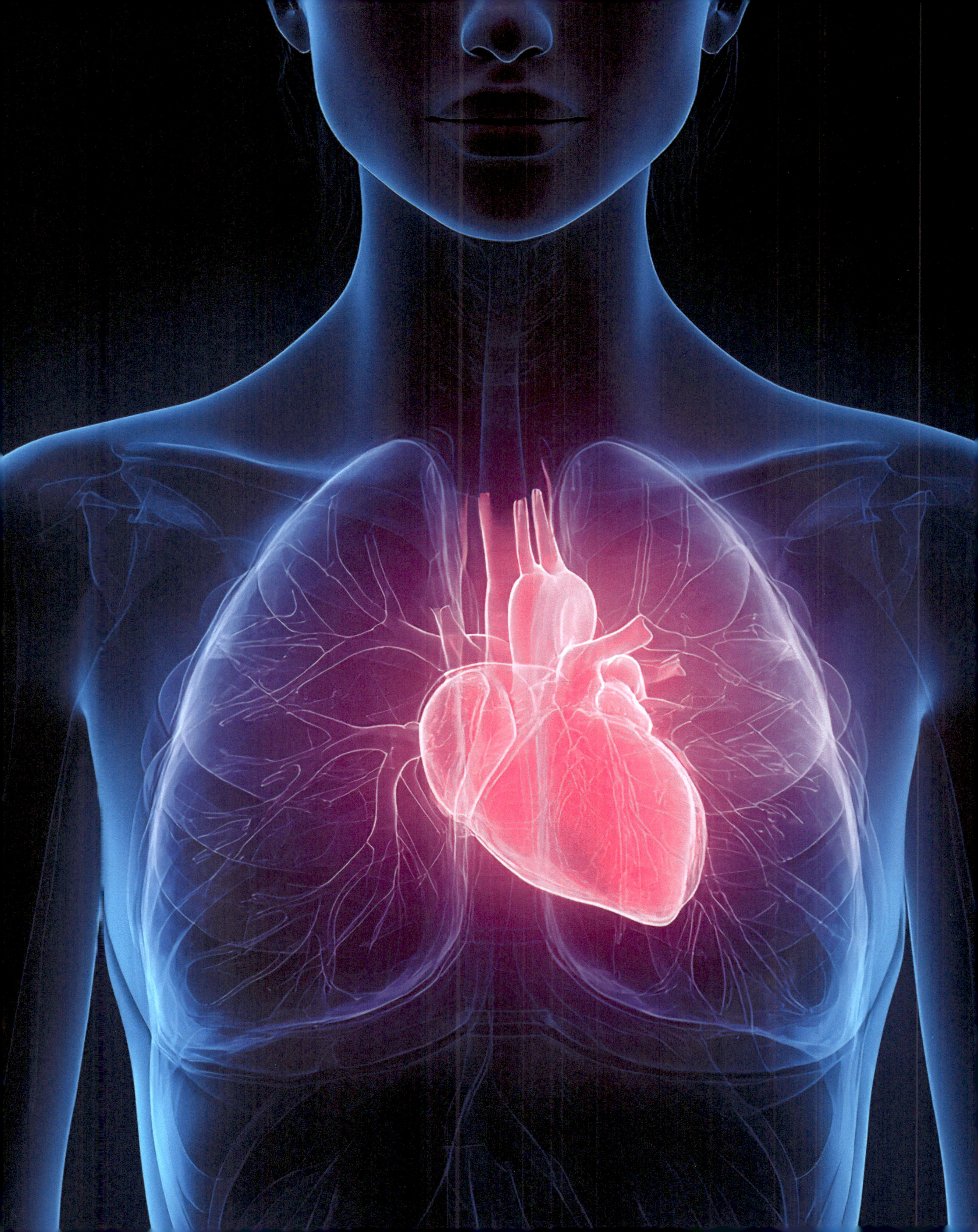

46 Testicular cancer

Table 46.1 Testicular cancer staging.

Stage	Discussion
Stage 0	Germ cell neoplasia in situ (GCNIS), abnormal cells in the testicle. Microscopically cells look abnormal, only in the seminiferous tubules. No spread into other parts of the testicle. Can become an invasive cancer.
Stage 1	The earliest stage of testicular cancer. Cancer is only in the testicle and has not spread to nearby lymph nodes or other organs. Stage 1: split into stage 1A and 1B depending on the size of tumour. Stage 1S: raised levels of markers in blood after surgery. Stage 1A: Cancer still within the testicle, has not grown into nearby lymph nodes or blood vessels. Tumour markers are normal (S0). Stage 1B: Cancer has grown outside the testicle into nearby structures. Has not spread to lymph nodes or distant organs. Tumour markers are normal (S0). Stage 1S: Cancer might have spread outside the testicle. At least one tumour marker level is raised (S1, S2 or S3).
Stage 2	Cancer cells have spread from the testicle into nearby lymph nodes in the abdomen or pelvis. Normal or slightly raised levels of markers in the blood (S0 or S1). Stage 2 testicular cancer is split into 2A, 2B and 2C. Depends on how many lymph nodes cancer has spread to and size of lymph nodes. All stage 2 cancers might have grown outside the testicle into nearby structures; they have not spread to distant lymph nodes or organs. Tumour marker levels normal or slightly raised (S0 or S1). Stage 2A: Cancer has spread to no more than 5 nearby lymph nodes. These lymph nodes are all 2cm or smaller in size. Stage 2B means one of the following. Cancer has spread: • to at least one nearby lymph node which is larger than 2cm but no larger than 5cm • to more than 5 nearby lymph nodes, but these are all smaller than 5cm • through the outside covering of the lymph node Stage 2C: Cancer has spread to at least one nearby lymph node which is larger than 5cm.
Stage 3	Cancer has spread to lymph nodes or other organs. Split into 3A, 3B and 3C depends on where the cancer has spread to and levels of markers in the blood. Stage 3A: tumour marker level is normal (S0) or slightly raised (S1). Cancer has spread to: • distant lymph nodes • lungs Stage 3B: one of the following. Cancer has spread to: • Nearby lymph nodes and a moderately high tumour marker level (S2) • Lungs or distant lymph nodes and a moderately high marker level (S2) Stage 3C: means one of the following: • the same as stage 3B but a very high tumour marker level (S3) • cancer has spread to another body organ, such as liver or brain, tumour markers are any level (S0, S1, S2 or S3)

Figure 46.1 Pelvic and para-aortic lymph nodes.

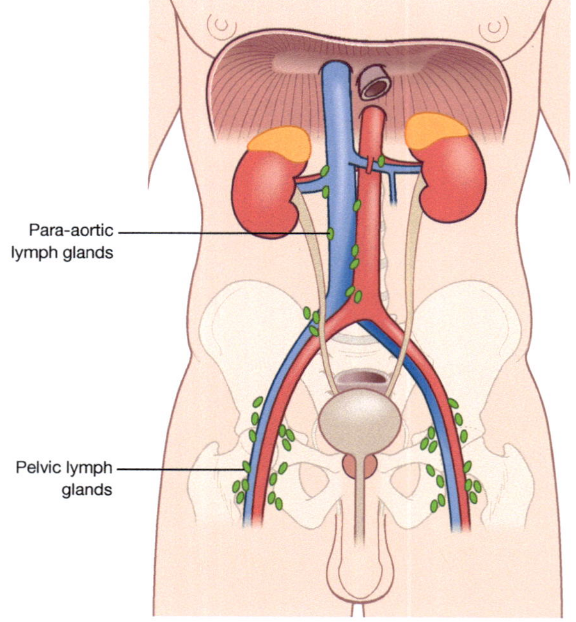

Source:
Peate, Wild & Nair, *Nursing Practice: Knowledge and Care*, 2014

Testicular cancer is rare, accounting for 1% of male tumours in the UK. Around 2,400 men in the UK are diagnosed with testicular cancer annually. Although testicular cancer is rare, it is more common in men in their early 30s; it then becomes less common as men get older. Trans women can also develop testicular cancer if they have not undergone an orchidectomy.

With timely diagnosis, testicular cancer is highly treatable and usually curable. Testicular cancers are sensitive to chemotherapy and, even when metastatic, are often curable. It is the most treatable form of urological cancer.

Testicular cancer

Approximately 50% of all cases occur in men under the age of 35, and testicular cancer rarely occurs before puberty. It is the most common cancer affecting men aged 15–44 years. The incidence of testicular cancer has increased over recent decades, although the reasons for this remain unclear.

Pathophysiology

The majority of testicular tumours arise from germ cells. Testicular germ cell tumours (TGCTs) are classified as seminomas or non-seminomatous germ cell tumours (NSGCTs), with seminomas slightly more common than non-seminomas. Rare non-germ cell tumours include Sertoli–Leydig cell tumours, accounting for less than 5% of cases.

Recognised risk factors include cryptorchidism (undescended testis), previous testicular cancer, family history and male infertility. Other reported associations include testicular microlithiasis (tiny calcifications within the seminiferous tubules of the testis), Klinefelter's syndrome and low birth weight. Most TGCTs display chromosomal abnormalities, reflecting a genetic susceptibility. First-degree relatives of men with testicular cancer are at increased risk, especially siblings and sons.

Testicular cancers follow a characteristic metastatic pattern, initially spreading to the retroperitoneal lymph nodes, with potential subsequent involvement of the lungs, mediastinum and, rarely, the liver.

Signs and symptoms

Any lump or firm area within the testis should be considered malignant until proven otherwise.

Localised disease

The most common presenting symptom of testicular cancer is a painless swelling or nodule in one testis, with a lump palpable in nearly all cases. On physical examination, the mass is firm and cannot be separated from the testis. In men with atrophic testes (testes that are abnormally small and often soft), the tumour may present as an enlargement of the testis. Some men may experience a dull ache or a heavy sensation in the lower abdomen or scrotum or report a dragging sensation. Occasionally, a tumour is discovered after scrotal trauma, which prompts self-examination; the trauma itself is not considered a cause of malignancy.

Metastatic disease

In metastatic testicular cancer, symptoms arise from lymphatic or haematogenous spread. A neck mass may be present due to supraclavicular lymph node involvement. Gastrointestinal symptoms such as anorexia, nausea or abdominal discomfort may occur. Bulky retroperitoneal disease (large metastatic lymph node masses in the retroperitoneum) can present as lower back or flank pain, while cough, chest pain, haemoptysis or shortness of breath may indicate mediastinal lymphadenopathy or lung metastases.

Gynaecomastia may occur in men with germ cell tumours that produce human chorionic gonadotropin (hCG), such as choriocarcinoma. Rarely, high levels of hCG can induce hyperthyroidism due to structural similarities between hCG and thyroid-stimulating hormone (TSH).

Men presenting with a scrotal swelling should be examined carefully, with efforts made to differentiate intratesticular masses from other intrascrotal swellings. Scrotal ultrasound is the first-line investigation to determine whether a lump arises from the testis or another intrascrotal structure.

Investigations

The initial evaluation of suspected testicular cancer begins with clinical examination and testicular ultrasound. Ultrasound is the first-line imaging modality to identify intratesticular masses and assess the contralateral testis if indicated. Serum tumour markers – including alpha-fetoprotein (AFP), beta-human chorionic gonadotropin (β-hCG) and lactate dehydrogenase (LDH) – should be measured at presentation, as they are valuable for diagnosis, staging and monitoring response to treatment.

Definitive diagnosis requires histological confirmation following radical inguinal orchidectomy, which also allows for pathological staging. Once a testicular tumour is confirmed, cross-sectional imaging with CT of the thorax, abdomen and pelvis is performed to assess for retroperitoneal and distant metastases.

Tumour markers:

- AFP: produced by yolk sac elements; not elevated in pure seminomas.
- β-hCG: produced by trophoblastic elements; may be mildly elevated in seminomas and markedly elevated in choriocarcinoma or mixed germ cell tumours.
- LDH: reflects tumour burden, particularly in advanced disease, but is nonspecific.

Staging is commonly used to stage testicular cancer (see Table 46.1, Cancer Research UK staging). Internationally, tumour, node and metastases staging is also widely applied.

Management

The management of testicular cancer depends on the histological type and stage, guided by national protocols. Refer to a specialist centre with a multidisciplinary team to ensure optimal care. Initial treatment is typically a radical inguinal orchidectomy, which involves the removal of the testis, tunica albuginea and spermatic cord. At the time of surgery, men should be offered a testicular prosthesis, and fertility preservation through sperm banking should be discussed with those who may require chemotherapy or radiotherapy.

In men with NSGCTs, retroperitoneal lymph node dissection (RPLND) may be performed following orchidectomy for both staging and therapeutic purposes. Surgery carries potential risks, including infertility and ejaculatory dysfunction.

For those presenting with metastatic disease and markedly elevated tumour markers, chemotherapy may be started promptly, even prior to orchidectomy, when the diagnosis is clear. Chemotherapy is indicated for extratesticular disease, high-risk NSGCT and recurrent or relapsed tumours following initial treatment. Men with seminoma may require adjuvant radiotherapy to the retroperitoneal lymph nodes, depending on stage and risk factors (see Figure 46.1).

Comprehensive care also includes long-term follow-up, surveillance for recurrence and supportive measures, such as ongoing fertility counselling and psychosocial support.

Clinical considerations

Health education and promotion are essential in testicular cancer. Men, especially those aged 15–44 years, should be encouraged to perform regular testicular self-examination, seeking prompt medical review for any lumps or changes. Awareness of risk factors such as cryptorchidism, family history, infertility and prior testicular cancer supports early detection. Discussions on fertility preservation, including sperm banking and psychosocial support, including prosthesis options and coping strategies, are important.

The female reproductive system

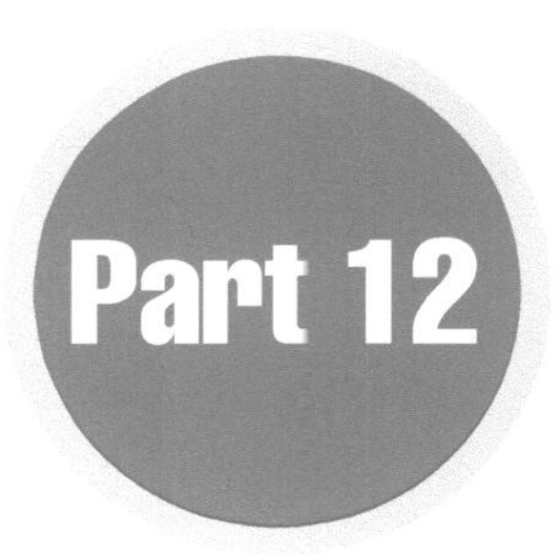

Chapters

47 Cancer of the vulva

Figure 47.1 The vulva.

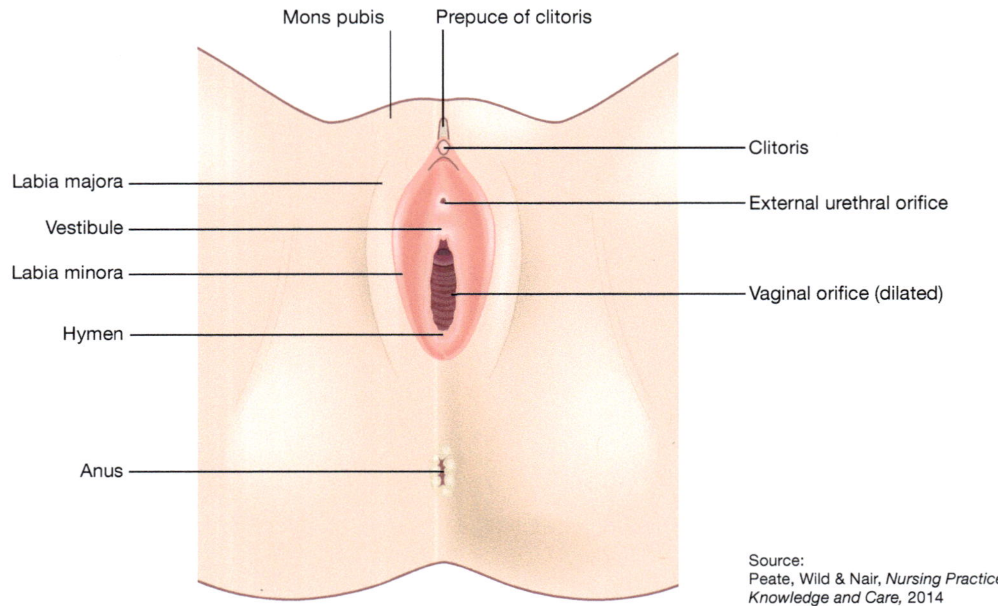

Source:
Peate, Wild & Nair, *Nursing Practice: Knowledge and Care,* 2014

Table 47.1 FIGO Staging of cancer of the vulva.

Stage	Discussion
I	Tumour confined to the vulva
IA	Tumour size less than or equal to 2 cm and stromal invasion less than or equal to1 mm
IB	Tumour size greater than 2 cm or stromal invasion greater than 1 mm
II	Tumour of any size with extension to lower one-third of the urethra, lower one-third of the vagina, lower one-third of the anus with negative nodes
III	Tumour of any size with extension to upper part of adjacent perineal structures, or with any number of nonfixed, nonulcerated lymph node
IIIA	Tumour of any size with disease extension to upper two-thirds of the urethra, upper two-thirds of the vagina, bladder mucosa, rectal mucosa, or regional lymph node metastases less than or equal to 5 mm
IIIB	Regional lymph node (inguinal and femoral lymph nodes) metastases greater than 5 mm
IIIC	Regional lymph node (inguinal and femoral lymph nodes) metastases with extracapsular spread
IV	Tumour of any size fixed to bone, or fixed, ulcerated lymph node metastases, or distant metastases
IVA	Disease fixed to pelvic bone, or fixed or ulcerated regional lymph node (inguinal and femoral lymph nodes) metastases
IVB	Distant metastases

The vulva

The vulva is a collective term referring to the external female genitalia and the surrounding skin (see Figure 47.1). It includes:

- The mons pubis
- The labia majora and labia minora
- The clitoris
- The external urethral meatus and vaginal introitus

Cancer of the vulva

Vulvar cancer most commonly arises from the labia majora, labia minora or clitoris, with the majority being squamous cell carcinomas. It is one of the five main gynaecological malignancies, although it remains relatively uncommon compared with cancers of the cervix, endometrium and ovary. In approximately three-quarters of cases, the tumour originates in one of the labia.

The global incidence of vulvar cancer is not precisely known; however, the incidence of pre-invasive disease (vulvar intraepithelial neoplasia [VIN]) has increased significantly over the past decade, particularly among younger women. This trend may, in the future, contribute to a rise in invasive disease. In the UK, around 1,400 people are diagnosed each year.

Vulvar carcinoma demonstrates a bimodal age distribution. In younger women, human papillomavirus (HPV)-associated high-grade squamous intraepithelial lesions are a common precursor, often linked to infection with HPV types 16 and 18. In contrast, vulvar cancer in older women is more frequently HPV-independent, arising in a background of chronic inflammatory or degenerative conditions, such as lichen sclerosus or chronic irritation.

Smoking is a significant cofactor, increasing the risk of VIN. Other risk factors include multiple sexual partners and a history of HPV infection, both of which are associated with increased viral exposure.

Pathophysiology

The majority of vulvar cancers (around 90–95%) are squamous cell carcinomas. Other, less common histological types include melanomas, adenocarcinomas (often arising from Bartholin's glands), basal cell carcinomas and sarcomas. The labia majora are the most frequent site of origin, accounting for about 50% of cases, followed by the labia minora (approximately 20%). The clitoris and Bartholin's glands are less commonly affected. Vulvar cancer typically spreads slowly and locally, initially involving adjacent tissues and subsequently metastasising to the inguinal and femoral lymph nodes before potentially reaching the pelvic nodes.

In many women, the development of VIN and invasive vulvar cancer is associated with infection by high-risk HPV types, particularly HPV 16, 18, 31, 33 and 45. These oncogenic types are also linked to cervical intraepithelial neoplasia and cervical cancer. The pathogenesis of HPV-related transformation involves integration of viral DNA into the host genome and disruption of tumour suppressor pathways, although the process is not yet fully understood.

Signs and symptoms

Diagnosis of vulval carcinoma is frequently delayed. Many women do not seek medical attention for several months after the onset of symptoms, and additional delays may occur following initial presentation to a clinician. In some cases, biopsy is deferred while lesions are treated empirically with topical therapies. Any persistent, unexplained, or clinically suspicious vulval lesion should be biopsied to exclude malignancy.

The most common presenting symptom is pruritus (itching), often associated with a vulvar lesion or a mass that the woman has noticed herself. Other symptoms include pain, bleeding, ulceration or discharge. However, early vulvar cancer may be asymptomatic and only detected through careful inspection of the vulva during examination. Bleeding, pain and discharge are more commonly associated with advanced disease.

The pattern of spread depends largely on the histological differentiation of the tumour. Well-differentiated squamous cell carcinomas tend to spread superficially along the epithelium with minimal invasion, whereas poorly differentiated or anaplastic lesions are more likely to be deeply invasive. Local spread may involve adjacent structures such as the vagina, urethra or anus, while lymphatic spread typically involves the inguinal and femoral lymph nodes, followed by the deep pelvic nodes. Approximately 5% of cases metastasise to distant sites.

Investigations

The definitive diagnosis of vulvar cancer is established by biopsy. Any suspicious vulvar lesion is biopsied to confirm malignancy and determine histological type. A punch biopsy is often sufficient to obtain a representative tissue sample, particularly when multiple or dysplastic lesions are present.

For staging purposes, investigations are directed at assessing local invasion and potential metastases. These may include cystoscopy or proctoscopy if there is suspicion of involvement of the urethra, bladder, rectum or anus. Cross-sectional imaging, typically CT or MRI of the pelvis and abdomen, is used to evaluate nodal spread, particularly when inguinal lymph nodes are enlarged or suspicious. CT thorax is preferred over chest X-ray to assess pulmonary metastases.

In selected cases, sentinel lymph node biopsy may be performed to assess pelvic nodal involvement, reducing the need for extensive lymph node dissection. Vulvar colposcopy can help identify abnormal areas and guide biopsy, although it is more challenging than cervical colposcopy due to the large surface area and variable appearance of vulvar intraepithelial lesions.

Blood tests are primarily supportive and preoperative. These typically include a full blood count to assess for anaemia, renal and liver function tests to guide treatment planning and contrast imaging, and coagulation profiles prior to surgery. There are currently no disease-specific serum tumour markers for vulvar carcinoma.

Staging

Accurate staging of vulvar cancer is essential, as it informs the clinician about the size of the tumour, depth of invasion and potential spread to local or distant sites. Information from biopsy, imaging and nodal assessment contributes to staging, and treatment decisions are guided primarily by the cancer stage.

In the UK, vulvar cancer is usually staged according to the Fédération Internationale de Gynécologie et d'Obstétrique (FIGO) system. This system classifies the disease into four main stages, based on tumour size, depth of invasion and regional or distant spread (see Table 47.1).

Management

The primary treatment for vulvar cancer is surgery, with the type and extent of excision determined by the location, size and depth of the primary lesion as well as the risk of lymph node involvement. The goal is to achieve complete removal of cancerous tissue while minimising functional and cosmetic impact; however, in some cases, extensive surgery may be unavoidable. Sentinel lymph node biopsy or inguinofemoral lymphadenectomy is performed to assess nodal involvement and guide further treatment.

In selected patients, primary radiotherapy or chemoradiation may be offered when surgery would result in unacceptable urinary or faecal morbidity, or when the patient prefers a non-surgical approach. Chemoradiation is also used in advanced or unresectable disease for local and regional control or palliative purposes to relieve symptoms and improve quality of life.

> **Clinical considerations**
>
> Early detection of vulvar cancer is essential to improve outcomes. Encourage women to seek prompt medical attention for any persistent vulvar symptoms, including pruritus, pain bleeding, lumps, ulceration or non-healing lesions. Offering information on vulvar anatomy and health can help women recognise abnormal changes; awareness of risk factors may prompt closer vigilance. Clinicians should ensure a supportive, non-judgemental environment, emphasising that all persistent or unusual vulvar lesions should be biopsied, as delays in diagnosis are common and may compromise prognosis.

 48 Menorrhagia

Box 48.1   Issues to be addressed during the history-taking phase.

- Exclusion of pregnancy (the most common cause of irregular bleeding in women of reproductive age and the first diagnosis that should be excluded before further testing or drug therapy)
- Quantity and quality of bleeding
- Age
- Pelvic pain and pathology
- Menses pattern from menarche
- Sexual activity
- Contraceptive use (intrauterine device (IUD) or hormones)
- Presence of hirsutism (polycystic ovarian syndrome)
- Galactorrhoea (pituitary tumour)
- Systemic illnesses (hepatic or renal failure, or diabetes)
- Symptoms of thyroid dysfunction
- Excessive bruising or known bleeding disorders
- Current medications (hormones or anticoagulants)
- Previous medical or surgical procedures or diagnoses

Table 48.1   Risk factors and menorrhagia.

Category	Risk factors	Notes
Hormonal / Endocrine	Anovulation, Polycystic Ovary Syndrome, Thyroid disorders (hypothyroidism, hyperthyroidism), Hyperprolactinaemia	Hormonal imbalances disrupt normal endometrial shedding, leading to prolonged or heavy bleeding.
Structural / Anatomical	Uterine fibroids (leiomyomas), Adenomyosis, Endometrial polyps, Congenital uterine anomalies	Structural changes increase endometrial surface area or interfere with contraction, causing heavier bleeding.
Haematological / Coagulation	Von Willebrand disease, Platelet function disorders, Coagulopathies	Impaired clotting prolongs menstrual bleeding.
Iatrogenic / Medications	Anticoagulants (warfarin, heparin, Direct Oral Anticoagulants), Hormonal contraception (e.g., levonorgestrel intrauterine device), Tamoxifen	Medications can alter coagulation or endometrial stability.
Systemic / Chronic Conditions	Liver disease, Kidney disease, Obesity	Systemic illness affects hormone metabolism, coagulation, or endometrial function.
Lifestyle / Demographic	Age (perimenopause), High BMI, Smoking	Hormonal fluctuations with age or adiposity contribute to menorrhagia.
Infections / Inflammatory	Pelvic inflammatory disease, Endometritis	Local inflammation disrupts normal endometrial shedding.

Heavy menstrual bleeding refers to menstrual blood loss that interferes with a woman's physical, emotional, social or material quality of life; it may occur alone or with other symptoms. While historically defined as menstrual blood loss exceeding 80 mL per cycle, current clinical practice focuses on the impact on quality of life. The primary aim of any intervention is to improve the quality of life.

Menorrhagia

The average menstrual cycle lasts 21–35 days, with menstrual bleeding typically lasting 3–7 days. Menstrual blood loss is usually heaviest during the first few days, and it then gradually decreases toward the end of the period. The normal menstrual blood loss is approximately 30–40 mL per cycle.

Other commonly used definitions include:

- Metrorrhagia – bleeding at irregular intervals.
- Menometrorrhagia – heavy and/or prolonged bleeding that occurs at irregular intervals.
- Polymenorrhoea – menstrual bleeding occurring at intervals that are shorter than 21 days.
- Dysfunctional uterine bleeding – abnormal uterine bleeding in the absence of structural or systemic pathology.
- Dysmenorrhoea – painful menstruation.

Menorrhagia, or heavy menstrual bleeding, is subjective and is best defined by the woman and its impact on the woman: it refers to menstrual loss that exceeds what she feels she can reasonably manage, interfering with her physical, emotional, social or material quality of life.

Pathophysiology

Heavy menstrual bleeding results from structural, endometrial, systemic and iatrogenic factors that disrupt normal endometrial shedding and haemostasis.

1 Endometrial (non-structural) causes – abnormal uterine bleeding – endometrial.
   - Approximately half of women with heavy menstruation have no structural uterine pathology, previously referred to as dysfunctional uterine bleeding.
   - The most common mechanism is hormonal imbalance, particularly anovulatory cycles, which are most frequent at the extremes of reproductive life.
   - Pathophysiology: absence of ovulation → lack of progesterone → unstable endometrium → irregular, prolonged or heavy bleeding.
   - Other endometrial causes may involve local abnormalities in endometrial haemostasis, vascular regulation or inflammation.
2 Structural uterine causes – abnormal uterine bleeding, polyp, adenomyosis, leiomyoma, malignancy and hyperplasia
   - Fibroids (leiomyomas): increased endometrial surface area and abnormal vascularisation.
   - Endometrial polyps: fragile vasculature prone to bleeding.
   - Adenomyosis: endometrial tissue within the myometrium → heavy, painful bleeding.
   - Endometrial hyperplasia or carcinoma: excessive proliferation → abnormal bleeding.
   - Endometritis/pelvic inflammatory disease: inflammation disrupts normal endometrial function.
3 Systemic causes
   Coagulopathies (disorders of blood clotting), liver or kidney disease, hypothyroidism → impaired haemostasis or altered hormone metabolism → heavy bleeding.
4 Iatrogenic causes (caused by medical treatment or intervention)
   Intrauterine devices (IUDs): copper IUDs may increase menstrual blood loss, while hormonal IUDs usually reduce it.
   - Certain medications, including anticoagulants, can exacerbate bleeding.

Signs and symptoms

Symptoms reported by the woman with menorrhagia may often be more instructive than laboratory tests. It is essential to undertake a detailed patient history. Box 48.1 outlines some essential issues that should be addressed in the history-taking phase.

The physical examination should be modified in order to meet the needs of the woman. The clinician should observe for signs of severe anaemia, which may confirm the patient's history of very heavy bleeding and prompt immediate inpatient care. Obesity is an independent risk factor for endometrial cancer (see Table 48.1). Adipose tissue is ideal for oestrogen conversion. Signs of androgen excess (hirsutism) may be PCOS, leading to anovulatory bleeding. Ecchymosis is usually a sign of trauma or a bleeding disorder; purpura is also a sign of trauma or a possible bleeding disorder. Uterine size, shape and contour should be assessed. Adnexal tenderness (these are structures adjacent to the uterus) or masses could indicate ovarian cancer; intermenstrual bleeding may be its only symptom. Finding an adnexal mass should prompt an immediate pelvic ultrasound.

Investigations

A full blood count is essential, as menorrhagia is a common cause of iron deficiency anaemia in women. Thyroid function tests and other endocrine investigations may be indicated if there is clinical suspicion of hormonal irregularities. Assessment for bleeding disorders should be considered when the history suggests excessive or unusual bleeding.

Endometrial biopsy may be performed to exclude endometrial cancer or atypical hyperplasia, particularly in women over 45 years old or those with risk factors. Transvaginal ultrasound is the first-line diagnostic tool for evaluating structural abnormalities such as fibroids or polyps. Cervical screening or infection testing should be undertaken according to age, risk factors and local guidelines.

Management

The management of menorrhagia should be individualised, with the woman at the centre of all decisions. Medical therapy is considered the first-line treatment tailored to the patient's age, coexisting medical conditions, family history and desire for fertility. If initial medical therapy is ineffective, a second medical option should be considered before referral for surgical intervention. Shared decision-making is essential for ensuring the woman is fully informed about the benefits, risks and implications of each option.

Correction of iron deficiency is an important first step; women with heavy menstrual bleeding are at risk of anaemia. Oral iron supplementation should be provided to restore haemoglobin levels and optimise overall health prior to considering more invasive interventions.

The levonorgestrel-releasing intrauterine system (LNG-IUS) is regarded as first-line medical therapy. This long-acting device reduces menstrual blood loss by thinning the endometrium and is typically left in place for at least 12 months. For women in whom the LNG-IUS is unsuitable or unacceptable, alternatives include tranexamic acid, non-steroidal anti-inflammatory drugs such as mefenamic acid, and the combined oral contraceptive pill, all of which can reduce menstrual blood loss to varying degrees. Short-term courses of gonadotropin-releasing hormone (GnRH) analogues may also be considered in preparation for surgical interventions, particularly in women with large fibroids, although there is no consensus on the most effective regimen.

Surgical management is considered when medical therapy fails, is contraindicated, or is declined. The choice of procedure is influenced by uterine size, the underlying pathology and the woman's fertility wishes. Endometrial ablation is recommended and involves the destruction of the endometrium and superficial myometrium. This procedure preserves the uterus but is contraindicated in women with large fibroids, suspected malignancy or those who have not completed their family. Other uterus-preserving options include hysteroscopic myomectomy for submucosal fibroids and uterine artery embolisation for women wishing to retain their uterus.

For women who do not wish to preserve their uterus, hysterectomy represents the definitive surgical management option. Vaginal hysterectomy is generally preferred due to a shorter recovery time, but abdominal hysterectomy may be necessary in certain cases, with ovarian conservation maintained when appropriate.

Throughout all stages of management, the woman's preferences, fertility goals and overall well-being should guide clinical decisions. Regular follow-up is essential to monitor treatment efficacy, correct anaemia and address any ongoing symptoms, ensuring that care remains patient-centred and responsive to her needs.

49 Breast cancer

Figure 49.1 The female breast.

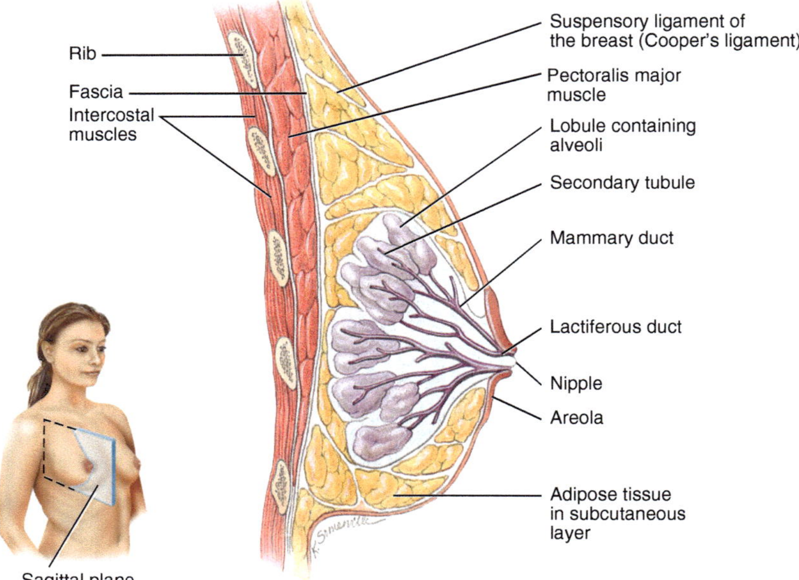

Box 49.1 Risk factors.

- Age (increases with age)
- Reproductive history
- Endogenous and exogenous hormones
- Breast density
- Previous breast disease
  - the genes BRCA1, BRCA2 and TP53 mutations carry very high risk. Family history, a first-degree relative, is the most widely recognized breast cancer risk factor
- Non-reproductive lifestyle factors

Table 49.1 Breast cancer staging.

Stage	Discussion
0	Stage 0 refers to carcinoma in situ (ductal carcinoma in situ or lobular carcinoma in situ), which is confined to ducts or lobules with no invasion.
I	Stage 1 is divided into 2 stages:
IA	Cancer is 2 cm or smaller. It has not spread outside the breast.
IB	Cancer is not found in the breast tissue or is 2 cm or smaller. Tiny numbers of cancer cells have spread to lymph nodes in the axilla (micrometastases).
II	Stage 2 is divided into 2 stages:
IIA	Cancer cannot be found in breast tissue or is 2 cm or smaller. It has also spread to 1 to 3 lymph nodes in the axilla or near the sternum. Or Cancer is between 2 and 5 cm and it has not spread to the lymph nodes in the axilla or near the sternum.
IIB	Cancer is between 2 and 5 cm, has spread to 1 to 3 lymph nodes in the armpit. Or Cancer is bigger than 5 cm, has not spread to the lymph nodes.
III	Stage III breast cancer is sometimes called locally advanced breast cancer. Cancer has spread to the lymph nodes, skin of the breast or the chest muscle. Skin may be red, swollen or have broken down, causing an ulcer. Some breast cancers spreading to the skin may be inflammatory breast cancer.
IIIa	Cancer cannot be found in the breast or it is 5 cm or smaller. It has spread to 4 to 9 lymph nodes in the axilla. Or The cancer is bigger than 5 cm. It has spread to up to 3 lymph nodes in the axilla or near the sternum.
IIIb	Cancer has spread into tissue nearby, such as the skin of the breast and the intercoastal muscle. It may have spread to 1 to 9 lymph nodes in the axilla.
IIIc	Cancer may be any size or it cannot be found in the breast. It has spread into tissue nearby, such as the skin of the breast and the intercoastal muscle. It has spread to 10 or more lymph nodes in the axilla. Cancer has spread to lymph nodes below the sternum and above or below the clavicle. It has spread to 4 or more lymph nodes in the axilla.
IV	Stage IV breast cancer is also called secondary or metastatic breast cancer. Cancer has spread to other parts of the body, such as the bones, liver or lungs.

Globally, breast cancer is the most frequently diagnosed life-threatening cancer in women and is the leading cause of cancer death among women. Breast cancer can be discovered while *in situ* (localised) or as a malignant neoplasm (spreading). Although breast cancer is far more common in women, men can also develop the disease.

The female breasts

An adult woman's breasts are milk-producing glands located on the anterior chest wall, resting on the pectoralis major muscles and attached to the chest wall by Cooper's ligaments, which provide support and maintain the contour of the breast. Each breast contains 15–20 lobes arranged radially, each composed of multiple lobules containing glands that produce milk in response to hormonal stimulation (see Figure 49.1).

Many early breast cancers are asymptomatic, particularly those detected through screening programmes. Larger tumours may present as a painless mass, and pain or discomfort is rarely a symptom of breast cancer.

A substantial proportion of breast cancer cases in the UK are associated with factors that influence oestrogen exposure, including reproductive history, hormonal therapy, obesity, alcohol intake and physical activity. Breast cancer risk is predominantly linked to modifiable lifestyle and environmental factors (see Box 49.1, risk factors).

Pathophysiology

Breast cancer most commonly begins in the epithelial cells of the breast ducts, known as ductal carcinoma, or in the small glandular units at the ends of the ducts, called lobular carcinoma. Some cancers remain confined within the ducts or lobules, referred to as in situ carcinoma, while others become invasive, breaking through the walls of the ducts or lobules and spreading into the surrounding fatty tissue of the breast.

The development of breast cancer is driven by genetic changes within the breast cells. These changes can affect genes that normally control cell growth, division and repair. Mutations in oncogenes can cause cells to grow uncontrollably, while changes in tumour suppressor genes remove the normal 'brakes' on growth. Faulty DNA repair genes allow additional genetic errors to accumulate, further increasing the risk of malignant transformation. As a result, the affected breast cells divide excessively, avoid programmed cell death (apoptosis) and gain the ability to invade surrounding tissues and form tumours.

Inherited genetic mutations also contribute to breast cancer in some women. Mutations in genes such as BRCA1, BRCA2 and TP53 increase susceptibility by making breast cells more likely to accumulate harmful mutations over time. Hereditary breast cancers often appear at a younger age, may affect both breasts and can have distinctive features compared with non-hereditary cancers.

There are also rarer forms of breast cancer. Paget's disease of the nipple occurs when cancer cells involve the nipple epithelium and is often associated with an underlying tumour deeper in the breast. Inflammatory breast cancer is an aggressive subtype in which cancer cells block the lymphatic vessels of the skin, causing rapid swelling, redness, warmth and thickening of the breast tissue.

Staging of the tumour

Tumour size, lymph node involvement and the presence of distant metastases are the key factors used to stage breast cancer (see Table 49.1). Diagnostic tests and investigations not only help confirm the diagnosis but can also provide important information about the stage of the disease. Accurate staging is crucial, as it guides the clinician in selecting the most appropriate treatment and helps predict prognosis.

Signs and symptoms

Many early breast cancers are asymptomatic, particularly when detected through routine breast screening programmes. When tumours grow larger, they often present as a painless lump in the breast. Pain or general breast discomfort is uncommon and occurs in only a small minority of women with malignant lesions.

Other signs may include nipple changes, such as retraction or inversion, and nipple discharge, which can be bloody, especially in cancers arising from the ducts. Alterations in the skin over the breast, including dimpling, thickening or changes in contour, may also be observed. Recognising these features is important, as early detection improves treatment outcomes and prognosis.

Investigations

Assessment of suspected breast cancer begins with a detailed history and physical examination, including careful inspection and palpation of the breasts and evaluation of the axillary and cervical lymph nodes. Further investigations are then undertaken to confirm the diagnosis, characterise the tumour and determine the stage of disease, which is essential for guiding treatment decisions. All investigations should follow local and national clinical guidelines.

The cornerstone of diagnosis is the triple assessment, which combines clinical examination, imaging and biopsy. Imaging usually includes mammography, which is most effective in less dense breasts and routinely performed in women over 40 years, and ultrasound, which is particularly useful in younger women or those with dense breast tissue and for evaluating palpable lumps. Magnetic resonance imaging (MRI) may be indicated in women with dense breasts, a strong family history or BRCA mutations, silicone implants, multifocal or multicentric disease, or when the primary tumour is not clearly identified but axillary lymph nodes are positive. MRI is also useful for assessing the extent of disease prior to surgery.

Biopsy is essential for confirming a diagnosis. Image-guided core needle biopsy is the preferred method, providing tissue for both histological examination and receptor testing before surgery. Fine-needle aspiration may be used selectively, mainly for palpable lymph nodes. In rare cases, an excisional or incisional biopsy may be performed if the core biopsy is inconclusive or when complete removal of a small lesion is required.

Investigations for staging are guided by tumour characteristics, clinical features and symptoms. These may include blood tests, such as a full blood count and liver function tests, and imaging of the chest, abdomen and pelvis with CT if distant metastases are suspected. Bone scintigraphy may be performed if there is concern about bone involvement, and PET-CT can be used in selected cases to detect occult metastatic disease.

Together, these investigations provide a complete picture of the tumour, including its size, nodal involvement and presence of distant metastases, which are critical for accurate staging, treatment planning and prognostication.

Management

Treatment of breast cancer must be patient-centred, taking into account the woman's individual needs, preferences and values. Where appropriate, discussions may involve family members, provided the patient has consented to this. Prognosis depends on both the biological characteristics of the tumour, including size, grade, hormone receptor and HER2 status (these are key molecular characteristics of breast cancer) and the patient, as well as on the timeliness and appropriateness of therapy.

For early-stage breast cancer, surgery remains the primary treatment, and in selected low-risk cases, surgery alone may be curative. However, adjuvant therapies such as radiotherapy, hormone therapy, chemotherapy or targeted therapy are often recommended based on tumour biology and patient factors to reduce the risk of recurrence. The goals of surgery are to completely remove the tumour with clear margins, reduce the risk of local recurrence, and allow pathological assessment of the tumour and axillary lymph nodes, which provides important prognostic information.

Adjuvant therapy is used to treat micrometastatic disease, cancer cells that have spread beyond the primary tumour but have not yet formed detectable metastases. Adjuvant treatment may include radiotherapy, chemotherapy, endocrine therapy and targeted biological agents, depending on tumour biology and patient factors. The purpose of adjuvant therapy is to reduce the risk of recurrence and improve breast cancer-specific survival, thereby lowering both morbidity and mortality associated with the disease.

Clinical considerations

Early detection of breast cancer improves survival, as many tumours are asymptomatic initially. Mammography is the primary screening tool, with ultrasound or MRI used for younger women, dense breasts or high-risk individuals. Encourage patients to attend screening and report new breast changes promptly, as early diagnosis allows for more effective treatment and better outcomes.

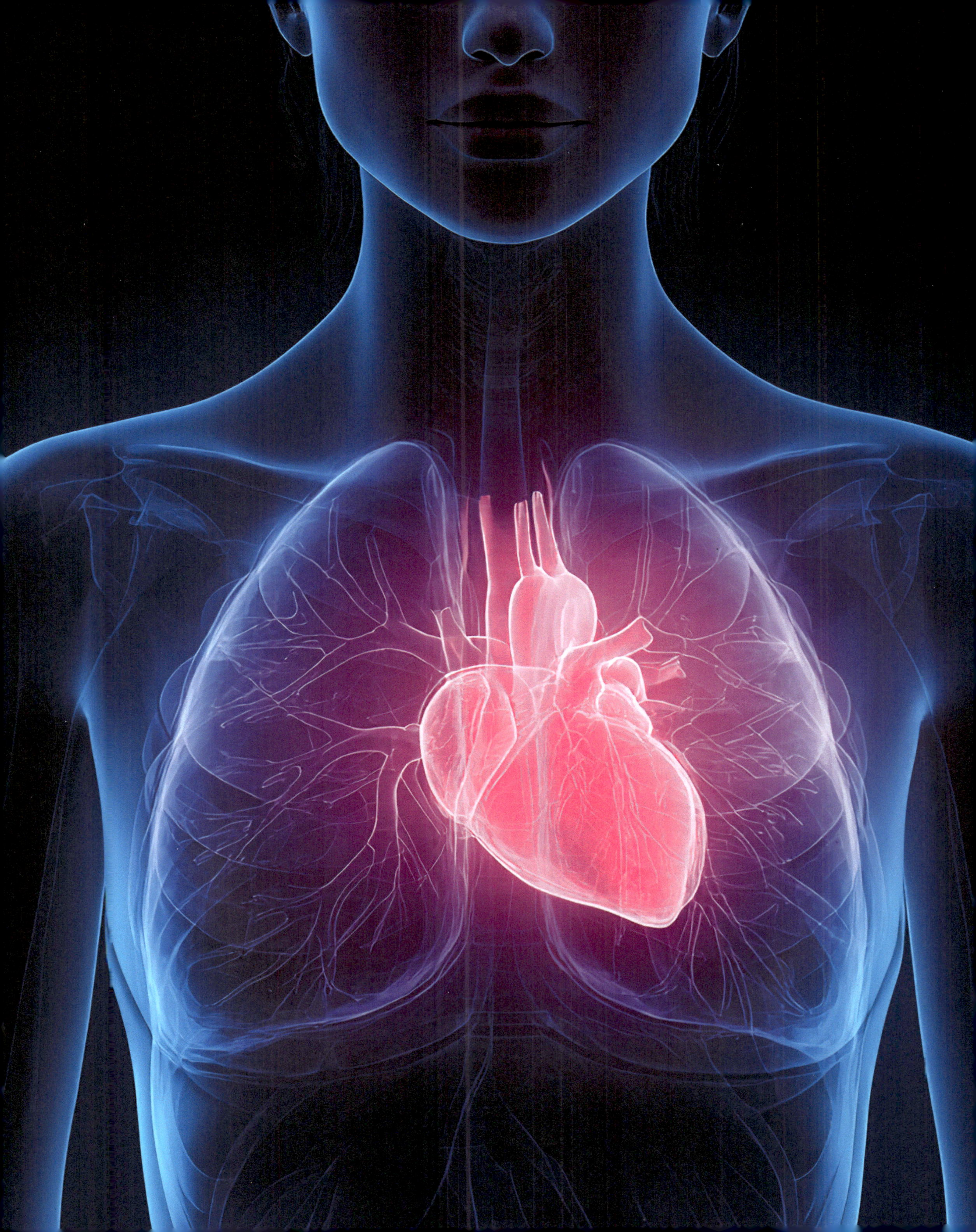

50 Cervical cancer

Figure 50.1 Squamocolumnar junction of the cervix.

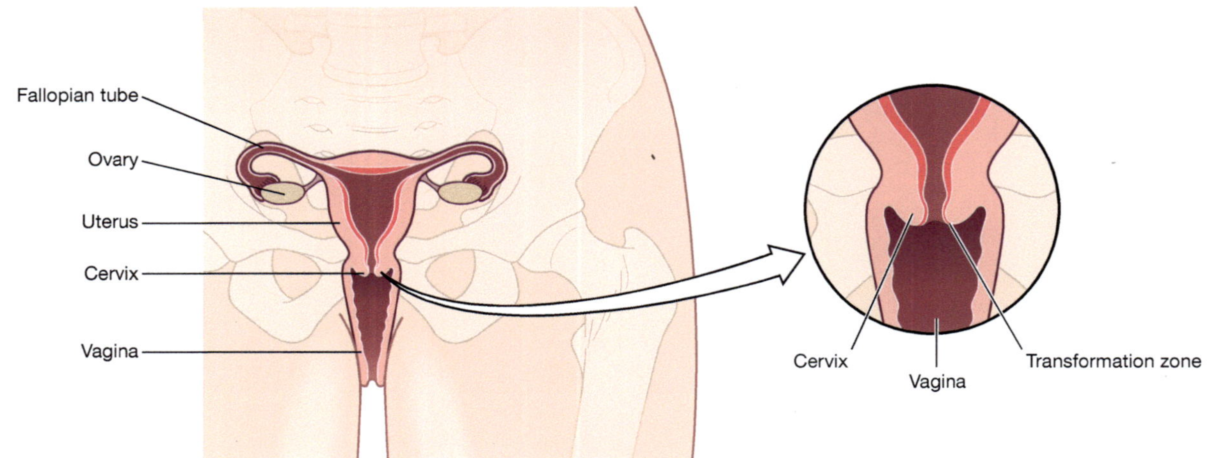

Figure 50.2 Cervical intra-epithelial neoplasia.

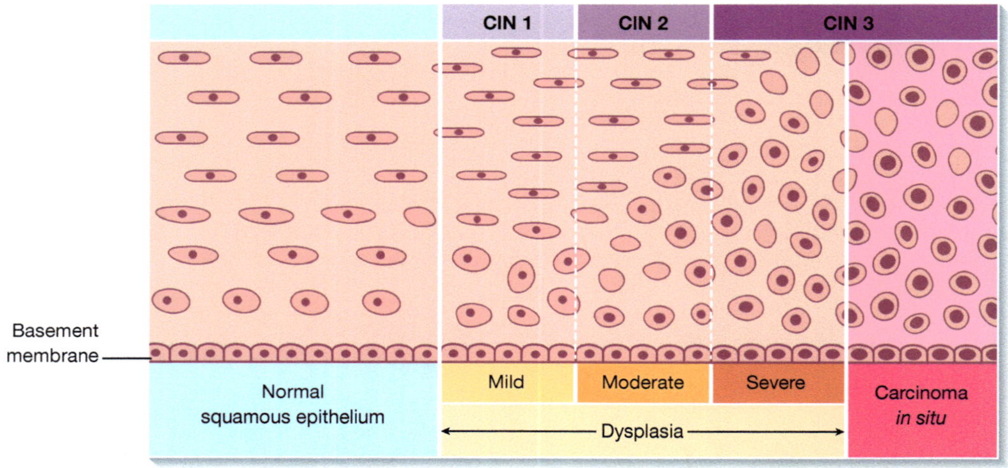

Figure 50.3 Cone biopsy.

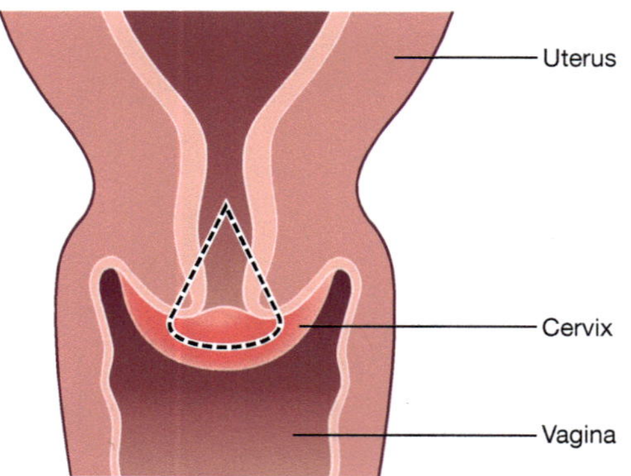

Cervical cancer

Cervical cancer is one of the few preventable cancers and remains a significant global health concern. It is the fourth most common cancer in women worldwide and a leading cause of cancer-related death in many low- and middle-income countries. The widespread implementation of cervical screening programmes and human papillomavirus (HPV) vaccination has substantially reduced the incidence and mortality of cervical cancer by enabling early detection and prevention.

Persistent infection with high-risk human papillomavirus (HPV), particularly types 16 and 18, is a necessary cause of cervical cancer. Additional risk factors include early sexual activity, multiple sexual partners, high parity, cigarette smoking, low socio-economic status and a history of sexually transmitted infections such as herpes simplex virus or genital warts. Women who are immunosuppressed, for example, due to HIV infection or immunosuppressive therapy, are also at increased risk. Regular participation in cervical screening remains critical for reducing the risk of invasive disease.

Pathophysiology

Cervical cancer is most commonly classified as squamous cell carcinoma, followed by adenocarcinoma, with mixed and other rare types accounting for a smaller proportion of cases. Most cervical cancers arise from pre-invasive epithelial abnormalities that may progress to invasive carcinoma if untreated. Persistent infection with high-risk HPV, particularly types 16 and 18, is the primary cause of cervical cancer. HPV promotes the neoplastic transformation of epithelial cells, most frequently occurring at the squamocolumnar junction of the cervix (see Figure 50.1). Neoplastic transformation means normal cells lining a tissue (epithelial cells) have changed into abnormal cells that can grow uncontrollably and form a tumour.

Pre-invasive disease is categorised as cervical intraepithelial neoplasia (CIN) grades 1 to 3, with CIN 3 corresponding to carcinoma in situ, in which the full thickness of the epithelium is replaced by dysplastic cells without invasion of the basement membrane (see Figure 50.2). Progression from CIN to invasive cancer typically takes between 10 and 20 years. Cervical screening, through cytology (sometimes called the smear test) or HPV testing, is particularly effective at detecting these pre-invasive lesions, as the cervix may appear normal to the naked eye in early disease. Most women with early stage cervical cancer are asymptomatic, whereas advanced disease can present with abnormal bleeding, discharge or pain.

Invasive cervical cancer spreads primarily through direct local invasion and via the lymphatic system, with haematogenous dissemination (cancer spreading through the bloodstream) occurring in later stages. Local extension usually involves the endocervix, vaginal fornices, parametrial tissues and, eventually, adjacent organs such as the main body of the uterus (uterine corpus), bladder or rectum. Lymphatic spread typically follows a stepwise progression through pelvic and para-aortic nodes, while haematogenous spread can lead to distant metastases in the lungs, liver, bones or other organs. Tumours may appear exophytic or ulcerative, and the risk of metastasis increases with tumour size and extent.

Signs and symptoms

Cervical screening detects many pre-invasive lesions and early stage cancers before symptoms develop. The first symptoms of established cervical carcinoma often include an abnormal vaginal discharge, which may vary in amount and character and can be intermittent or continuous. In the early stages, vaginal bleeding may occur spontaneously or following sexual intercourse (postcoital bleeding). Some women may dismiss light or irregular bleeding as a menstrual variation. Occasionally, severe vaginal bleeding may occur, necessitating emergency hospital admission. Other early features can include vaginal discomfort and mild urinary symptoms.

As the disease advances, symptoms may result from local invasion or distant spread. Late manifestations can include painless haematuria, persistent urinary frequency, rectal bleeding, altered bowel habits, lower limb swelling (oedema), pelvic or lower back pain and hydronephrosis leading to renal impairment, which may indicate pelvic wall involvement. Pelvic discomfort or poorly localised dull pain in the suprapubic or sacral regions is also common in more advanced stages.

On physical examination, findings may be subtle or even normal in early disease. The cervix may show leukoplakia (white) or erythematous (red) areas, which represent abnormal epithelial changes. With disease progression, the cervix and upper vagina may develop an irregular, friable or ulcerated appearance due to tumour growth or erosion. On rectal examination, there may be a palpable mass or bleeding, indicating posterior extension. Bimanual palpation may reveal pelvic fullness or a fixed mass suggestive of parametrial spread. Lymphatic or vascular obstruction can lead to unilateral or bilateral leg oedema. Evidence of distant metastases may include hepatomegaly from liver involvement or pleural effusion and respiratory symptoms due to pulmonary metastases.

Investigations

If cervical cancer is suspected, a range of investigations is undertaken to confirm the diagnosis and determine the stage of the disease. Colposcopy allows detailed visual examination of the cervix under magnification to identify abnormal epithelial changes. Targeted biopsies are taken for histological confirmation.

When colposcopy identifies a lesion requiring excision, a large loop excision of the transformation zone (LLETZ) may be performed under local anaesthetic. This procedure uses a thin, electrically heated wire loop to remove the abnormal area of cervical tissue. A needle excision of the transformation zone (NETZ) is a similar technique, using a straight wire for more precise excision of the affected tissue.

A cone biopsy (cervical conisation) may be indicated when the abnormal area cannot be fully visualised with colposcopy or when early invasive disease is suspected. This is usually carried out under general anaesthetic, though local anaesthetic may sometimes be used (see Figure 50.3).

Additional investigations are performed to assess the extent of disease and guide staging. These typically include full blood count, renal and liver function tests, and cross-sectional imaging such as MRI (to evaluate local pelvic spread) and CT or PET-CT (to detect nodal or distant metastases). Cystoscopy may be performed to assess bladder involvement, and proctoscopy if rectal invasion is suspected.

The FIGO 2018 staging system incorporates findings from imaging and pathology to provide a more accurate assessment of disease extent.

Management

The management of cervical cancer depends on the stage of disease, the patient's age, general health and fertility wishes.

Treatment may involve surgery, radiotherapy, chemotherapy or a combination of these modalities. Early stage disease is often treated surgically, typically by radical hysterectomy with pelvic lymph node assessment. For locally advanced disease, concurrent chemoradiotherapy is the standard of care, usually combining external beam radiotherapy with intracavitary brachytherapy and cisplatin-based chemotherapy. The choice and extent of treatment are guided by tumour stage, comorbidities and multidisciplinary team discussion and, above all, the woman's wishes.

Clinical considerations

Cervical cancer is largely preventable through HPV vaccination and regular cervical screening. Vaccination protects against high-risk HPV types, particularly 16 and 18, and is most effective when it is given before sexual debut. Screening detects pre-invasive changes and early cancers, which are often asymptomatic. HPV vaccination combined with screening is the cornerstone of prevention and early detection.

The endocrine system

Chapters

51 Diabetes mellitus

Figure 51.1 Overview of the pathophysiology related to abnormal glucose metabolism in type 2 diabetes mellitus.

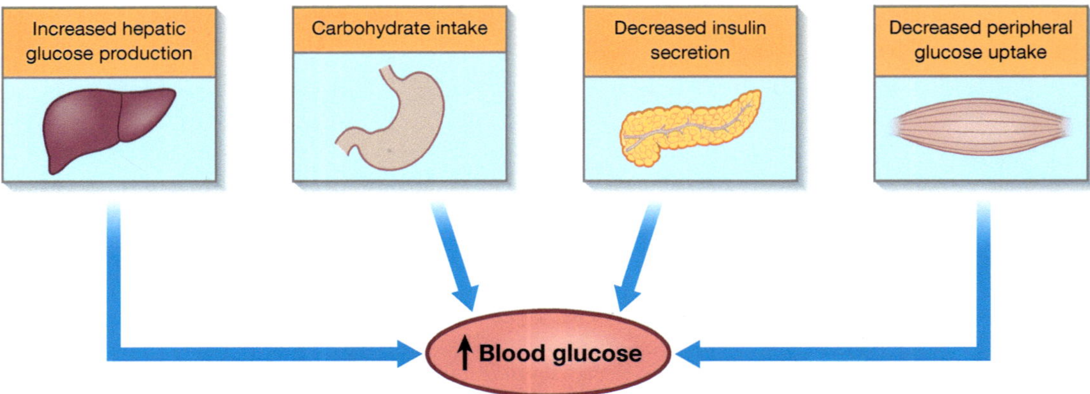

Figure 51.2 Key symptoms of diabetes.

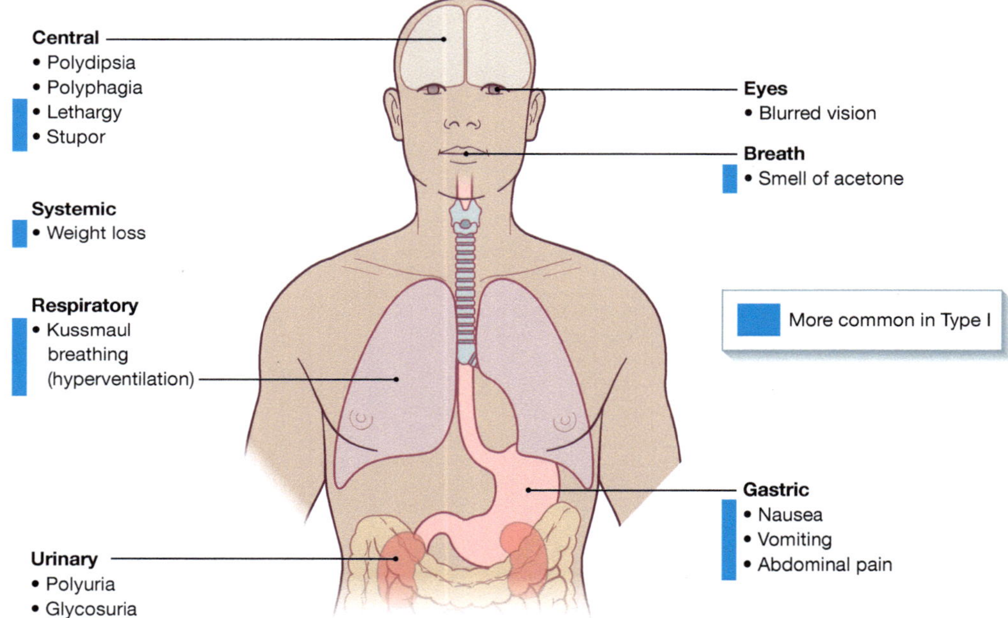

Table 51.1 A classification of three types of diabetes mellitus.

Type	Features	Cause	Treatment
Type 1	Total lack of insulin	Autoimmune	Insulin
Type 2	Insensitivity to insulin and deficiency in secreting insulin	Obesity and genetics	Diet, exercise, hypoglycaemic agents and transporter stimulating drugs
Gestational	Diagnosed during pregnancy	Increased metabolic demands, family history of diabetes and decreased insulin sensitivity	Diet, insulin and hypoglycaemic agents

Diabetes mellitus

Diabetes mellitus is a metabolic disorder caused by a deficiency or diminished effectiveness of endogenous insulin. The main types of diabetes mellitus are:

- Type 1 diabetes mellitus: results from autoimmune destruction of pancreatic β-cells, leading to an absolute deficiency of insulin.
- Type 2 diabetes mellitus: results from insulin resistance combined with a relative insulin deficiency; circulating insulin levels are often normal or elevated in the early stages.
- Gestational diabetes mellitus: occurs during pregnancy in women without previously diagnosed diabetes; it may increase the risk of developing type 2 diabetes later in life.
- Maturity-onset diabetes of the young (MODY): comprises several forms of diabetes resulting from monogenic defects of β-cell function, leading to impaired insulin secretion.
- Secondary diabetes mellitus: accounts for approximately 1–2% of all diabetes cases. Causes include pancreatic disease, endocrine disorders, certain medications, congenital lipodystrophy, acanthosis nigricans and various genetic syndromes.

Diabetes mellitus is characterised by hyperglycaemia, disordered metabolism and long-term complications predominantly affecting the vascular system (see Table 51.1).

Type 1 Diabetes mellitus

This condition results from a combination of genetic susceptibility and an autoimmune process that leads to the gradual destruction of the pancreatic β-cells, resulting in absolute insulin deficiency. Possible triggers include viral infections, dietary factors, environmental toxins and emotional or physical stress.

Those individuals with type 1 diabetes will always require insulin therapy and are at risk of developing diabetic ketoacidosis. The highest incidence occurs among people of Caucasian or Northern European ancestry, with Scandinavian populations showing the greatest prevalence.

Type 2 Diabetes mellitus

Type 2 diabetes mellitus typically presents in adults over the age of 30 years, although it is increasingly being diagnosed in children and adolescents. The condition is strongly associated with excess body weight, physical inactivity and genetic predisposition.

The condition is caused by a combination of insulin resistance and impaired insulin secretion, and it develops gradually over time. People with type 2 diabetes may initially be managed with lifestyle modification and oral hypoglycaemic agents, but insulin therapy may eventually be required. Type 2 diabetes is more prevalent among individuals of South Asian, African, African-Caribbean, Polynesian, Middle Eastern and American Indian ancestry.

Pathophysiology of type 2 diabetes

Type 2 diabetes mellitus is characterised by a combination of peripheral insulin resistance and inadequate insulin secretion by the pancreatic β-cells.

Insulin resistance, associated with elevated levels of free fatty acids and pro-inflammatory cytokines in the plasma, leads to reduced glucose uptake by skeletal muscle, increased hepatic glucose production and enhanced lipolysis. Over time, the β-cells fail to compensate for this resistance, resulting in progressive hyperglycaemia.

Type 2 diabetes is considered an islet paracrinopathy: the normal reciprocal relationship between the glucagon-secreting α-cells and the insulin-secreting β-cells becomes disrupted. This dysregulation results in inappropriate hyperglucagonaemia, which further contributes to increased hepatic glucose output and sustained hyperglycaemia.

For type 2 diabetes to develop, both insulin resistance and β-cell dysfunction must be present. Although most overweight individuals exhibit some degree of insulin resistance, diabetes occurs only in those whose β-cells cannot augment insulin secretion sufficiently to maintain normal glucose levels. Consequently, insulin levels (concentration) may be elevated, but they are insufficient to overcome the insulin resistance and normalise blood glucose (see Figure 51.1).

Signs and symptoms

Individuals with diabetes mellitus may present with a range of symptoms related to hyperglycaemia and its metabolic consequences. Common manifestations across all types of diabetes include polyuria (frequent urination), polydipsia (excessive thirst), lethargy and recurrent infections, such as furuncles (boils), urinary tract infections or pruritus vulvae.

Type 1 diabetes mellitus often develops more acutely, with a relatively short duration of symptoms. In addition to the general features, individuals may present with weight loss, dehydration, ketonuria and hyperventilation (Kussmaul breathing). These features reflect the absolute insulin deficiency and rapid metabolic derangements characteristic of type 1 diabetes.

In contrast, type 2 diabetes mellitus usually develops more gradually, and many individuals remain asymptomatic for years. When symptoms do occur, they are often milder and may include polyuria, polydipsia, fatigue and recurrent infections. The gradual onset of type 2 diabetes often delays diagnosis, allowing chronic hyperglycaemia and its complications to develop silently.

Both types of diabetes may be associated with acute complications, such as diabetic ketoacidosis in type 1 diabetes or hyperosmolar hyperglycaemic state in type 2 diabetes, as well as chronic microvascular and macrovascular complications affecting the eyes, kidneys, nerves and cardiovascular system (see Figure 51.2).

Investigations

Diabetes mellitus can be diagnosed based on one abnormal plasma glucose measurement in the presence of typical diabetic symptoms, such as thirst, polyuria, recurrent infections, weight loss, drowsiness or coma. The diagnostic thresholds are:

- Random plasma glucose greater than or equal to 11.1 mmol/L
- Fasting venous plasma glucose greater than or equal to 7.0 mmol/L

In individuals who are asymptomatic, a diagnosis requires two fasting venous plasma glucose measurements in the abnormal range.

Alternatively, diabetes can be diagnosed using an oral glucose tolerance test (OGTT), with a 2-hour venous plasma glucose greater than or equal to 11.1 mmol/L following the ingestion of 75 g of anhydrous glucose.

The World Health Organization (WHO) also recommends that glycated haemoglobin (HbA1c) may be used as a diagnostic test. An HbA1c of 6.5% or higher is considered the cut-off for diagnosing diabetes.

Management

The primary goals in caring for people with diabetes mellitus are to alleviate symptoms and prevent, or slow, the development of complications. Microvascular complications, such as retinopathy and nephropathy, can be reduced through optimisation of glycaemic control and blood pressure management, while macrovascular complications, including coronary, cerebrovascular and peripheral vascular disease, are addressed through management of lipids and hypertension, smoking cessation and, in selected individuals, antiplatelet therapy. Control of glycaemia also plays a central role in reducing metabolic and neurological complications.

Management must be individualised, taking into account the type of diabetes, comorbidities, lifestyle and patient preferences. Contemporary national guidelines provide structured frameworks. Optimising glycaemic control while minimising adverse effects, such as hypoglycaemia, is a key component of care. Attention must also be given to other modifiable risk factors, including early detection and treatment of hypertension, lipid management and consideration of antiplatelet therapy. Regular monitoring for complications, including cardiovascular disease, foot problems, retinopathy, nephropathy and neuropathy, is essential, and timely interventions can reduce progression and improve outcomes.

A global assessment of cardiovascular risk is vital to guide the intensity of interventions and to personalise management strategies for each individual with diabetes.

Clinical considerations

Diabetes mellitus is associated with microvascular and macrovascular complications. Microvascular complications, including retinopathy, nephropathy and neuropathy, which can lead to vision loss, chronic kidney disease and foot ulceration. Macrovascular complications, such as coronary, cerebrovascular and peripheral arterial disease, increase the risk of heart attack, stroke and limb ischaemia. Acute metabolic emergencies include diabetic ketoacidosis, typically in type 1 diabetes, and hyperosmolar hyperglycaemic state, which is more common in type 2 diabetes.

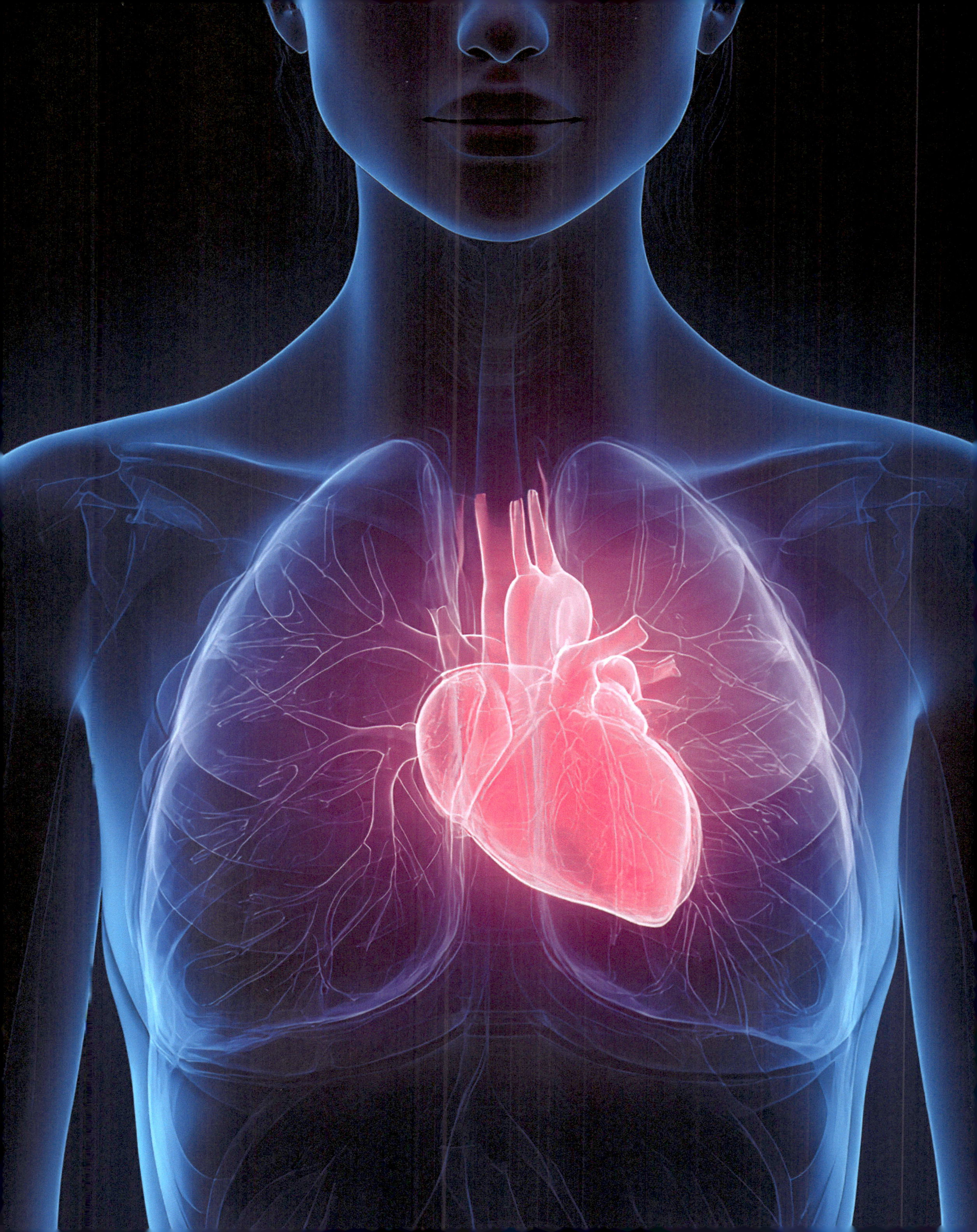

52 Adrenal insufficiency

Figure 52.1 The adrenal glands.

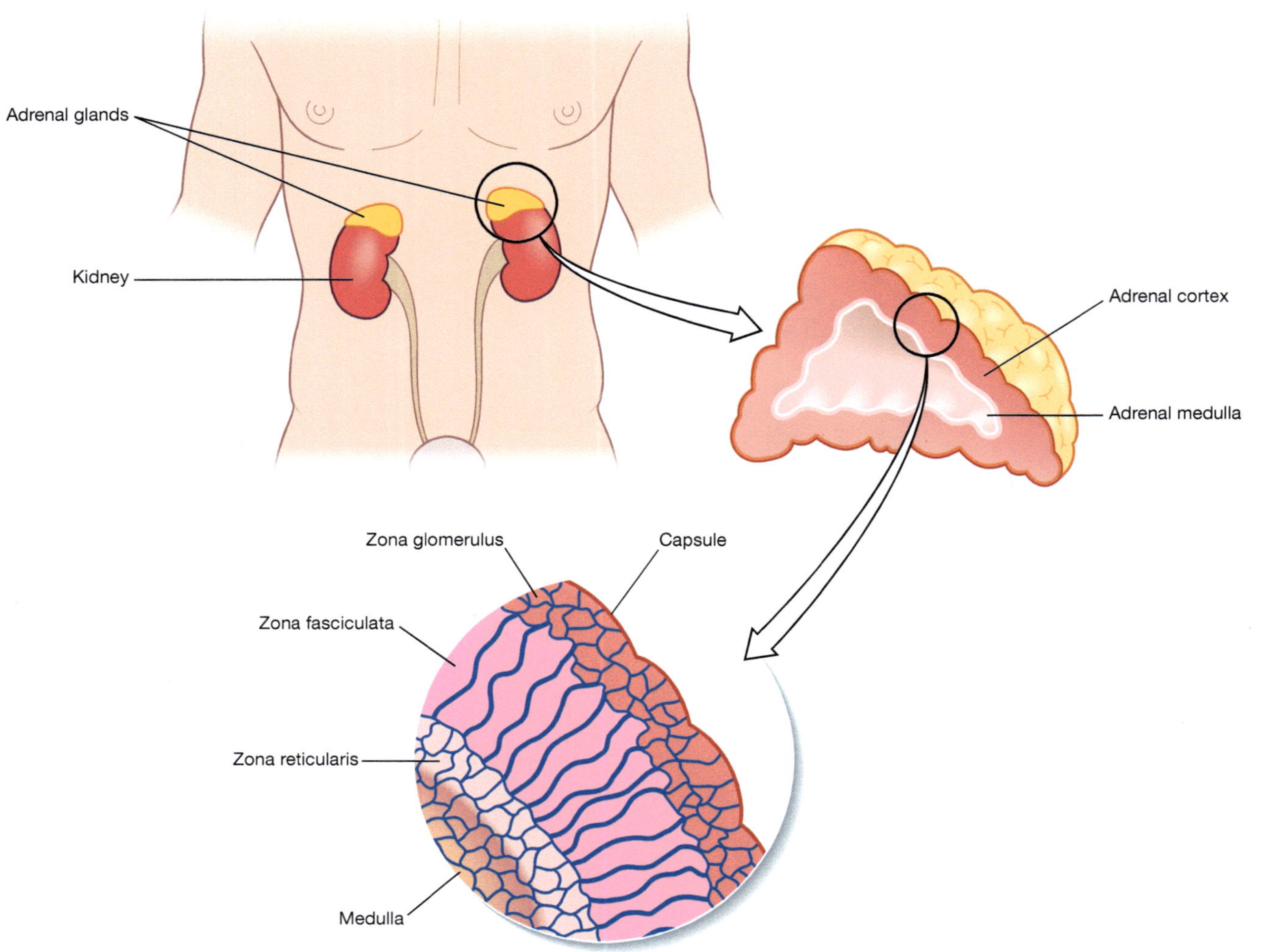

Box 52.1 Abnormal findings in adrenal insufficiency.

Sodium – reduced
Chloride – reduced
Bicarbonate – reduced
Potassium – increased
Uraemia
Hypoglycaemia
Abnormal liver function tests
Calcium – increased in 5–10%
Normocytic anaemia
Lymphocytosis
Moderate eosinophilia

The adrenal glands

The adrenal glands are located at the superior poles of the kidneys and consist of two distinct regions: the adrenal medulla and the adrenal cortex. The medulla functions as a neuroendocrine organ, working with the central nervous system to secrete epinephrine and norepinephrine in response to sympathetic stimulation.

The adrenal cortex is anatomically divided into three zones: the zona glomerulosa, zona fasciculata and zona reticularis. The outer zona glomerulosa secretes aldosterone, a mineralocorticoid that regulates sodium and potassium balance and thus contributes to fluid and electrolyte homeostasis. The zona fasciculata and zona reticularis secrete glucocorticoids (e.g. cortisol) and androgens.

Adrenocorticotropic hormone (ACTH) primarily stimulates the zona fasciculata to synthesise and secrete cortisol, which regulates carbohydrate, protein and lipid metabolism. Aldosterone secretion is mainly controlled by the renin–angiotensin–aldosterone system, although ACTH can exert a transient stimulatory effect. The adrenal cortex also produces smaller quantities of other corticosteroids with glucocorticoid, mineralocorticoid or mixed activity (see Figure 52.1).

Pathophysiology

Adrenal insufficiency occurs when there is a reduction in adrenal hormone output, particularly glucocorticoids and/or mineralocorticoids (these are two main classes of steroid hormones that are produced by the adrenal cortex).

Primary adrenal insufficiency arises from an intrinsic defect of the adrenal glands, which results in inadequate production of steroid hormones despite elevated ACTH levels from the pituitary. Autoimmune destruction of the adrenal cortex is the most common cause, which is known as Addison's disease. Both glucocorticoid and mineralocorticoid secretion are impaired in primary insufficiency.

Secondary adrenal insufficiency occurs due to inadequate pituitary or hypothalamic stimulation of the adrenal glands, leading predominantly to glucocorticoid deficiency, while mineralocorticoid secretion is usually preserved. A common cause is suppression of the hypothalamic–pituitary–adrenal (HPA) axis by exogenous glucocorticoids – taking glucocorticoid medications (steroids) from outside the body, such as prednisolone, hydrocortisone or dexamethasone, can suppress the body's natural hormone regulation system, which is the HPA axis. If there is rapid withdrawal of steroids or sudden physiological stress, this can precipitate an adrenal crisis, as cortisol production cannot immediately meet the body's increased demands.

Signs and symptoms

Adrenal insufficiency often develops gradually; its clinical presentation can be subtle and non-specific, which may delay recognition and diagnosis. Individuals typically experience generalised fatigue and weakness, which may be accompanied by weight loss.

In primary adrenal insufficiency, hyperpigmentation of the skin is a characteristic feature. It is often most noticeable in areas exposed to friction or pressure, such as the palmar creases, knuckles, elbows and knees, and may also be apparent on the oral mucosa. In people with darker skin, pigmentation changes may be subtle or diffuse, making examination of high-friction and mucosal areas particularly important.

Cardiovascular manifestations include hypotension and orthostatic hypotension, which can lead to syncope. Gastrointestinal symptoms are common and may include anorexia, nausea, vomiting, diarrhoea and salt craving, reflecting the electrolyte disturbances, particularly hyponatraemia, associated with mineralocorticoid deficiency. Musculoskeletal complaints such as myalgia and arthralgia are also reported.

Neuropsychiatric symptoms, including depression and lethargy, may be present; women may experience menstrual irregularities. Because these features are often mild or gradual in onset, they may be overlooked until a minor infection or physiological stress triggers a disproportionate response, resulting in prolonged illness or adrenal crisis.

Investigations

History and physical examination are essential, clinical features of adrenal insufficiency – fatigue, weakness and weight loss are often non-specific. Laboratory findings may include hyponatraemia and, in primary adrenal insufficiency, hyperkalaemia, with occasional anaemia. These abnormalities are not exclusive to adrenal insufficiency and can occur in a variety of other conditions.

The diagnosis is usually confirmed with the short Synacthen test (SST), also known as the ACTH stimulation test or cosyntropin test. This assesses the ability of the adrenal glands to produce cortisol in response to ACTH.

In primary adrenal insufficiency, the adrenal cortex itself is damaged, resulting in impaired secretion of glucocorticoids and mineralocorticoids. Biochemical hallmarks include hyponatraemia, hyperkalaemia and elevated ACTH levels.

In secondary adrenal insufficiency, the defect lies in pituitary or hypothalamic ACTH production; cortisol secretion is reduced but mineralocorticoid secretion is usually preserved, and potassium levels are typically normal.

Additional investigations may be indicated. These can include an electrocardiogram (ECG), abdominal imaging (CT or MRI) to assess adrenal morphology, and, in selected cases, a 24-hour urine collection to evaluate adrenal steroid metabolites. Abnormalities observed in adrenal insufficiency are illustrated in Box 52.1.

Management

Adrenal crisis is a life-threatening emergency that may be precipitated by physical stress, such as infection or surgery, or by emotional stress in individuals with adrenal insufficiency.

When an adrenal crisis is suspected, emergency hospital admission is required, and treatment should be initiated immediately, even before formal confirmation of the diagnosis. The SST can be performed once the patient is stabilised to confirm adrenal insufficiency.

Glucocorticoid replacement is the mainstay of treatment. In acute crises, hydrocortisone is administered parenterally. Patients with confirmed adrenal insufficiency who have been advised by their clinician may increase their usual glucocorticoid dose, typically doubling it, during intercurrent illness until recovery. If unable to take oral medication, parenteral administration should be initiated promptly under medical guidance. If oral administration is not possible, parenteral hydrocortisone is required.

Long-term hormone replacement therapy is only indicated in patients with confirmed adrenal insufficiency.

Secondary adrenal insufficiency can result from pituitary failure (panhypopituitarism) or from suppression of the HPA axis by steroids or certain medications, such as sodium valproate.

Other causes include pituitary or hypothalamic tumours, metastases, craniopharyngioma, tuberculosis, postpartum pituitary necrosis, trauma and surgery or radiotherapy. Hormone replacement therapy may be required until the underlying cause is definitively treated, for example, following surgical removal of a pituitary tumour.

Patient education is a critical component of care and should emphasise the importance of wearing a medical alert bracelet, carrying a steroid emergency card, and understanding stress dosing during illness or surgery.

Clinical considerations

Patients with confirmed adrenal insufficiency should wear a medical alert bracelet and carry a steroid emergency card at all times. This ensures that healthcare providers are immediately aware of the patient's condition in an emergency.

During periods of physical stress, illness or surgery, glucocorticoid doses may need to be temporarily increased, but only under the guidance of a clinician. Patients should also be trained to self-administer parenteral hydrocortisone if they are unable to take oral medication and should seek prompt medical attention if symptoms of adrenal crisis develop.

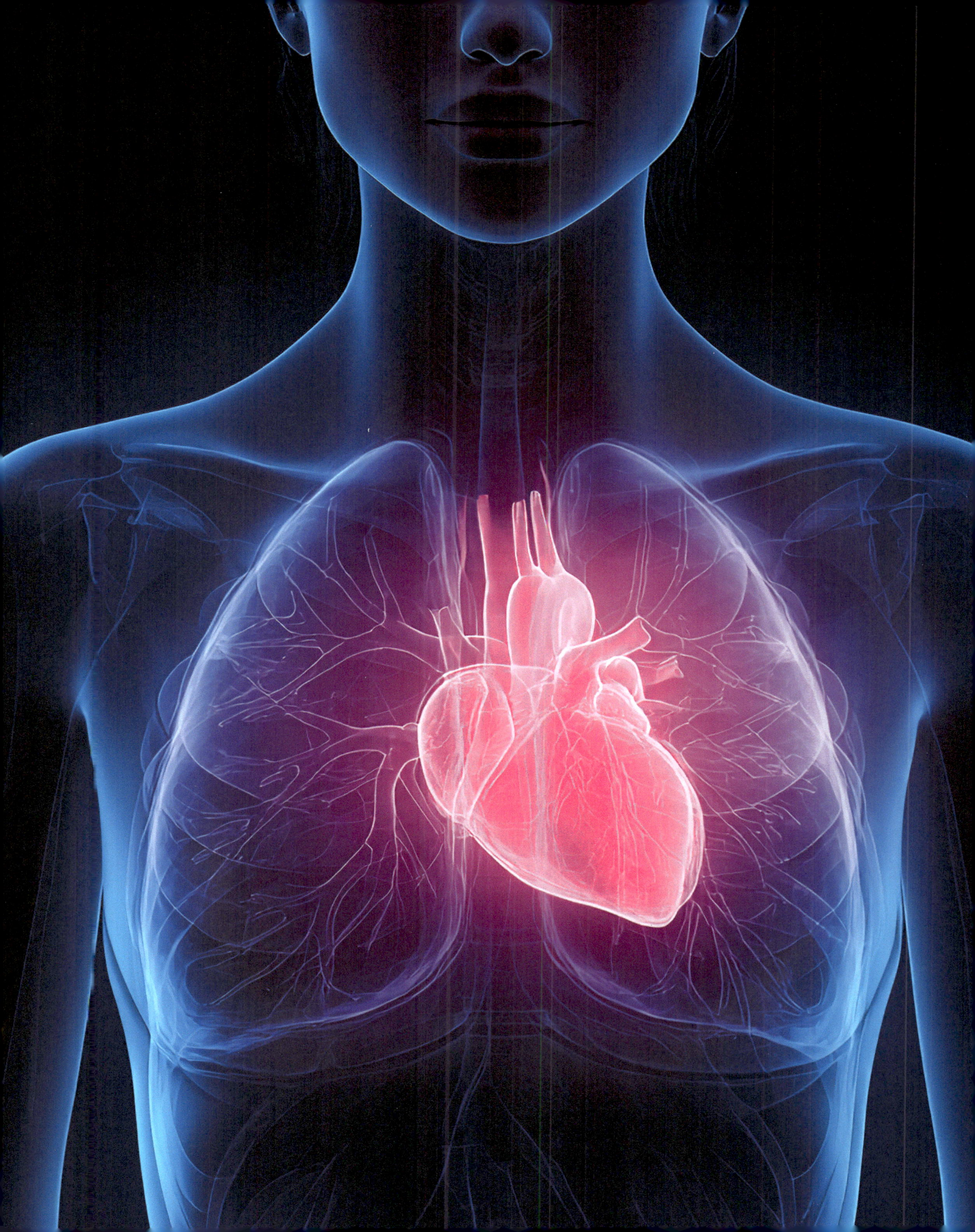

53 Cushing syndrome

Figure 53.1 Cushing's syndrome.

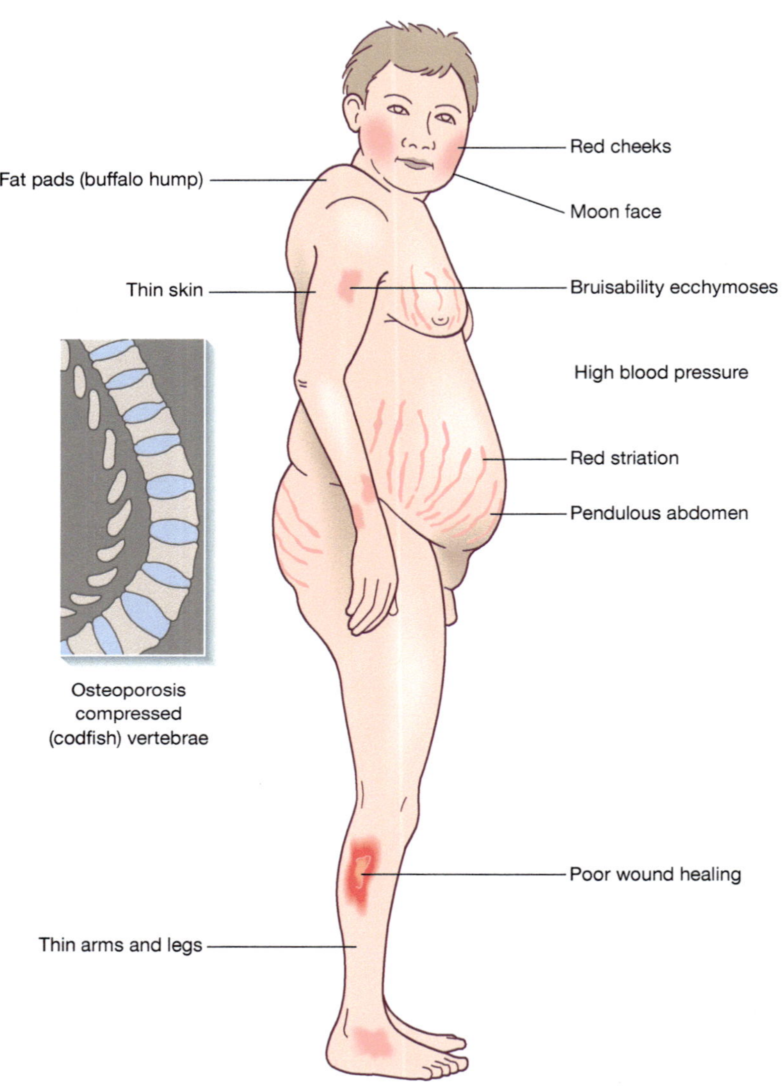

Cushing's syndrome results from excess levels of the glucocorticoid cortisol. It can arise from a variety of causes, and investigation is required to determine the underlying source of the cortisol excess.

Cushing's syndrome

Glucocorticoids

Glucocorticoids are a class of steroid hormones; along with mineralocorticoids and sex hormones, they have a central role in reducing inflammation throughout the body. Cortisol is the primary endogenous glucocorticoid and is produced by the adrenal glands; it regulates inflammation and influences carbohydrate, protein and lipid metabolism. Synthetic glucocorticoids, such as prednisone, dexamethasone and hydrocortisone, replicate these effects and are often more potent than natural cortisol. These medications act by entering cells and binding to glucocorticoid receptors, which modulate gene expression to suppress pro-inflammatory proteins and enhance anti-inflammatory proteins. Through these mechanisms, glucocorticoids are crucial in controlling inflammatory responses, immune activity and metabolic processes.

Pathophysiology

Cushing syndrome results from prolonged exposure to elevated levels of glucocorticoids, either endogenous or exogenous. In adrenocorticotropic hormone (ACTH)-dependent disease, excessive ACTH stimulates the adrenal cortex, overwhelming normal hypothalamic–pituitary–adrenal feedback. The most common cause is Cushing's disease, which is due to an anterior pituitary adenoma. Ectopic ACTH production from non-pituitary tumours, such as small-cell lung carcinoma or carcinoid tumours, accounts for other ACTH-dependent cases. Excess ACTH drives bilateral adrenal hyperplasia and persistent cortisol secretion.

In ACTH-independent disease, cortisol is secreted autonomously by adrenal adenomas or carcinomas or results from prolonged exogenous glucocorticoid therapy. In these cases, hypothalamic–pituitary feedback remains intact but is unable to suppress cortisol overproduction. Chronic glucocorticoid excess affects multiple systems, including carbohydrate, protein and lipid metabolism, the immune system and cardiovascular function, producing the characteristic features of Cushing syndrome, although other adrenal steroids may also be elevated in some cases.

Signs and symptoms

The clinical manifestations of Cushing syndrome arise from prolonged exposure to excessive glucocorticoids, and a thorough history and physical examination are essential for diagnosis (see Figure 53.1). In women, features may include menstrual irregularities, amenorrhoea, infertility and a decrease in libido, whereas men can often present with reduced sex drive and erectile dysfunction. Weight gain, particularly in the truncal region, a plethoric face ('moon face') and supraclavicular fat pads are common, alongside thin, fragile skin, easy bruising and purple striae.

Musculoskeletal effects may include proximal muscle weakness, osteoporosis and an increased risk of fractures, while metabolic complications often involve hyperglycaemia, insulin resistance and dyslipidaemia. Psychological manifestations range from depression and anxiety to cognitive impairment and emotional lability.

Patients with ACTH-producing pituitary tumours (Cushing disease) may also experience headaches, polyuria, nocturia, visual disturbances or galactorrhoea, and if the tumour exerts a mass effect, additional hormone deficiencies may develop, including growth hormone deficiency, hypothyroidism, hyperprolactinaemia or hypogonadism.

A rapid onset of glucocorticoid excess, especially when accompanied by virilisation (the development of male physical characteristics as a result of excessive androgen production) in women or feminisation in men, may suggest adrenal carcinoma as the underlying cause. Due to the significant morbidity and mortality associated with Cushing syndrome, early recognition, timely investigation and prompt management are critical to improve outcomes.

Investigations

Diagnosis of Cushing syndrome requires a combination of investigations, as no single test is definitive. Initial screening tests include the 24-hour urinary free cortisol, the 1 mg overnight low-dose dexamethasone suppression test and late-night salivary cortisol measurement. These tests help confirm cortisol excess.

Baseline investigations should include a full blood count and assessment of serum electrolytes, as hypokalaemia and metabolic alkalosis may occur.

Once hypercortisolism is confirmed, further investigations are performed to determine the underlying cause. These include plasma ACTH measurement, the high-dose dexamethasone suppression test and, when indicated, inferior petrosal sinus sampling to differentiate pituitary from ectopic ACTH secretion. MRI of the pituitary and CT imaging of the chest and abdomen may then be used to identify the source of ACTH or cortisol overproduction.

Management

Management of Cushing syndrome is guided by the underlying cause and aims to normalise cortisol levels, thereby reducing the morbidity and mortality that are associated with chronic glucocorticoid excess.

The definitive treatment for endogenous Cushing syndrome is surgical resection of the causative tumour. This may involve transsphenoidal surgery for pituitary adenomas (Cushing disease), adrenalectomy for adrenal tumours, or resection of ectopic ACTH-secreting tumours when feasible. Pituitary radiotherapy may be considered in cases of persistent hypercortisolism following surgery, and bilateral adrenalectomy may be required when cortisol levels remain uncontrollable.

Medical therapy is indicated for patients who are acutely unwell, awaiting surgery, have inoperable or unidentified tumours, are unfit for surgery, or have persistent hypercortisolism postoperatively. Drugs such as ketoconazole, metyrapone and mitotane reduce cortisol synthesis by inhibiting adrenal steroidogenesis (they block the biochemical pathways inside the adrenal glands that produce cortisol). These agents may also be used as long-term therapy in selected cases.

Because of the metabolic effects of hypercortisolism, including tissue fragility, impaired wound healing, hypertension and diabetes mellitus, perioperative management requires careful planning with the patient at the centre of all that is done.

54 Hyperthyroidism

Figure 54.1 Location of the thyroid gland.

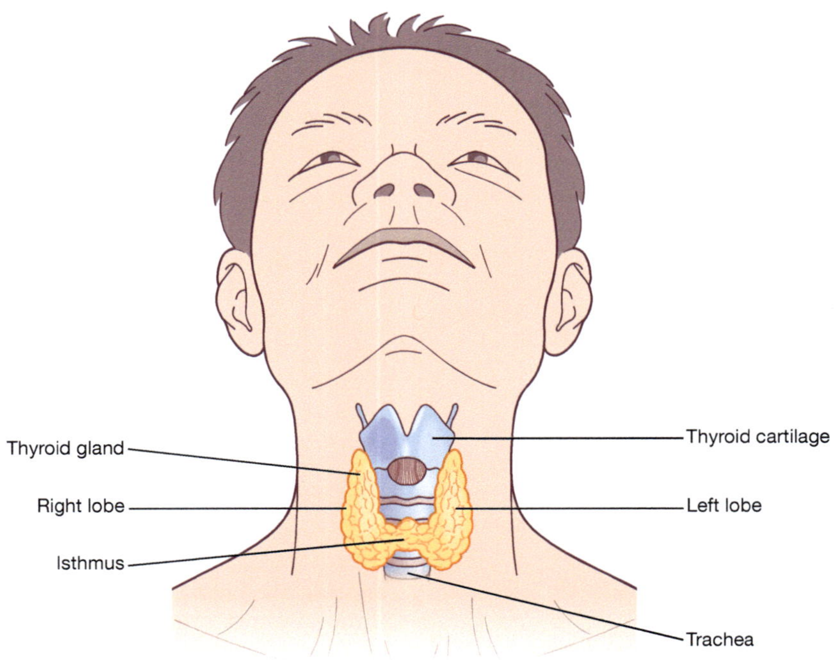

Figure 54.2 Hypothalamic-pituitary-thyroid axis feedback.

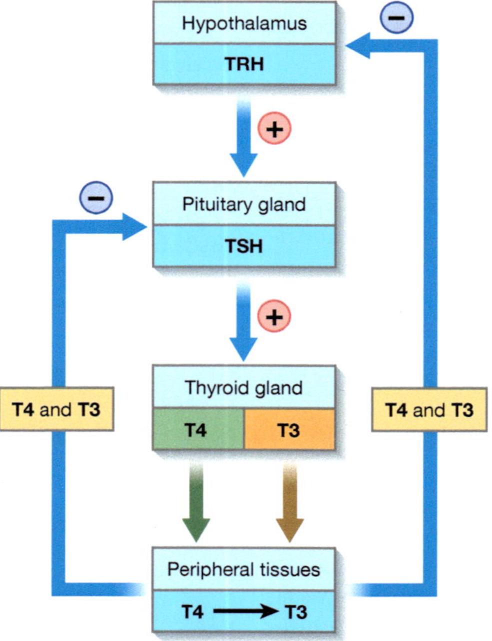

The thyroid gland

The thyroid gland is a highly vascular, butterfly shaped organ located in the lower anterior neck, anterior to the trachea, with two lateral lobes connected by a narrow isthmus (see Figure 54.1). In its normal state, the gland is usually non-palpable. The recurrent laryngeal nerves run posteriorly in the tracheo-oesophageal groove, while the external branch of the superior laryngeal nerve lies close to the superior poles, making careful anatomical knowledge essential during thyroid surgery.

The thyroid synthesises and secretes two primary hormones, thyroxine (T4) and triiodothyronine (T3), in response to thyroid-stimulating hormone (TSH) from the anterior pituitary, which is itself regulated by thyrotropin-releasing hormone (TRH) from the hypothalamus. T4 is produced in greater amounts than T3 and functions as a prohormone, converted peripherally in the liver, kidney and other tissues into the more active T3. Most circulating thyroid hormone is protein-bound to thyroxine-binding globulin, transthyretin and albumin; only the free fraction is biologically active.

Thyroid hormones regulate basal metabolic rate, protein, carbohydrate and lipid metabolism, and influence thermoregulation, growth and organ development. Negative feedback by free T3 and T4 on the hypothalamus and pituitary modulates TRH and TSH secretion, maintaining hormonal balance (see Figure 54.2). Adequate thyroid hormone levels are critical for normal brain development during infancy and childhood. Dysfunction, whether hypo- or hyperthyroidism, can have widespread systemic effects, highlighting the gland's central role in maintaining metabolic and physiological homeostasis.

Hyperthyroidism

Hyperthyroidism encompasses disorders in which the thyroid gland produces and secretes excess thyroid hormones, resulting in thyrotoxicosis, a hypermetabolic clinical state. The most common causes include diffuse toxic goitre (Graves' disease), toxic multinodular goitre and toxic adenoma.

Hyperthyroidism may be classified as primary or secondary. In primary hyperthyroidism, the pathology originates within the thyroid gland itself. Secondary hyperthyroidism occurs when the thyroid is overstimulated by elevated circulating TSH, usually due to pituitary disease. Rarely, excessive TRH from the hypothalamus can cause tertiary hyperthyroidism.

Pathophysiology

Graves' disease is an autoimmune disorder with a genetic predisposition, arising from the interplay between inherited susceptibility and environmental triggers. Certain genes increase the likelihood of developing Graves' disease, and the specific genes or variants involved can differ depending on a person's ethnic background. Environmental and lifestyle factors, such as smoking, high dietary iodine intake, thyroid trauma or surgery, the postpartum period, and certain medications (including amiodarone and highly active antiretroviral therapy), can act as triggers, initiating the autoimmune process in genetically susceptible individuals.

The hallmark of Graves' disease is the presence of thyrotropin receptor autoantibodies (TRAb) in the circulation. These antibodies bind to and activate the TSH receptor on thyroid follicular cells, providing continuous stimulation independent of pituitary regulation. This leads to increased thyroid hormone synthesis and release, enhanced iodine uptake, accelerated thyroglobulin and protein production, and thyroid gland hyperplasia, producing a characteristic diffuse goitre.

The resulting excess circulating free thyroid hormones cause thyrotoxicosis, a hypermetabolic state that affects nearly every organ system. At the cellular level, thyroid hormones increase transcription of target genes, raising the basal metabolic rate and altering energy use, cardiovascular function, thermoregulation and neuropsychiatric function. Understanding this pathophysiology underpins both the diagnosis and targeted treatment of Graves' disease.

Signs and symptoms

The presentation of thyrotoxicosis is highly variable, reflecting the systemic effects of excess thyroid hormone. Increased sympathetic nervous system activity produces anxiety, hyperactivity, tremor, palpitations and hyperreflexia, which are more prominent in younger patients. Older adults often present with cardiovascular manifestations, including dyspnoea, atrial fibrillation or angina, while classic sympathetic symptoms may be subtle or absent, a pattern sometimes referred to as apathetic hyperthyroidism.

The hypermetabolic state leads to heat intolerance, increased perspiration and variable weight changes. Weight loss is common, even with increased appetite, although some patients may gain weight if caloric intake rises. Fatigue is frequently reported, particularly in the late afternoon or evening, and insomnia, irritability and emotional lability are common. Muscle weakness, particularly of the proximal muscles, can further limit daily activities.

Other clinical features may include goitre, fine hair, warm, moist skin and, in Graves' disease, ophthalmopathy or pretibial myxoedema. The onset of symptoms is usually gradual, often developing over weeks to months, which may delay recognition. Importantly, the severity of clinical manifestations does not always correlate with biochemical thyroid hormone levels, and careful clinical assessment, including a detailed history and physical examination, is essential for diagnosis and management.

Investigations

A thorough medical history is essential when evaluating patients with suspected thyrotoxicosis. Clinicians should assess the duration and severity of symptoms, as well as past medical and family history, which, together with physical examination findings, guide diagnosis. Graves' disease, an autoimmune disorder, often occurs in individuals with a personal or family history of autoimmune conditions, such as rheumatoid arthritis, vitiligo or pernicious anaemia. Additional relevant history includes exposure to iodine-deficient regions or dietary patterns affecting thyroid function.

A careful review of medications and supplements is important, as substances such as amiodarone, iodinated contrast or supplements containing seaweed or thyroid extracts may precipitate or worsen thyrotoxicosis in susceptible individuals.

Laboratory assessment begins with thyroid function tests. Suppressed TSH is the initial indicator of primary hyperthyroidism, confirmed by elevated free T4 or T3. Detection of TSH-TRAb supports a diagnosis of Graves' disease.

Imaging studies further characterise the thyroid. Ultrasound assesses gland morphology, nodularity and vascularity, while radioactive iodine uptake scans differentiate hyperfunctioning 'hot' nodules from non-functioning 'cold' areas. Integrating history, examination, laboratory results and imaging enables clinicians to confirm thyrotoxicosis and identify its underlying cause, guiding appropriate management.

Management

Management of thyrotoxicosis begins with symptom control. Beta-blockers are commonly used to reduce palpitations, tremor and anxiety, with non-selective agents like propranolol also decreasing peripheral conversion of T4 to T3. Calcium-channel blockers may be considered in patients unable to tolerate beta-blockers. Definitive treatment consists of:

- Antithyroid drugs: carbimazole is the first choice; propylthiouracil is reserved for specific situations such as early pregnancy.
- Radioiodine therapy: selectively used in adults and occasionally in teenagers, depending on local guidance.
- Surgery: subtotal or near-total thyroidectomy, indicated for large goitres, malignancy risk or contraindications to other treatments.

Clinical considerations

Effective management of Graves' disease depends on concordance to antithyroid medications, such as carbimazole or propylthiouracil. Consistent use controls thyrotoxicosis, alleviates symptoms and reduces the risk of complications. Poor concordance can lead to persistent hyperthyroidism, relapse and reduced likelihood of remission.

Patients require regular thyroid function monitoring to guide dose adjustments and should be informed about potential side effects and the need to report symptoms such as rash, fever or jaundice. Symptomatic treatments, such as beta-blockers, should also be used as prescribed.

The musculoskeletal system

Chapters

 55 Osteoarthritis

Figure 55.1 Osteoarthritis.

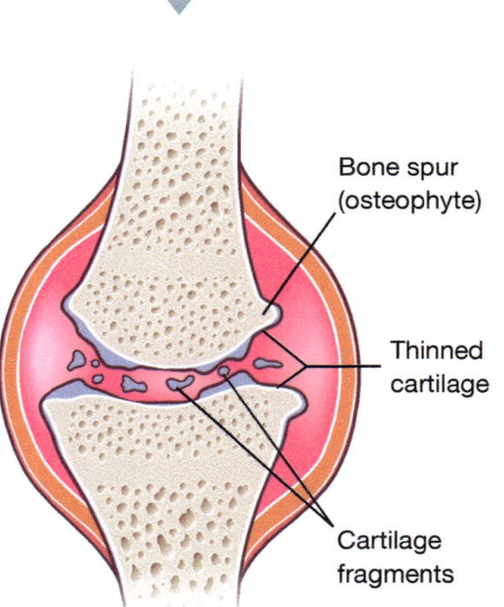

Figure 55.2 Classification of joints.

Type of joint	Examples		Structure
Hinge	Elbow, knee	Humerus / Trochlea / Trochlear notch / Ulna	
Pivot	Radius and ulna, the atlas and axis	Radial notch / Head of radius / Annular ligament / Radius / Ulna	
Ball and socket	Hip, shoulder	Acetabulum of hip bone / Head of femur	
Saddle	The carpometacarpal joints of the thumb	Radius / Ulna / Trapezium / Metacarpal of thumb	
Condyloid	The radiocarpal and metacarpophalangeal joints of the hand	Radius / Ulna / Scaphoid / Lunate	
Gliding	Intertarsal and intercarpal joints of the hands and feet	Navicular / Second cuneiform / Third cuneiform	

Source: Peate, Wild & Nair, *Nursing Practice: Knowledge and Care,* 2014

Joints

Synovial joints are composed of articular cartilage, subchondral bone, a synovial membrane, synovial fluid and a fibrous joint capsule. Articular cartilage is composed of chondrocytes embedded in an extracellular matrix rich in type II collagen and proteoglycans. This structure distributes mechanical load, maintains low contact stress and provides smooth articulation, protecting underlying bone. Synovial fluid, produced by synoviocytes, contains hyaluronic acid, which ensures lubrication, shock absorption and nutrient delivery to the avascular cartilage.

Joints can be classified functionally as synarthroses (immovable), amphiarthroses (slightly moveable) and diarthroses (freely moveable), or structurally as synovial, fibrous and cartilaginous. Osteoarthritis (OA) primarily affects diarthrodial (synovial) joints, where movement and load contribute to cartilage stress (see Figure 55.1).

Risk factors include age, genetic predisposition, joint injury, obesity, and repetitive mechanical stress. Biomechanical and biochemical processes combine, leading to cartilage degradation, synovial inflammation and subchondral bone sclerosis. Loss of cartilage increases friction, and osteophyte formation alters joint shape, contributing to pain, stiffness and reduced mobility.

Understanding joint anatomy and the early pathophysiology of OA is essential for recognising clinical features, planning management strategies and implementing preventative measures to slow disease progression.

OA is the most common type of joint disease and represents a degenerative disorder of the synovial joints. It arises from the biochemical breakdown of articular cartilage, leading to cartilage loss, subchondral bone changes and the formation of osteophytes (bone spurs). OA is not limited to cartilage; it affects the entire joint organ, including the subchondral bone, synovium, ligaments and periarticular muscles (see Figure 55.2). Early changes in OA include cartilage softening, fibrillation (in this context fibrillation refers to the development of tiny cracks or fraying on the surface of the articular cartilage) and altered load distribution, which can accelerate joint degeneration.

Pathophysiology

OA is the most common joint disorder; it represents a degenerative, whole-joint disease. It primarily affects weight-bearing joints; these include the knees, hips and spine, as well as the distal interphalangeal joints, though any synovial joint may be involved. OA can be isolated to a single joint, or it may affect multiple joints; this can cause pain, stiffness, reduced mobility and functional limitations, with significant psychosocial and socioeconomic consequences.

Risk factors include increasing age, female sex, obesity, joint trauma, repetitive mechanical stress and genetic predisposition. Hormonal changes, such as decreased sex hormones, and previous inflammatory arthritis, metabolic disorders, haemoglobinopathies (these are genetic disorders affecting the structure or production of haemoglobin) or neuropathic disorders can contribute. Prior joint surgery, such as meniscectomy, and systemic conditions, including acromegaly or crystal deposition, may also increase susceptibility. These factors disrupt the balance between cartilage degradation and repair, triggering progressive joint degeneration.

Pathophysiologically, OA involves damage to multiple joint tissues. Articular cartilage undergoes focal degeneration, with loss of proteoglycans and disruption of the collagen network, reducing elasticity and water retention. The cartilage surface develops fissures and fibrillations, increasing friction accompanied by accelerating wear. Subchondral bone responds with sclerosis, cyst formation and osteophyte development, which alter stress distribution across the joint. Fragmentation of cartilage or osteophytes can produce loose intra-articular bodies; these contribute to mechanical symptoms such as locking and crepitus.

The synovium and synovial fluid are also affected in OA. Altered synovial fluid viscosity and decreased hyaluronic acid result in reduced lubrication and nutrient delivery to the avascular cartilage. The joint lining becomes mildly inflamed, and chemicals released by the cells break down cartilage and other joint tissues. Over time, the joint capsule, ligaments and periarticular musculature may thicken or adapt, further compromising the function of the joint.

OA is therefore a progressive disorder of joint tissue homeostasis, in which mechanical, biochemical and inflammatory processes interact. These changes highlight the clinical features of OA, including pain, stiffness, reduced range of motion and functional impairment. Understanding these mechanisms allows clinicians to interpret imaging findings, anticipate complications and implement targeted management strategies with the patient that are aimed at slowing disease progression, preserving joint mobility and improving the person's quality of life.

Signs and symptoms

OA typically develops gradually over years or decades, and early structural changes in the joint may occur without causing noticeable symptoms. Joints may appear normal initially, and patients may remain active without any obvious impairment. Pain is often the first symptom, usually described as a deep, achy discomfort that worsens with activity and improves with rest. Crepitus, which is a grating or crackling sensation during joint movement, may also be present.

Stiffness can develop, particularly after periods of inactivity, such as in the morning, though in OA it is usually brief and lasts less than 30 minutes. As the disease progresses, pain can occur even at rest and may become less responsive to simple analgesia. Reduced range of movement, joint swelling or synovitis, periarticular tenderness and bony enlargement or deformity may develop. Muscle weakness or wasting around the affected joint is also common, contributing to reduced joint stability and function.

Patients often reduce their activity as a result of the discomfort they are experiencing, which may increase susceptibility to complications related to immobility, such as cardiovascular deconditioning or reduced muscle mass. Understanding the gradual onset and progression of OA symptoms, along with characteristic clinical findings, is essential for early recognition, timely imaging and appropriate management to maintain joint function and quality of life.

Investigations

OA is primarily diagnosed through a detailed clinical assessment. Plain radiographs can demonstrate structural changes in more advanced disease, including joint space narrowing, osteophyte formation, subchondral sclerosis and cysts. MRI may be useful in selected cases to assess cartilage integrity, detect early joint changes or exclude other causes of joint pain. In patients with acutely swollen joints, joint aspiration may be performed to rule out inflammatory or infective arthritis, although it is not routinely required in typical OA.

Management

The goals of OA treatment are to relieve pain, maintain or improve joint function and enhance quality of life. Management is multi-modal, incorporating non-pharmacological approaches such as structured exercise, physiotherapy, weight management, patient education and use of supportive aids. Pharmacological therapy may include analgesics, non-steroidal anti-inflammatory drugs, topical agents or intra-articular corticosteroid injections for symptom relief. Treatment should be individualised according to symptom severity, comorbidities and patient preferences. National guidelines, such as those from the National Institute for Health and Care Excellence, provide evidence-based recommendations for the assessment and management of OA.

Clinical considerations

Maintaining mobility is key to managing osteoarthritis. Regular, low-impact exercise strengthens muscles, supports joint stability and reduces stiffness. Weight management and appropriate use of supportive aids help protect joints and slow disease progression. Patients should be encouraged to remain active within their limits, as prolonged rest can worsen stiffness and muscle weakness. Emphasise adherence to tailored exercise programmes to preserve function and quality of life.

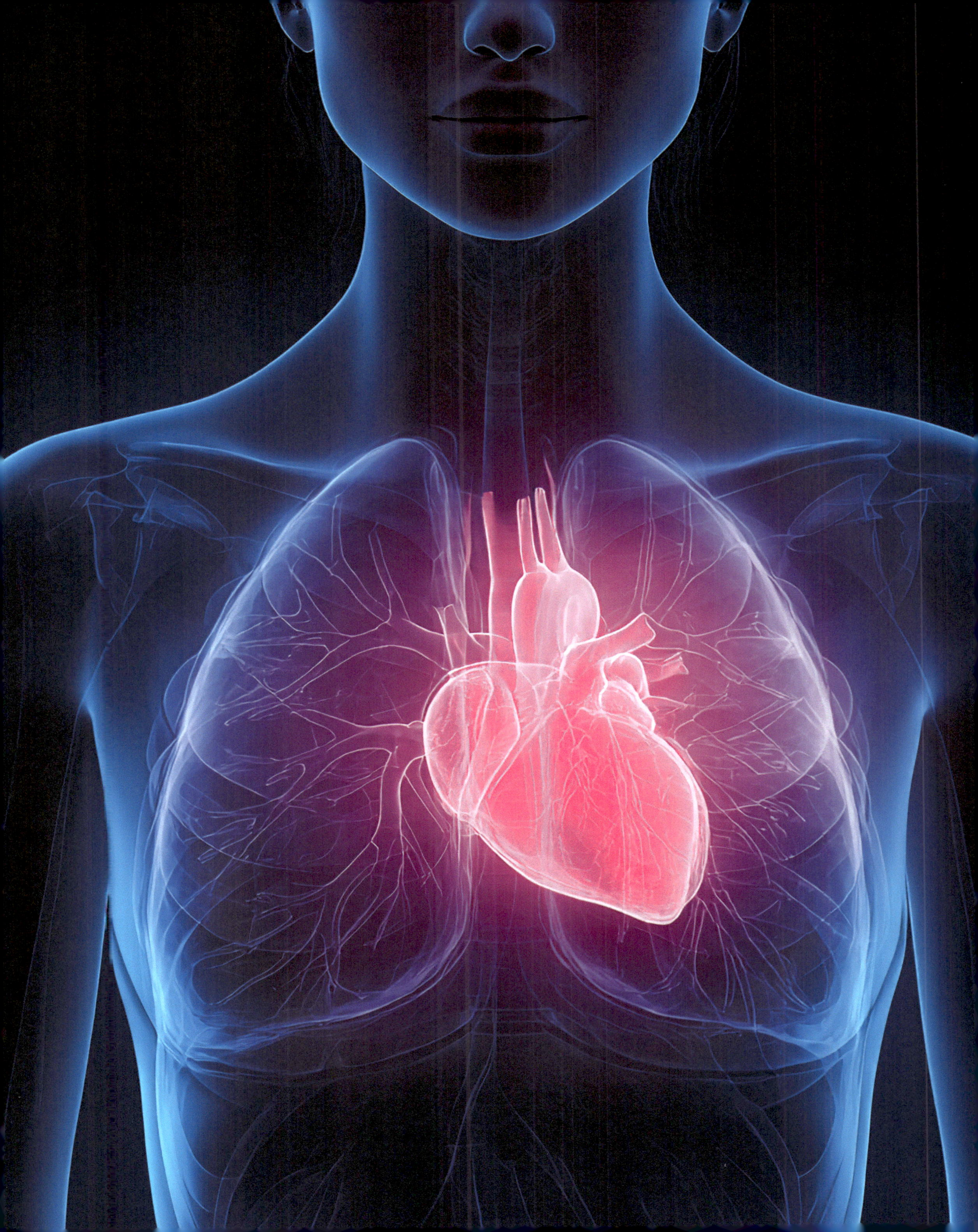

56 Osteoporosis

Figure 56.1   A healthy and an osteoporotic bone.

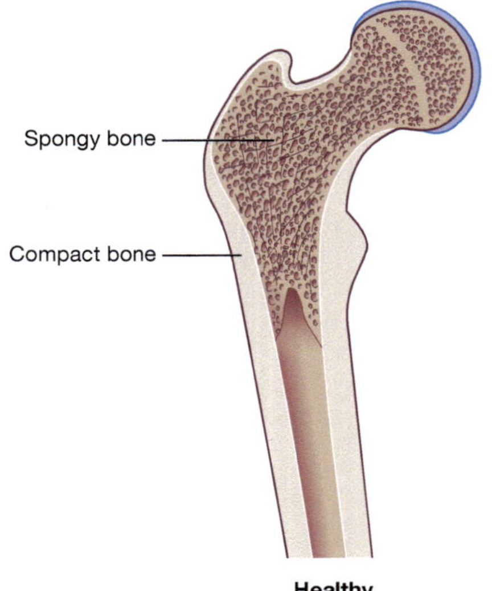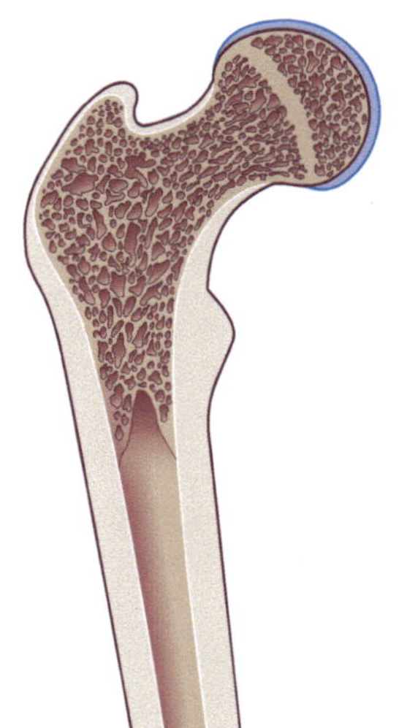

Table 56.1   Risk factors.

• Increasing age	• Corticosteroid therapy	• Anorexia nervosa	• Primary hyperparathyroidism
• Reduced BMD	• Cushing's syndrome	• Poor diet (calcium-deficient)	• Hyperthyroidism
• Parental history of hip fracture	• Ankylosing spondylitis	• Malabsorption syndromes (coeliac disease)	• Osteogenesis imperfecta
• Four or more units of alcohol daily	• Crohn's disease	• Prolonged immobilization	• Caucasian or Asian origin
• Rheumatoid arthritis	• Untreated premature menopause or prolonged secondary amenorrhoea	• Smoking	• Post-transplantation
• Female gender	• Low body mass (<19 kg/m^2)	• Primary hypogonadism (men and women)	• Chronic renal failure

Figure 56.2   Osteoporosis.

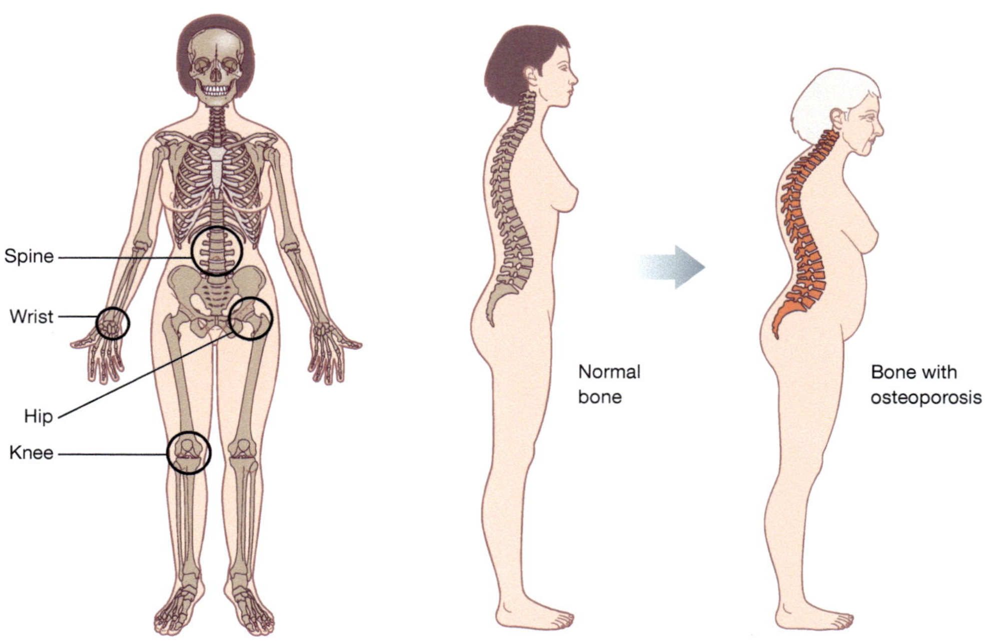

Osteoporosis

Osteoporosis is a chronic, progressive skeletal disorder of multifactorial aetiology, characterised by low bone mass and deterioration of bone microarchitecture, which together increase bone fragility and susceptibility to fracture (see Figure 56.1). The condition is often clinically silent until a fragility fracture occurs, commonly affecting the spine, wrist, hip or shoulder (see Figure 56.2). Such fractures can result in significant pain, loss of mobility, disability and reduced quality of life, emphasising the importance of early recognition and prevention.

Because osteoporosis may remain undetected for many years, its consequences are frequently underestimated and undertreated. Identifying individuals at risk, providing education and implementing preventive strategies, including lifestyle modification, fall prevention and optimisation of bone health, are central to mitigating morbidity. Secondary causes of osteoporosis, such as endocrine disorders, medication effects or chronic disease, should also be considered and addressed.

Bone mass peaks in early adulthood, typically around 30 years of age, when bone formation exceeds resorption. With ageing, this balance reverses, leading to progressive net bone loss. Bone mineral density (BMD), as defined by the World Health Organization, remains the standard for diagnosis, particularly in postmenopausal women and men aged 50 years and older. Osteoporotic fractures are defined as those resulting from low-energy mechanical forces that would not normally cause fracture.

Prevention, early diagnosis and management of osteoporosis are essential to reduce the burden of fractures and associated complications. Interventions aimed at maintaining bone strength, preserving mobility and minimising fall risk can significantly improve long-term outcomes and quality of life for affected individuals.

Pathophysiology

Osteoporosis is a systemic skeletal disorder, characterised by low bone mass and microarchitectural deterioration; this results in increased bone fragility and susceptibility to fractures. The condition arises from an imbalance in bone remodelling, in which bone resorption by osteoclasts exceeds bone formation by osteoblasts. Although bone remains normally mineralised, the loss of bone quantity and quality will compromise structural integrity.

Ageing is a major contributing factor, with reduced osteoblast number and activity over time. In postmenopausal women, oestrogen deficiency accelerates bone loss by promoting osteoclast survival and activity. Oestrogen modulates bone metabolism both directly, via receptors on osteoblasts, osteocytes and osteoclasts, and indirectly through cytokines and local growth factors. In men, age-related declines in sex hormones also contribute to bone loss, though this is typically at a slower rate.

Secondary factors can further exacerbate osteoporosis. Immobilisation, prolonged bed rest or reduced mechanical loading diminishes bone strength. Excess glucocorticoids, chronic inflammatory diseases, hyperthyroidism or hypogonadism disrupt bone remodelling. Adequate calcium and vitamin D are essential for bone homeostasis; deficiencies can induce secondary hyperparathyroidism, increasing bone resorption. Parathyroid hormone (PTH) responds to low serum calcium by mobilising calcium from bone, reducing renal excretion and stimulating active vitamin D production to enhance intestinal absorption, thereby maintaining calcium balance.

The pathophysiological changes preferentially affect trabecular bone, explaining why vertebral bodies, distal radius, hip and pelvis are common fracture sites. Microarchitectural deterioration includes thinning of trabeculae, increased cortical porosity and compromised connectivity, contributing to bone fragility. Cytokines, including interleukins and tumour necrosis factor-alpha, mediate low-grade inflammation that accelerates matrix degradation.

Fragility fractures are often the first clinical manifestation, occurring with minimal trauma. Vertebral fractures may be asymptomatic but lead to height loss and kyphosis, whereas hip fractures carry significant morbidity and mortality. Recognition of the underlying pathophysiology informs both preventive and therapeutic strategies, including weight-bearing exercise, optimisation of calcium and vitamin D intake and pharmacological interventions such as bisphosphonates, denosumab or anabolic agents, which aim to restore bone strength and reduce fracture risk.

Signs and symptoms

Osteoporosis develops gradually and is typically asymptomatic, often only becoming apparent after a fragility fracture. Many individuals may have few or no symptoms, or only minor risk factors, making early identification challenging. Fractures and reduced mobility can lead to chronic pain, loss of independence and a fear of falling, which may result in anxiety, depression and social isolation, highlighting the substantial psychological and quality-of-life burden associated with the condition (Table 56.1).

Investigations

Diagnosis of osteoporosis centres on the measurement of BMD using dual-energy X-ray absorptiometry (DEXA), which remains the gold standard for diagnosis and fracture risk assessment. In individuals with confirmed or suspected osteoporosis, screening blood tests should be performed to identify reversible secondary causes. These typically include full blood count, urea and electrolytes, liver and thyroid function tests, serum calcium, alkaline phosphatase, serum protein electrophoresis or immunoglobulins (with urinary Bence-Jones proteins) and, in men, testosterone and gonadotrophin levels.

Management

Management focuses on preventing fragility fractures through a combination of lifestyle modification and pharmacological therapy. Non-pharmacological strategies include regular weight-bearing and muscle-strengthening exercise, smoking cessation, moderation of alcohol intake, and ensuring adequate calcium and vitamin D intake, either through diet or supplementation.

Pharmacological interventions aim to reduce fracture risk rather than reverse established bone loss. First-line agents include bisphosphonates (e.g. alendronate, risedronate and zoledronic acid). Alternatives, depending on tolerance and clinical profile, include denosumab, selective oestrogen receptor modulators (e.g. raloxifene), PTH analogues (e.g. teriparatide) or hormone replacement therapy (HRT) in selected women. Secondary causes such as hyperthyroidism or hyperparathyroidism should be identified and treated.

Surgical options, including vertebroplasty and kyphoplasty, may be considered for selected patients with painful vertebral compression fractures unresponsive to conservative measures. Pain management should be optimised with appropriate analgesia, physiotherapy and supportive measures such as mechanical supports or thoracic orthoses to aid mobility and reduce discomfort. Hip protectors may be considered for frail individuals at high risk of falls.

Clinical considerations

Prevention focuses on maximising bone strength and reducing fracture risk. Adequate calcium and vitamin D, regular weight-bearing exercise and avoidance of smoking and excess alcohol are key. In older adults, fall prevention through balance training, vision checks and medication review is essential. Identifying secondary causes of bone loss, such as corticosteroid use or endocrine disorders, supports early intervention and reduces long-term complications.

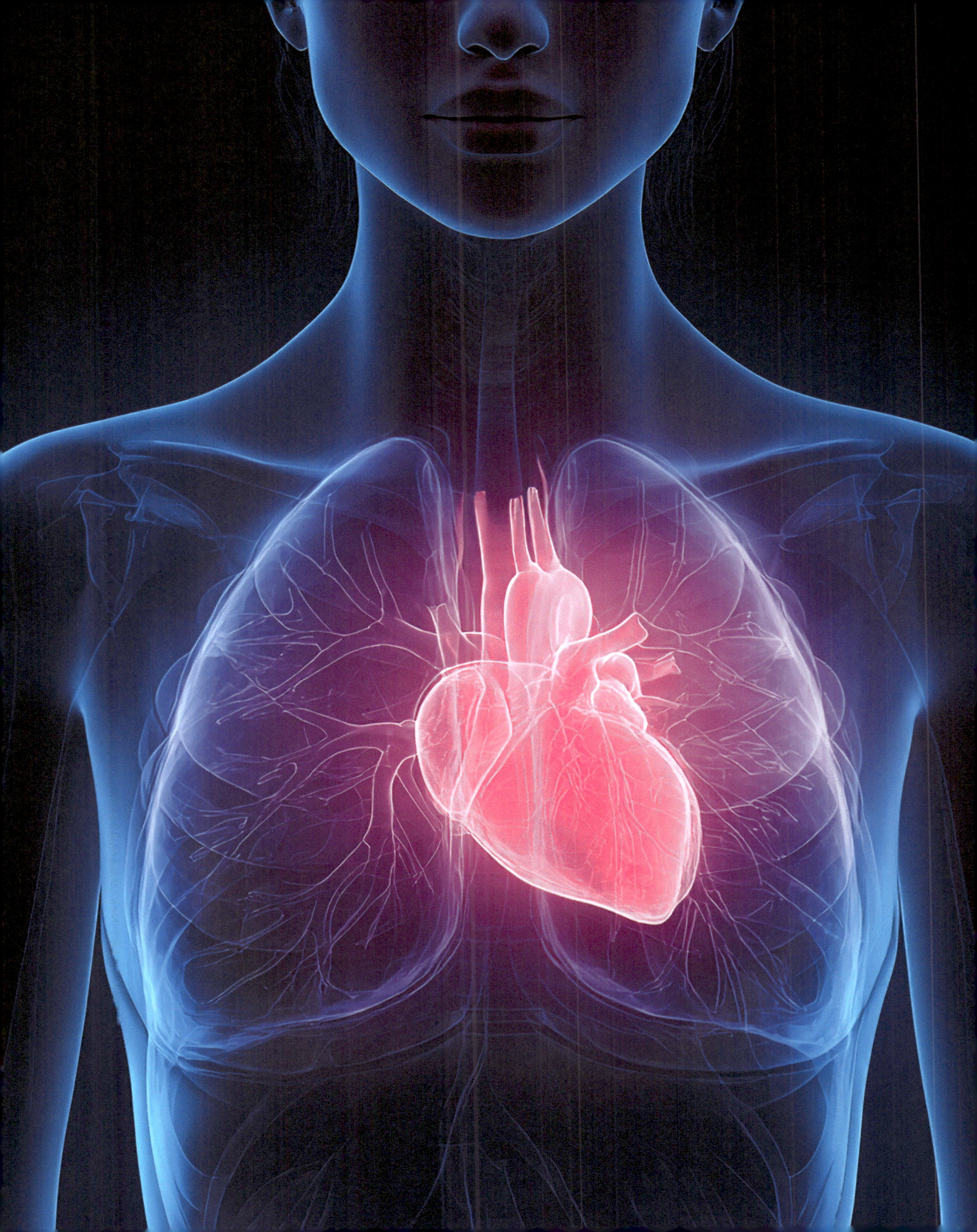

57 Osteomyelitis

Figure 57.1 Histology of bone.

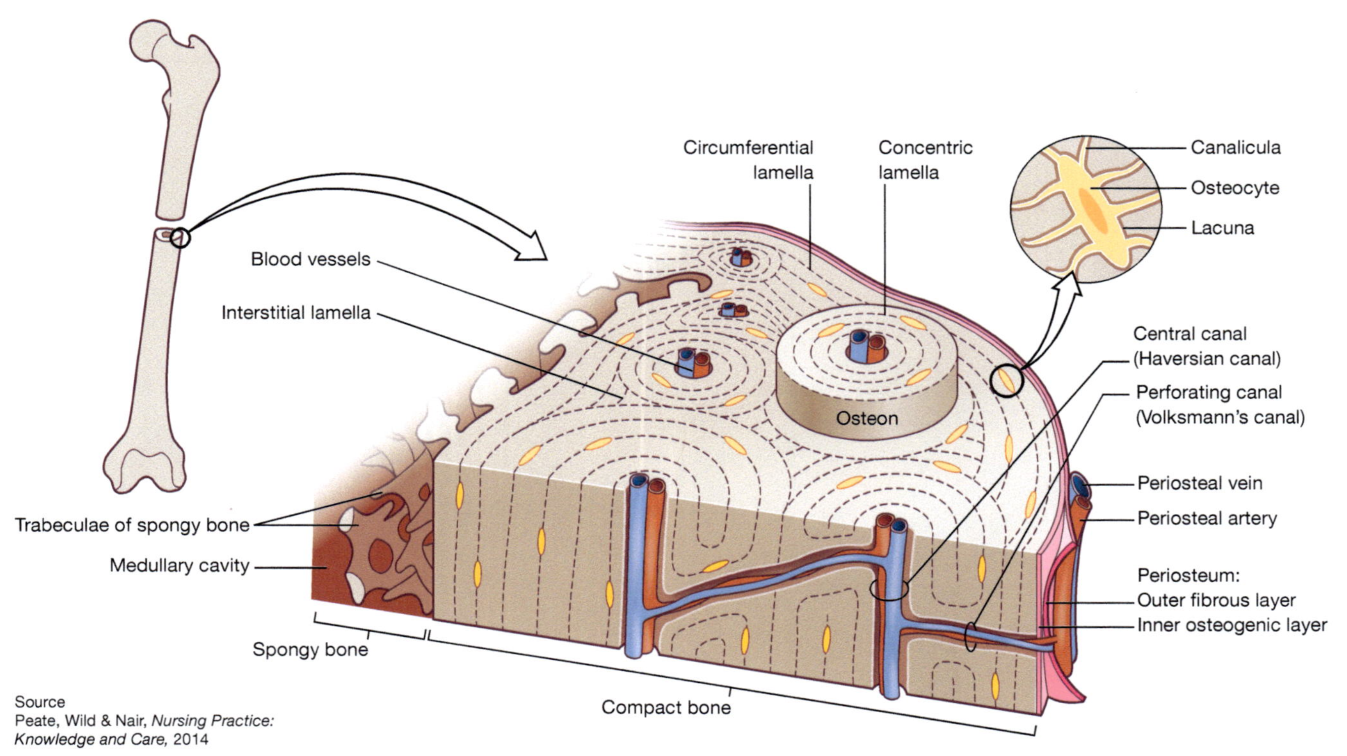

Source
Peate, Wild & Nair, *Nursing Practice: Knowledge and Care,* 2014

Figure 57.2 Bone infection in chronic osteomyelitis.

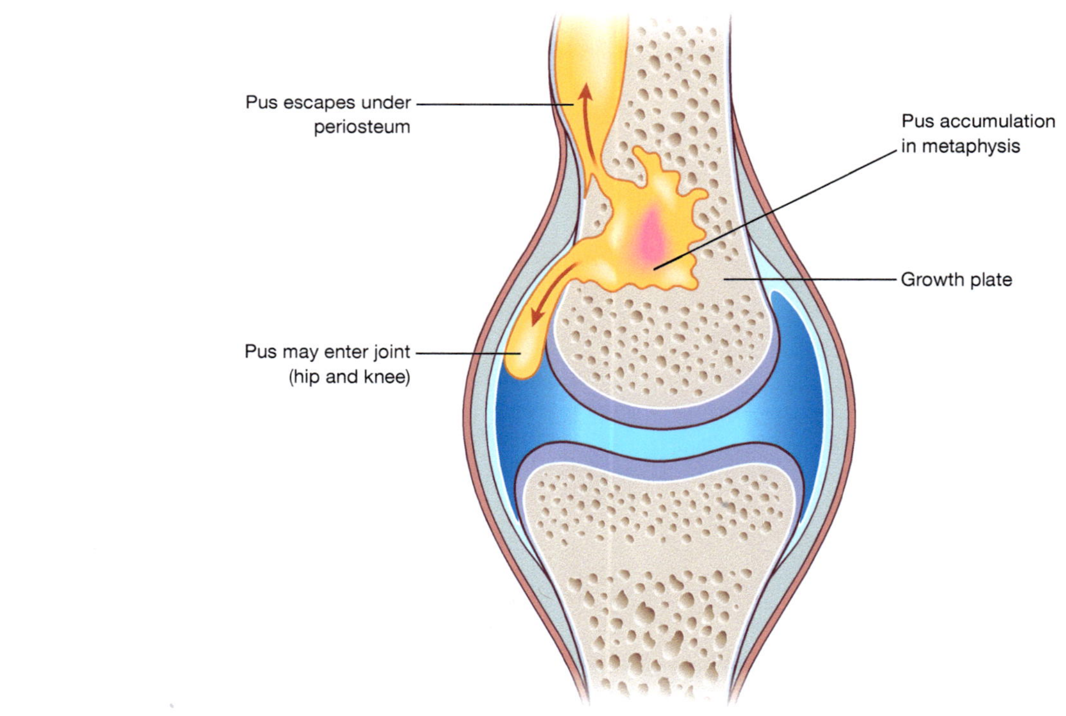

Osteomyelitis

Osteomyelitis refers to an infection of the bone, beginning in the bone marrow and potentially spreading to the cortex and periosteum through the Haversian canals, leading to inflammatory destruction and, in severe cases, necrosis (see Figure 57.1). When a portion of dead bone separates from healthy bone, it is termed a sequestrum. This avascular fragment acts as a reservoir for infection because antibiotics cannot easily penetrate it. Any bone may be affected.

Bone is normally resistant to bacterial colonisation; however, trauma, surgery, the presence of foreign bodies or prosthetic implants can disrupt its integrity and predispose it to infection. Osteomyelitis may be acute or chronic, with chronic forms evolving over months or years and often associated with persistent inflammation, bone loss and deformity.

Osteomyelitis is commonly categorised by its route of infection. Haematogenous osteomyelitis occurs when bacteria spread through the bloodstream from a distant site, such as a urinary tract or skin infection. Direct (contiguous) osteomyelitis arises from direct inoculation of bacteria into bone (e.g. following trauma, surgery or prosthetic implantation). These cases often involve multiple organisms and more localised signs of infection, such as erythema, swelling, warmth and tenderness over the affected bone.

Early recognition is crucial, as delayed diagnosis increases the risk of bone necrosis, chronic infection and systemic complications. Diagnosis typically involves a combination of clinical assessment, laboratory investigations (elevated inflammatory markers), imaging studies such as X-ray, MRI or CT and microbiological confirmation via bone biopsy or aspirate. Management includes prompt initiation of targeted antibiotics, surgical debridement where necessary, and supportive care to preserve bone integrity and function. Chronic osteomyelitis often requires prolonged treatment and close monitoring to prevent recurrence.

Pathophysiology

Bone is normally resistant to microbial colonisation; infection occurs when this barrier is breached by trauma, surgery, foreign bodies, prosthetic material or a high inoculum of virulent microorganisms. The development and severity of osteomyelitis depend on a combination of factors, including the virulence of the infecting organism, the host's immune status and the location, structure and vascularity of the bone.

Acute osteomyelitis begins with bacterial colonisation of bone, most commonly by *Staphylococcus aureus*. The infection induces suppurative inflammation, leading to oedema, vascular congestion and thrombosis of small vessels. Compromised blood flow reduces the delivery of immune cells and antibiotics, allowing necrosis of bone. Necrotic bone fragments, sequestra, can serve as reservoirs for persistent infection, as they are avascular and inaccessible to systemic therapy.

If untreated or inadequately managed, acute osteomyelitis can progress to chronic disease. Chronic osteomyelitis is characterised by the formation of granulation tissue, persistent inflammatory infiltrates and attempts at repair by new bone deposition from surviving periosteum and endosteum. An involucrum, or encasing sheath of new bone, may form around necrotic bone. Irregular perforations in the involucrum allow purulent material to track into surrounding soft tissues, often forming chronic draining sinuses (see Figure 57.2).

Biofilm-forming bacteria, especially on prosthetic devices, play a critical role in chronic infection. Biofilms are highly structured bacterial communities embedded in a protective extracellular matrix, which shields microbes from host immune responses and antimicrobial agents, making eradication challenging. Osteomyelitis can also arise via haematogenous spread, particularly in children or immunocompromised adults, with distant foci of infection seeding the bone.

Throughout the disease, the interplay between microbial virulence, local bone vascular compromise, host immune response and structural bone characteristics determines the severity and chronicity of infection. Understanding these mechanisms underpins early recognition, targeted antimicrobial therapy and, where necessary, surgical intervention to remove necrotic bone and restore vascularised tissue.

Signs and symptoms

Acute haematogenous osteomyelitis usually presents with non-specific systemic symptoms such as fever, fatigue, lethargy or irritability, often accompanied by localised pain, swelling, warmth and erythema over the affected bone. Pain typically worsens with movement, and in some cases, mild or no pyrexia may be reported, sometimes following minor trauma. Vertebral involvement may cause chronic back pain, worse at rest or at night.

Contiguous osteomyelitis, associated with direct bone injury or surgery, presents similarly with local pain, erythema and fever, alongside a history of trauma or infection in adjacent tissues.

Chronic osteomyelitis may follow acute infection or develop insidiously. Patients may experience persistent localised bone pain, swelling, non-healing ulcers, reduced range of motion in nearby joints, fatigue and general malaise. Signs may be subtle, and systemic features are often absent.

Investigations

A full blood count should be performed, although the white cell count may be normal, especially in chronic cases. Inflammatory markers such as C-reactive protein (CRP) and erythrocyte sedimentation rate (ESR) should be measured, and blood cultures obtained. Any expressed pus, joint effusions or samples from potential primary infection sites (e.g. urine) should also be cultured.

Bone biopsy remains the gold standard for diagnosis and should be obtained through non-infected tissue. Microbiological identification guides targeted antibiotic therapy.

Magnetic resonance imaging (MRI) is the preferred imaging modality for early detection and assessment of osteomyelitis extent. Plain radiographs have limited sensitivity in early disease but can help identify chronic features such as sequestra, periosteal reaction and osteolytic changes.

Management

Management of osteomyelitis depends on whether the infection is acute or chronic, the bones involved, the severity of infection and patient-specific factors such as immune status and comorbidities. Acute osteomyelitis can often be managed with targeted antibiotic therapy alone, guided by culture and sensitivity results. In severe cases, empirical intravenous antibiotics should be initiated promptly, with subsequent adjustment according to microbiological findings.

Chronic osteomyelitis typically requires surgical debridement to remove necrotic bone and establish a clean environment for healing. Antibiotic therapy, usually for a minimum of 6 weeks, is administered parenterally and may be followed by an oral step-down regimen depending on the organism, site of the infection and clinical response. Biofilm-forming bacteria, particularly in prosthetic-associated infections, may necessitate prolonged therapy or combined surgical interventions.

Adjunctive measures include analgesia, immobilisation or splinting for long bones and optimisation of general health and nutrition to support bone healing. Multidisciplinary management is recommended, involving orthopaedic surgeons, infectious disease specialists, microbiologists and nursing teams.

Imaging, particularly MRI, guides both diagnosis and surgical planning, while plain radiographs may help assess chronic changes. Early and aggressive management is essential to prevent complications, including persistent infection, deformity or systemic spread. Identification of the causative microorganism through bone or soft tissue cultures remains the gold standard for guiding therapy.

Patient education is also key, including adherence to therapy, monitoring for recurrence and awareness of risk factors for future infections.

Clinical considerations

Long-term antibiotics are a cornerstone of osteomyelitis management, particularly in chronic or post-surgical cases. Therapy is typically administered intravenously for at least 6 weeks, often followed by oral step-down treatment, depending on the causative organism and site of infection. Close concordance to the prescribed regimen is essential to ensure eradication of infection and to reduce the risk of relapse. Monitoring for adverse effects, including renal, hepatic or haematological toxicity, is important throughout therapy. Regular assessment of clinical response and inflammatory markers helps guide treatment duration.

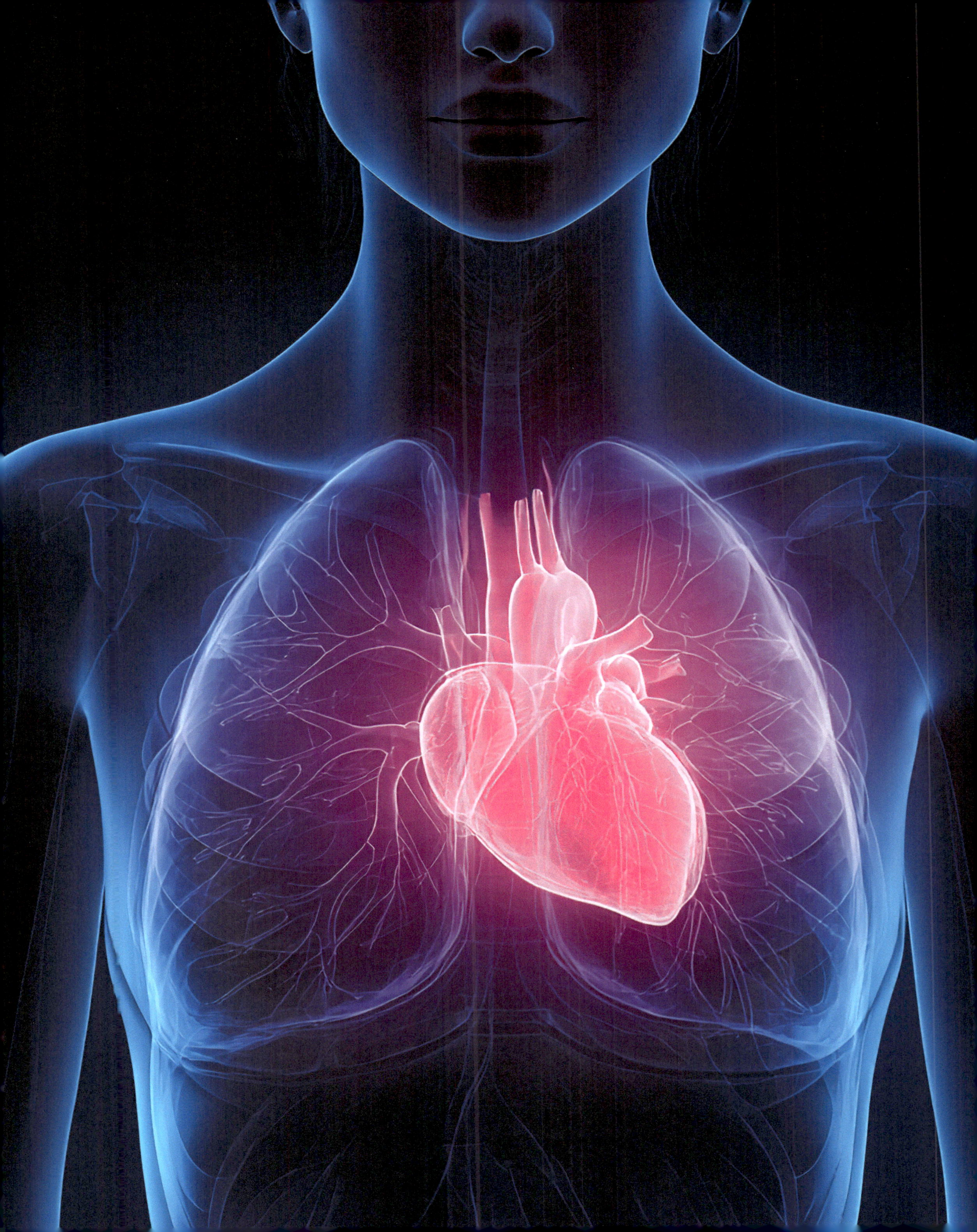

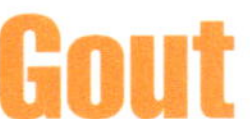

58 Gout

Figure 58.1 Locations of gout attack.

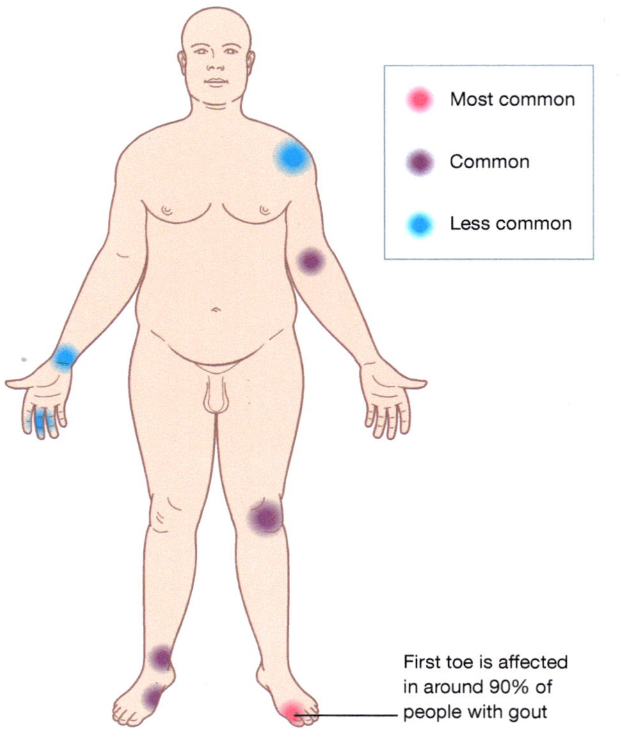

Figure 58.2 Gout.

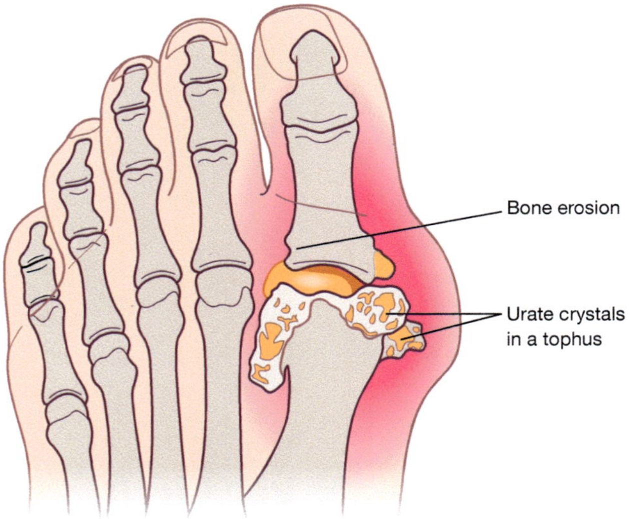

Figure 58.3 Complications of gout.

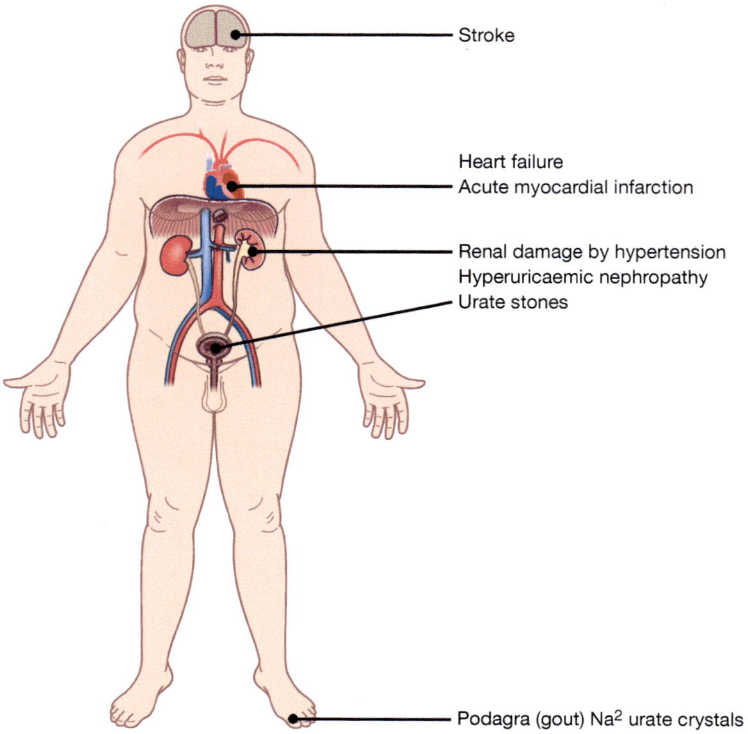

Gout

Gout is an acute inflammatory arthritis caused by the deposition of monosodium urate (MSU) crystals in joints and surrounding tissues. It typically presents with sudden, severe joint pain, swelling, redness and warmth, often affecting the first metatarsophalangeal joint. The disease exists along a spectrum, from isolated acute attacks to chronic tophaceous gout, which can cause joint deformity and tissue damage over time. Gout is extremely painful and can significantly impact the quality of life if untreated. Figure 58.1 shows the common locations of gout attacks.

Pathophysiology

Gout is a type of arthritis caused by tiny crystals called MSU crystals building up in the joints and surrounding tissues. This happens when there is too much uric acid in the blood, a condition called hyperuricaemia. Uric acid is a waste product formed when the body breaks down purines, substances found naturally in our cells and in certain foods. Normally, uric acid is removed from the body through the kidneys and, to a lesser extent, the gut. Hyperuricaemia occurs when the body produces too much uric acid or the kidneys cannot remove enough. It is important to know that high uric acid alone does not always cause gout; many people with high levels never develop symptoms, and blood levels may appear normal during an acute attack because the uric acid is temporarily deposited in the tissues.

Gout can be primary or secondary. Primary gout is the most common form and usually affects men between 30 and 60 years. It often happens because the kidneys do not remove enough uric acid. Genetics plays a role, with certain gene variants reducing uric acid excretion. Overproduction of uric acid can also cause gout (e.g. in people with certain cancers, after chemotherapy or during rapid tissue breakdown). Secondary gout has a known cause, such as kidney disease, diuretic medication, lead exposure, metabolic disorders or a diet very high in purines (however, a diet high in purines is contested).

A gout attack occurs when uric acid crystals form in the joint fluid. These crystals usually affect cooler, peripheral joints, such as the big toe (first metatarsophalangeal joint), midfoot or knee (see Figure 58.2). The crystals are recognised by the body's immune system as harmful, which triggers inflammation. Special immune cells, including macrophages, detect the crystals and activate inflammatory pathways, releasing substances such as interleukin-1β. This attracts white blood cells called neutrophils to the joint, causing pain, redness, swelling and warmth. Gout attacks can be triggered by sudden changes in uric acid levels, joint injury, surgery or alcohol intake.

If gout continues over time, uric acid crystals can form tophi – lumps of crystals surrounded by inflamed tissue. Tophi commonly appear on the ears, elbows, fingers and toes. If left untreated, they can damage bone and cartilage, causing joint deformities.

Several factors increase the risk of developing gout. These include being male, older age, obesity, insulin resistance, high blood pressure, kidney disease and abnormal cholesterol or triglyceride levels. Diet also plays a role: foods high in purines, such as red meat, organ meats, seafood and drinks high in fructose, as well as alcohol (especially beer and spirits), can raise the risk. Both lifestyle and genetic factors influence whether a person with high uric acid will develop gout.

It is important to distinguish gout from pseudogout, also called calcium pyrophosphate deposition disease. Pseudogout is caused by crystals of calcium pyrophosphate, usually affecting larger joints such as the knee or wrist. Risk factors include older age, osteoarthritis, metabolic problems (e.g. high parathyroid hormone, low magnesium or iron overload) and joint injuries. Unlike gout, genetics play a smaller role in pseudogout.

Understanding how gout develops helps guide treatment. Urate-lowering medications can prevent crystal formation, while anti-inflammatory drugs manage acute attacks. Early recognition of high uric acid, identifying modifiable risk factors and educating patients about diet and lifestyle are essential to prevent repeated attacks and long-term joint damage.

Signs and symptoms

Acute gout typically presents as sudden pain, swelling, tenderness and redness in a joint, often reaching its peak within 6–12 hours. The inflammation usually peaks within 24 hours and may be accompanied by mild pyrexia or malaise. Most attacks affect a single joint, commonly the first metatarsophalangeal joint, but atypical presentations can involve tendons (tenosynovitis) or bursae (bursitis) or mimic cellulitis.

Chronic gout can lead to the formation of tophi, firm, irregular nodules containing MSU crystals. These usually develop over years of recurrent attacks and high uric acid levels. Tophi are commonly found on extensor surfaces of fingers, hands, forearms, elbows, Achilles tendons and the ears, often appearing asymmetrical and with a chalky white appearance under the skin.

Synovitis, swelling and extreme tenderness with overlying erythema are typical during acute attacks, while tophi indicate long-standing disease. A definitive diagnosis requires identification of crystals in synovial fluid.

Investigations

Diagnosis of gout is primarily clinical but can be confirmed with targeted investigations. Typical presentations, such as sudden inflammation of the first metatarsophalangeal joint (podagra), hyperuricaemia or the presence of visible tophi, can allow a reasonably accurate clinical diagnosis. The gold standard for definitive diagnosis is identification of MSU crystals in synovial fluid obtained by joint aspiration. Gram staining and culture of synovial fluid are recommended to exclude septic arthritis, which can mimic acute gout.

Serum uric acid measurement is useful to support the diagnosis but has limitations: levels may be normal during an acute attack, and hyperuricaemia alone does not confirm gout. Renal uric acid excretion (24-hour urine collection) may help distinguish urate underexcretion from overproduction, but it is generally reserved for selected patients, particularly when planning urate-lowering therapy.

Imaging studies are increasingly used to support diagnosis, especially in atypical or chronic cases. Conventional radiographs are mainly helpful in chronic gout to detect bone erosions and joint damage. More advanced imaging, including ultrasound and dual-energy CT, can identify urate crystal deposits in joints and soft tissues, even before erosions develop, and are useful in less accessible sites.

Management

Pain relief is the main priority. The goal is to reduce pain and inflammation as quickly as possible. Short-term rest of the affected joint, ice packs and elevation can provide symptomatic relief while avoiding further trauma. Pharmacological treatment options include non-steroidal anti-inflammatory drugs (NSAIDs), colchicine or corticosteroids, selected based on the patient's comorbidities and the severity of the flare. Colchicine is most effective if started early, ideally within 36 hours of symptom onset.

In addition to managing acute symptoms, lifestyle measures should be addressed. These strategies support long-term urate control and help prevent recurrent attacks. Figure 58.3 shows the complications of gout.

Clinical considerations

Pain relief is the main goal during an acute gout flare. Short-term rest, ice packs and elevation can reduce swelling and discomfort. Pharmacological options include NSAIDs, colchicine (most effective within 36 hours) and corticosteroids if others are unsuitable. Long-term management focuses on lifestyle measures, hydration, weight control, regular exercise, moderation of alcohol and addressing comorbidities to prevent recurrence.

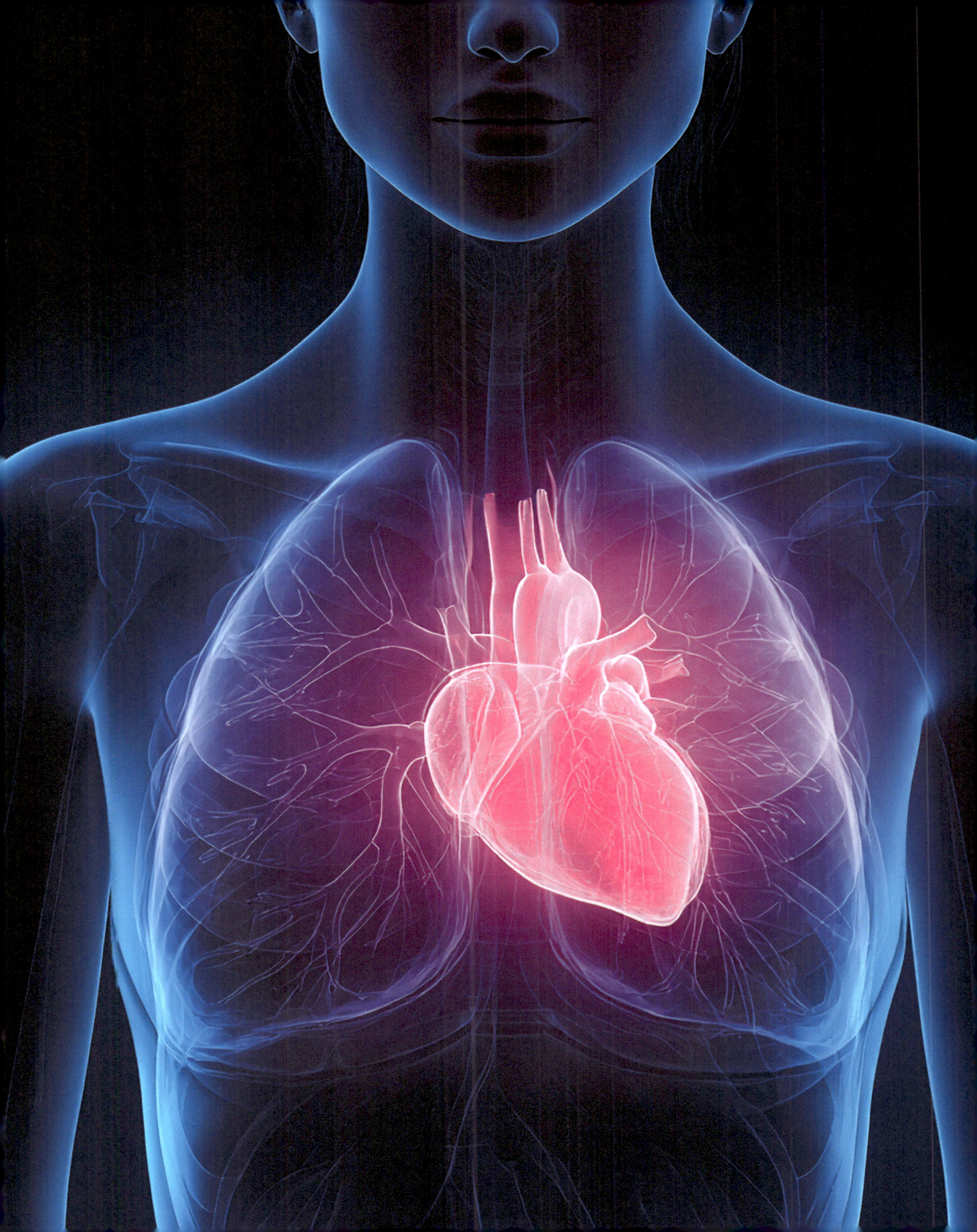

59 Rheumatoid arthritis

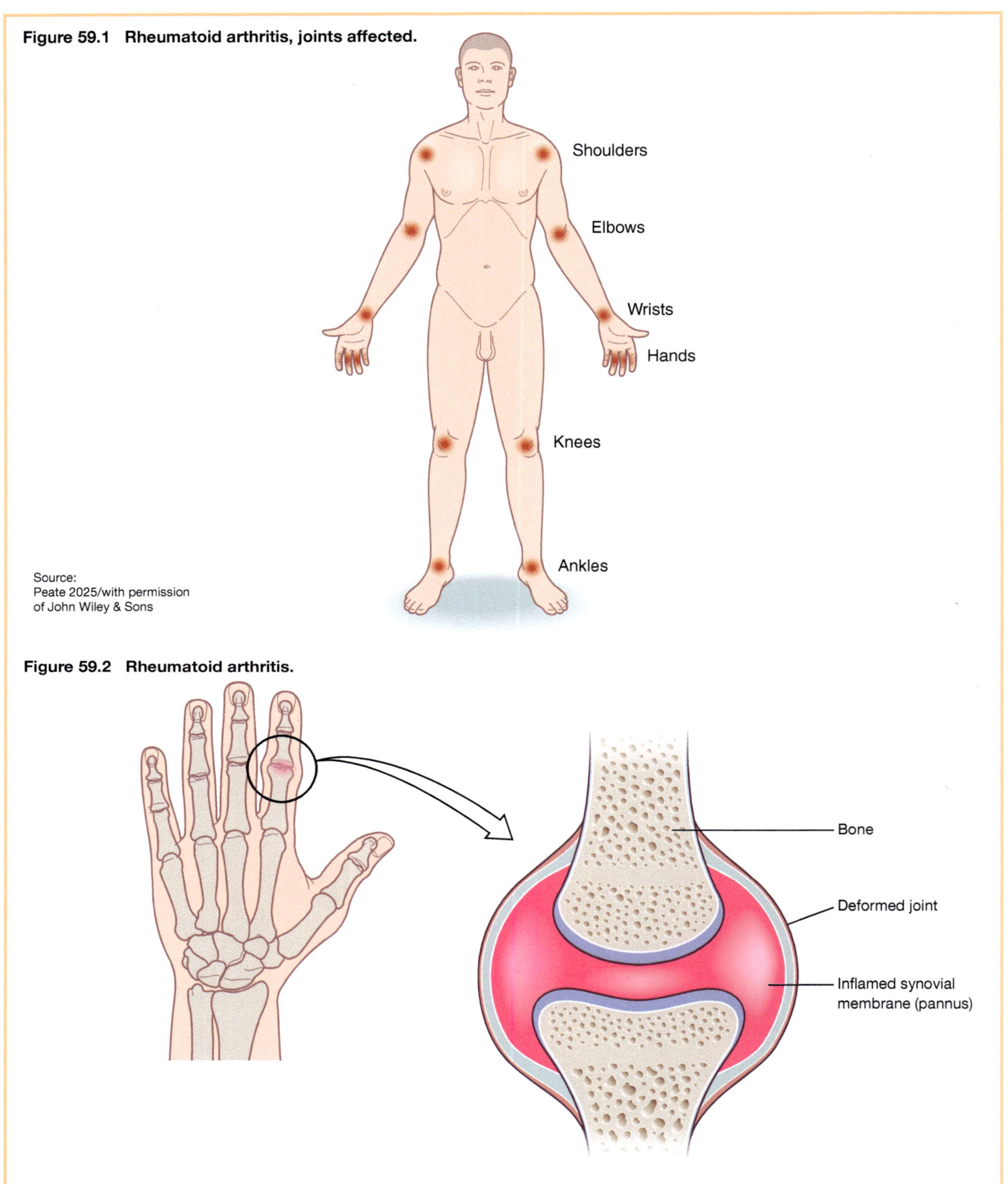

Rheumatoid arthritis (RA) is a chronic systemic autoimmune disease characterised by persistent synovial inflammation and joint destruction. It occurs in genetically susceptible individuals and may be triggered by environmental factors such as cigarette smoking, infection or trauma. Autoantibodies, including rheumatoid factor (RF) and anti-citrullinated protein antibodies (ACPA), play a central role in driving inflammation.

RA primarily affects the hands and feet, but any joint lined by synovium can be involved. Extra-articular manifestations may affect the skin, lungs, heart and eyes, and can significantly impact morbidity. Early recognition and treatment with disease-modifying anti-rheumatic drugs (DMARDs), including conventional, biologic and targeted synthetic agents, is essential to prevent joint damage, disability and long-term complications. Where mechanical joint damage has occurred, aids, appliances and sometimes surgery may be required.

Rheumatoid arthritis

While inflammation of the tissue surrounding the joints and inflammatory arthritis are typical features of RA, the disease can also cause inflammation and injury in other organs in the body (see Figures 59.1 and 59.2). Autoimmune diseases occur when the body's tissues are mistakenly attacked by the body's own immune system. The immune system contains a complex organisation of cells and antibodies that seek and destroy invaders of the body, particularly infections. Those with autoimmune diseases have antibodies in their blood that target their own body tissues, which can be associated with inflammation.

The RF is an antibody that is detectable in the blood of 80% of adults with RA. RF can be detected in the blood of normal people and of those with other autoimmune diseases that are not RA. In those with RA, high levels of RF can indicate a tendency towards more aggressive disease and/or a tendency to develop rheumatoid nodules and rheumatoid lung disease.

There is no known cure for RA.

Pathophysiology

RA is a chronic autoimmune disease that primarily affects women, with peak incidence in the fourth and fifth decades of life. The disease begins in the synovial membrane, which becomes inflamed and hyperplastic, forming a pannus that progressively invades cartilage, bone, ligaments and tendons. Early pathological events include synovial cell proliferation and endothelial activation, leading to persistent inflammation characterised by infiltration of CD4 T cells, B cells, monocytes/macrophages, fibroblasts, and neutrophils.

B cells produce autoantibodies, including RF and ACPA, which contribute to immune complex formation and complement activation. Inflammatory cells release cytokines, as well as proteolytic enzymes, driving tissue destruction. Osteoclast activation signalling leads to bone erosion, while ongoing synovial proliferation and inflammation gradually destroy cartilage and soft tissues, resulting in pain, swelling and joint deformity. These processes can also affect other organs, causing extra-articular manifestations such as rheumatoid nodules, interstitial lung disease, pericarditis, vasculitis and ocular involvement.

RA typically affects joints symmetrically, most commonly in the hands and feet, though any synovial joint may be involved. Genetic susceptibility, environmental triggers such as smoking or infection, and immune dysregulation propagate disease. Contemporary treatment strategies, including conventional and biologic DMARDs as well as targeted synthetic agents, aim to suppress these inflammatory pathways, reduce joint destruction and prevent systemic complications, highlighting the importance of early recognition and aggressive therapy.

Signs and symptoms

The characteristic feature of RA is persistent, symmetric polyarthritis (synovitis), most commonly affecting the hands and feet, though any joint lined by synovium may be involved. RA severity can fluctuate over time, and chronic disease leads to progressive joint destruction, deformity and functional impairment. Extra-articular manifestations may affect the skin, heart, lungs and eyes. Patients often experience fatigue, malaise, morning stiffness lasting over 30 minutes, weight loss and low-grade pyrexia. The duration of morning stiffness helps distinguish RA from osteoarthritis.

The onset is typically insidious, with systemic features such as pyrexia, malaise, arthralgia and weakness preceding visible joint swelling and inflammation. Early symptoms can impair daily activities, underlining the importance of prompt recognition and treatment to prevent long-term disability.

Investigations

Diagnosis of RA is primarily clinical, based on joint involvement, symmetry and chronicity. Investigations support the diagnosis, assess disease activity and help exclude other conditions. Routine laboratory tests include full blood count, CRP and ESR, while RF and ACPA are key autoantibody tests. Additional tests, such as liver function or synovial fluid analysis, may be indicated to rule out alternative diagnoses.

Radiographs of the hands and feet remain the first-line imaging modality to detect joint damage, but ultrasound or MRI can identify synovitis and early erosions before they are visible on X-ray, particularly in seronegative or early disease. Investigations should therefore be interpreted in the context of the clinical picture, and early specialist referral is recommended to guide treatment and prevent irreversible joint damage.

Management

The goals of RA treatment are to relieve pain, reduce inflammation, prevent structural joint damage and preserve function. Management combines pharmacological and non-pharmacological strategies. Symptomatic relief can be achieved with NSAIDs or short-term low-dose corticosteroids, though these do not prevent disease progression.

196

DMARDs, particularly methotrexate as first-line therapy, are used to slow or halt disease activity, improve symptoms and reduce extra-articular complications. If conventional DMARDs are insufficient, biologic or targeted synthetic DMARDs may be employed to modulate specific inflammatory pathways.

Non-pharmacological strategies include rest of inflamed joints during flares, physiotherapy, occupational therapy, patient education and exercise programmes to maintain mobility and function. Short-term corticosteroids can be used as a bridge while DMARD therapy takes effect, but long-term use is minimised due to side effects. Early, aggressive treatment aimed at disease suppression is essential to prevent joint deformity and maintain quality of life.

Clinical considerations

Maintaining independence and function is a key goal in RA management. Patients can benefit from joint protection strategies, such as using adaptive devices, pacing activities and avoiding repetitive strain. Physiotherapy and tailored exercises help preserve the range of movement, strengthen muscles and prevent stiffness, while occupational therapy supports safe performance of daily tasks and home or workplace adaptations. Alternating periods of rest with gentle movement prevents overuse without causing immobility. Information giving, advice and self-management skills enable patients to recognise flares, manage symptoms and adhere to treatment plans. When needed, assistive devices such as splints, braces or mobility aids can support independence and reduce pain.

The skin

Chapters

60 Atopic dermatitis

Figure 60.1 Pattern of lesions in children with atopic dermatitis.

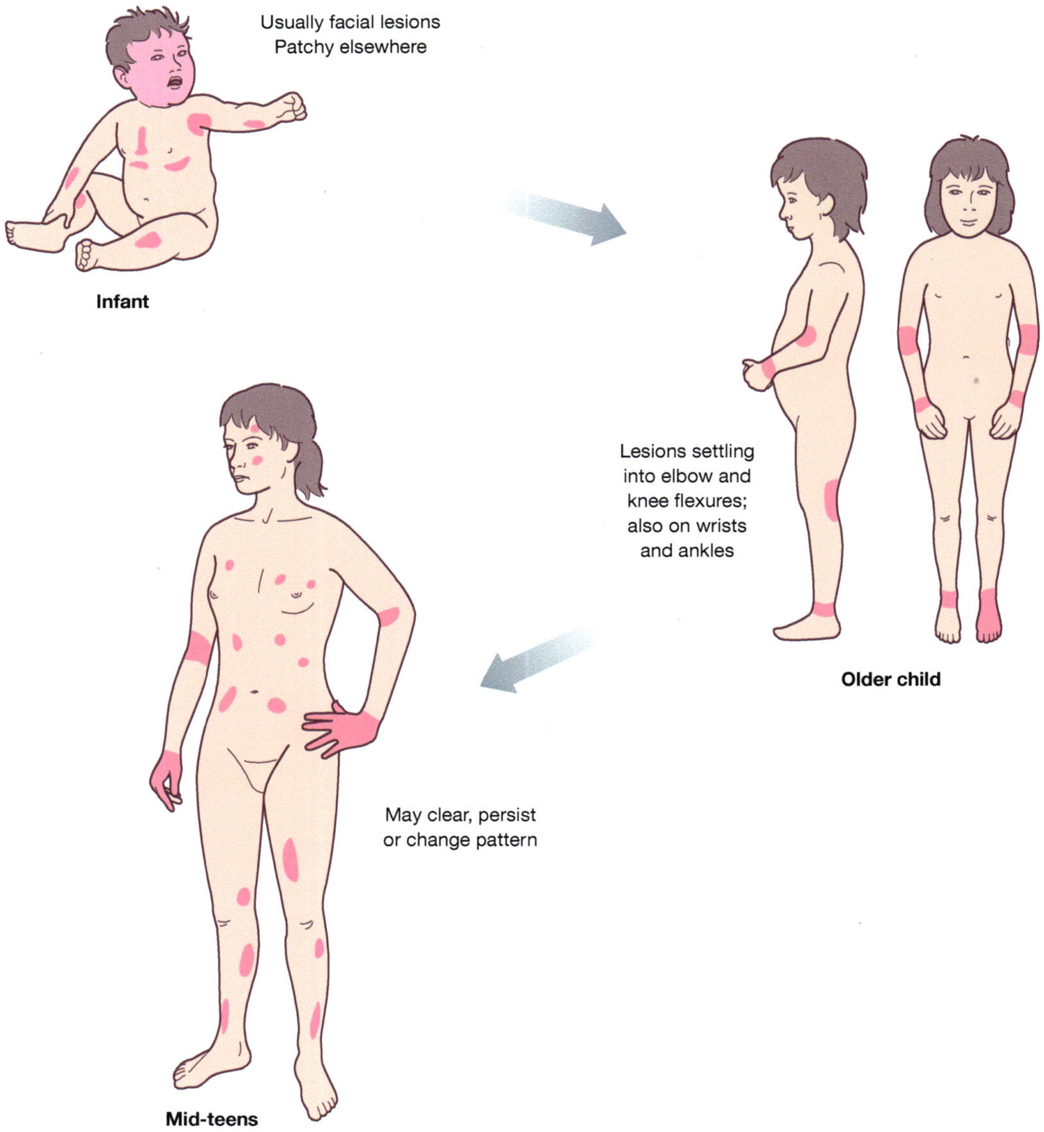

Table 60.1 Age-related signs of atopic dermatitis.

Infants	Childhood	Adulthood
Atopic dermatitis is usually noticed soon after birth.	Childhood xerosis is usually generalised, skin is flaky and rough.	Lesions become more diffuse, with an underlying background of erythema.
Xerosis occurs early, usually involving the whole body apart from the nappy area.	Lichenification is characteristic of childhood atopic dermatitis, signifying repeated rubbing of the skin seen mostly over the folds, bony protuberances and forehead.	The face is commonly involved and is dry and scaly.
Early lesions affect the antecubital and popliteal fossae, with erythema and exudation.		Xerosis is prominent.
Lesions usually localise over the following weeks to the cheeks, the forehead and scalp, and the extensors of the lower legs.	Lesions are eczematous and exudative. The antecubital and popliteal fossae and buttock-thigh are often affected.	Lichenification may be present.
Lesions are ill-defined, erythematous, scaly and eczematous patches and plaques.	Excoriations and crusting are common.	A brown macular ring around the neck is typical but not always present, representing localised deposition of amyloid.

Atopic dermatitis

Atopic dermatitis (eczema) is a chronic, relapsing-remitting inflammatory skin disease that is often associated with other atopic (immunoglobulin E (IgE)-mediated) conditions, such as IgE-mediated food allergy, asthma, urticaria and allergic rhinitis.

Atopic dermatitis is common, and its prevalence continues to rise globally, affecting both children and adults. Most cases present before the age of 5 years, with a higher prevalence among those who have an affected parent. The male-to-female ratio is approximately 1:1.4. The condition often develops during the first year of life and may undergo periods of remission, particularly during adolescence, although recurrence in early adulthood is not uncommon.

The pathophysiology involves complex interactions between genetic predisposition, immune dysregulation and environmental triggers. Skin barrier dysfunction and microbial dysbiosis, particularly colonisation with *Staphylococcus aureus*, play key roles in disease exacerbation. These factors contribute to chronic inflammation, pruritus and susceptibility to infection.

Atopic dermatitis has a considerable psychosocial impact on patients and their families, contributing to sleep disturbance, reduced quality of life and loss of school days in children. Psychological support, effective patient education and shared decision-making are therefore essential components of contemporary management.

Eczema herpeticum is a recognised complication of atopic dermatitis. It typically occurs following a primary herpes simplex virus infection but may also arise with recurrent infection. Vesicular lesions usually develop in areas of eczema and spread rapidly to involve both eczematous and unaffected skin. Lesions may become secondarily infected, requiring prompt antiviral and sometimes antibacterial treatment. Secondary bacterial infection with *S. aureus* or *Streptococcus pyogenes* is also common in individuals with atopic dermatitis and can exacerbate inflammation and skin damage.

Individuals with atopic dermatitis have an increased susceptibility to irritant and allergic contact dermatitis. Sensitisation to substances such as nickel and latex is more common than in the general population. Urticaria and acute anaphylactic reactions to foods also occur with greater frequency among those with atopic dermatitis, reflecting the broader atopic tendency.

Trigger factors

Environmental irritants and allergens that may exacerbate atopic dermatitis include soaps and detergents, shampoos, bubble baths, shower gels and washing-up liquids. *S. aureus* colonisation is a significant exacerbating factor, contributing to inflammation and disease flares. Extremes of temperature and humidity can also trigger symptoms; many patients experience improvement during the summer months and worsening in winter. Sweating induced by heat or exercise may provoke pruritus and exacerbate eczema, as can contact with abrasive fabrics such as wool.

Dietary factors may aggravate atopic dermatitis. Inhaled allergens, such as house dust mites, pollens, pet dander and moulds, may also act as trigger factors. Endogenous factors, including psychological stress, can worsen disease activity. Hormonal changes may influence disease expression, with some individuals experiencing premenstrual flare-ups or deterioration during pregnancy.

Pathophysiology

The pathophysiology of atopic dermatitis is not yet fully understood. Two principal hypotheses have been proposed to explain the development of inflammation characteristic of the disease.

The first proposes a primary immune dysfunction, leading to IgE sensitisation and secondary disturbance of the epithelial barrier. The second suggests a primary defect in the epithelial barrier, resulting in secondary immune dysregulation and subsequent inflammation.

In individuals with atopic dermatitis, there is an exaggerated activation of T lymphocytes and mast cells. In healthy skin, a balance exists between subsets of T helper (Th) cells. The immune dysfunction hypothesis proposes an imbalance between Th responses, resulting in the production of pro-inflammatory cytokines, such as interleukins, and increased IgE synthesis by B cells, accompanied by reduced interferon-gamma levels. In addition to T and B lymphocytes, other innate immune cells, including basophils, eosinophils and mast cells, contribute to the chronic inflammatory process.

The epidermal barrier dysfunction hypothesis suggests that individuals with atopic dermatitis have intrinsic defects in the skin barrier, allowing penetration of allergens, irritants and microbes. This disruption triggers the release of epithelial-derived cytokines, which in turn activate downstream immune pathways. Xerosis (dry skin) and ichthyosis are common clinical features reflecting impaired barrier function.

Mutations in the filaggrin gene, which encodes a key structural protein of the stratum corneum, represent the strongest known genetic risk factor for atopic dermatitis. Loss of filaggrin function leads to reduced natural moisturising factors, increased transepidermal water loss and enhanced entry of environmental allergens and pathogens. These effects contribute to cutaneous inflammation, heightened sensitivity and the potential progression to other atopic conditions, the so-called atopic march.

It remains uncertain whether primary immune dysregulation leads to secondary barrier breakdown or whether barrier defects precede and drive immune activation. Current evidence suggests that both mechanisms interact in a self-perpetuating cycle of inflammation, barrier dysfunction and pruritus.

Signs and symptoms

The hallmark symptom of atopic dermatitis is pruritus, which may begin within the first weeks of life but typically becomes more noticeable as the characteristic itch–scratch cycle develops during early infancy. The condition usually follows a relapsing–remitting course, with flares and periods of remission that are often triggered by environmental or endogenous factors.

Primary clinical signs include xerosis, lichenification and eczematous lesions, with excoriations and crusting commonly observed. The morphology and distribution of lesions vary with age. In infants, lesions predominantly affect the face, scalp, trunk and extensor surfaces. In older children, flexural areas such as the antecubital and popliteal fossae are more commonly involved, whereas in adults, the face, hands and flexural regions are most frequently affected (see Figure 60.1).

The diagnosis of atopic dermatitis is based on a combination of features, including a chronic or relapsing course, pruritus, typical eczematous morphology with age-dependent distribution, early age of onset, xerosis and a personal or family history of atopic disease, such as asthma, hay fever or eczema. Table 60.1 summarises the age-related clinical features of atopic dermatitis.

Investigations

Investigations are rarely necessary to establish the diagnosis of atopic dermatitis, which is primarily clinical. Measurement of total or specific IgE may indicate an atopic tendency but does not confirm the diagnosis. Historically, specific IgE (sIgE) was assessed using the radioallergosorbent test (RAST), but in modern practice these have largely been replaced by enzyme-linked sIgE assays or component-resolved diagnostics. Allergy testing is generally reserved for cases in which coexisting food allergy or other atopic conditions are suspected, and routine testing is not recommended for most patients.

Management

National guidelines provide clear recommendations for the management of atopic dermatitis. Known irritants and allergens should be avoided; regular, liberal use of emollients forms the foundation of treatment. Patients are advised to wear soft, non-irritant clothing and to minimise stress, as well as avoid extremes of temperature.

Topical corticosteroids are prescribed to reduce inflammation and allow healing, using the lowest-potency preparation sufficient to control disease, applied according to a reactive or proactive regimen to minimise side effects. Topical calcineurin inhibitors (pimecrolimus and tacrolimus) may be considered for areas at risk of corticosteroid-induced damage (e.g. face, flexures) or for patients not adequately controlled with corticosteroids.

Oral antihistamines may be used, primarily to aid sleep in patients with severe nocturnal pruritus. Antibiotic therapy is reserved for cases with clinically evident secondary bacterial infection.

For patients with moderate to severe atopic dermatitis unresponsive to topical therapy, newer systemic and targeted therapies, including biologics and Janus kinase inhibitors, may be considered in line with specialist guidance.

Clinical considerations

Emollients are the foundation of therapy for atopic dermatitis, helping to restore the skin barrier and reduce the frequency of flares. While generally safe and well-tolerated, some precautions should be observed. Emollients, particularly ointments, are highly flammable; patients should avoid open flames, smoking or using heating pads immediately after application. Excess emollient on floors or surfaces may create a slipping hazard, so any spills should be wiped promptly.

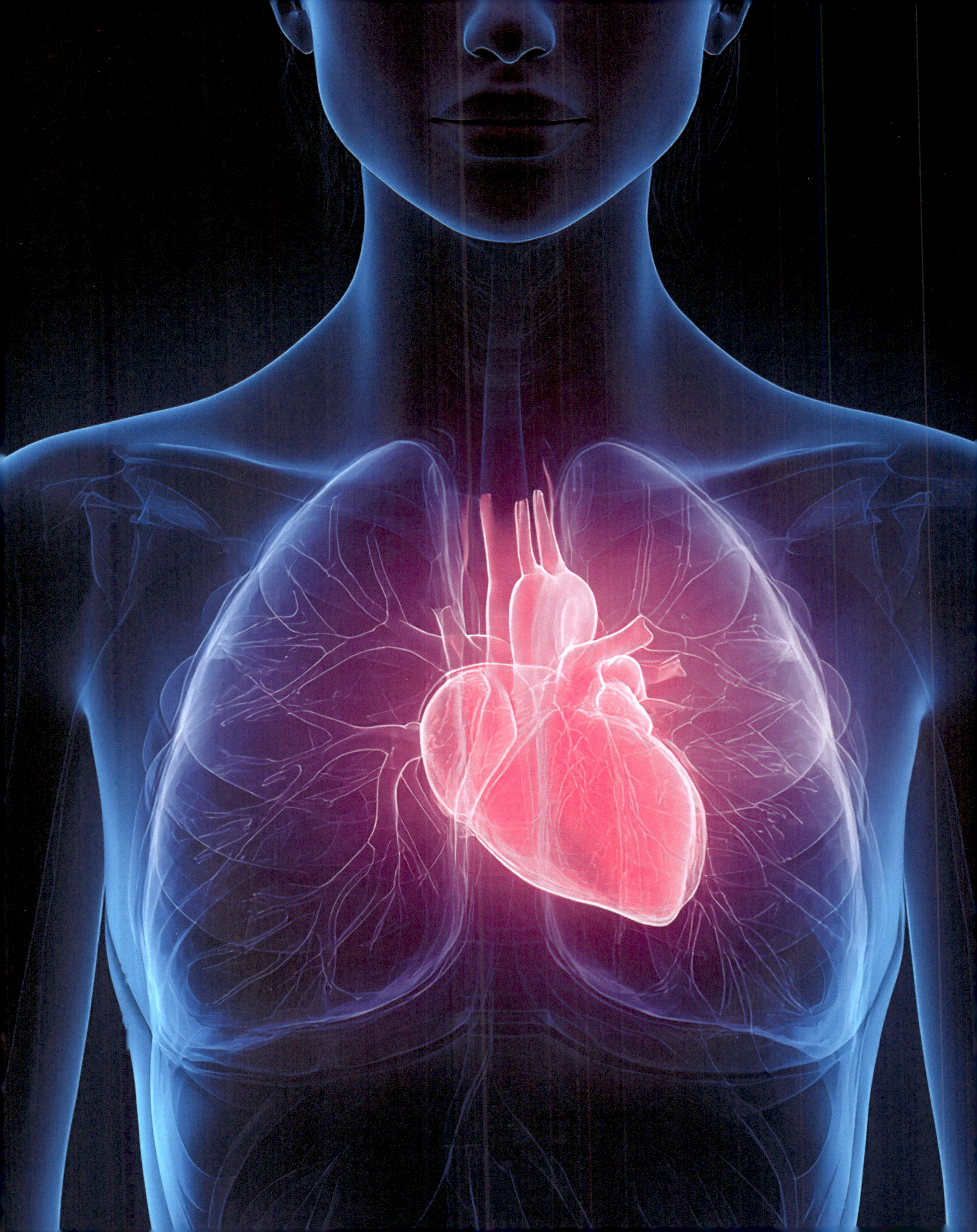

61 Psoriasis

Figure 61.1 Psoriasis locations.

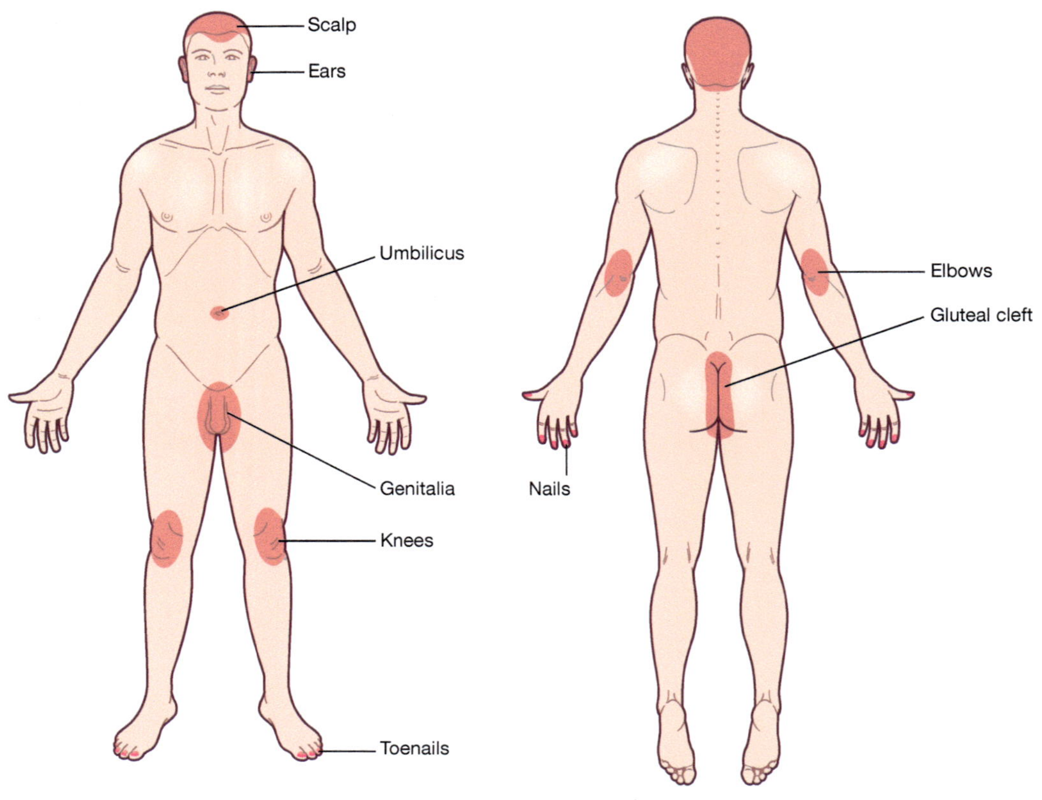

Figure 61.2 Normal skin and psoriasis.

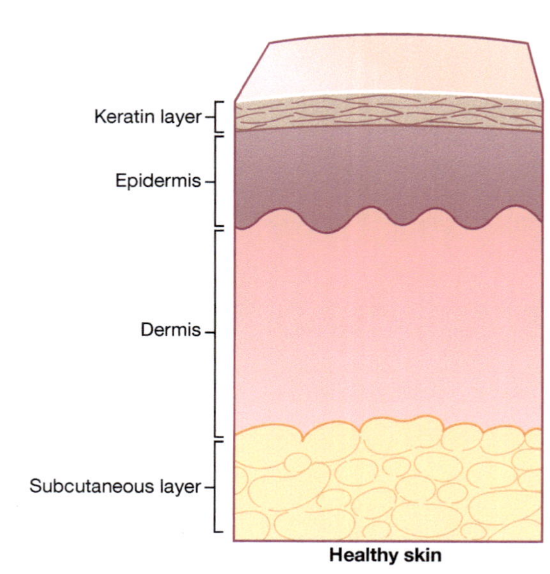

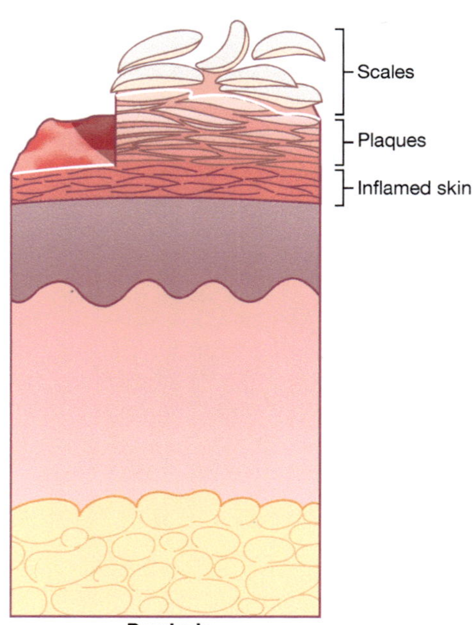

Psoriasis

Psoriasis, most commonly in the form of plaque psoriasis (psoriasis vulgaris), is a chronic, immune-mediated, inflammatory skin disease characterised by the formation of inflamed, raised plaques that shed scales due to hyperproliferation of epidermal keratinocytes. The epidermal cell turnover is accelerated, occurring 6–9 times faster than normal. Psoriasis is a complex, multifactorial condition involving genetic predisposition, immunological dysregulation and environmental triggers. Activated T lymphocytes release cytokines, which stimulate keratinocyte proliferation and the expression of dermal adhesion molecules, further amplifying local inflammation.

The disease most commonly affects the elbows, knees, scalp, lumbosacral areas, intergluteal clefts and glans penis (see Figure 61.1). The prevalence in the UK is approximately 1.3–2.2%, the highest among white populations. Psoriasis can occur at any age, with the first presentation usually before 35 years; it is uncommon in children. Plaque psoriasis is the most frequent clinical form, and a significant proportion of patients develop psoriatic arthritis.

Severity is classified according to body surface area affected: mild (less than 2%), moderate (2–10%) and severe (more than 10%). Psoriasis follows a chronic, relapsing–remitting course, with flares often triggered by systemic or environmental factors such as infections or psychological stress. The condition is non-contagious but has multisystem implications, including an increased risk of cardiovascular and metabolic comorbidities. It can significantly impact quality of life, psychosocial well-being and, indirectly, long-term health outcomes.

Pathophysiology

Psoriasis is a chronic, immune-mediated, inflammatory skin disease, most commonly manifesting as plaque psoriasis (also called psoriasis vulgaris), with raised, inflamed plaques that are covered by silvery, micaceous scales. Other types of psoriasis include guttate, inverse, erythrodermic and pustular psoriasis and psoriatic arthritis.

The condition is multifactorial, arising from a combination of genetic predisposition, environmental triggers and immune dysregulation. Environmental factors such as sunlight, trauma (Koebner phenomenon; patients with psoriasis should avoid unnecessary skin trauma, as even minor injuries can provoke new lesions), infection, stress, hormonal changes, drugs, smoking and alcohol may trigger or exacerbate the disease. Streptococcal infection is particularly associated with guttate psoriasis. In many patients no obvious trigger is identifiable.

Pathophysiologically, psoriasis involves infiltration of activated T lymphocytes into the dermis and epidermis. These cells release cytokines, which stimulate keratinocyte hyperproliferation and further immune activation; this then creates a self-perpetuating inflammatory loop.

Histologically (this is the study of skin under the microscope), in psoriatic skin, the epidermis is thicker, the skin cells are dividing and moving to the surface too quickly, and they do not mature properly; therefore, the outer layer of the skin (stratum corneum) retains nuclei that it normally loses during cell maturation. This is what forms the raised and scaly plaques that are characteristic of psoriasis.

Epidermal cells fail to produce sufficient lipids; this will lead to a poorly adherent stratum corneum, which accounts for the characteristic silvery scales. Vascular engorgement and dermal inflammation contribute to the erythematous, raised appearance of plaques (see Figure 61.2).

Signs and symptoms

Psoriasis is a chronic, immune-mediated inflammatory skin disease with multiple clinical forms. Plaque psoriasis, the most common type, presents with erythematous, raised plaques covered by silvery scales, often symmetrically distributed on the elbows, knees, scalp and lumbosacral area. Lesions are frequently pruritic and occasionally painful and may arise at sites of trauma through the Koebner phenomenon, which reflects/is in response to local immune activation. Guttate psoriasis appears as small, drop-like red lesions on the trunk, arms or legs, is often triggered by streptococcal infection and is thinner than plaque psoriasis. Inverse psoriasis involves bright red, smooth, shiny patches affecting flexural areas such as the axillae, groin and inframammary regions, with minimal scaling due to moisture. Erythrodermic psoriasis is a rare, severe form that is characterised by widespread redness, scaling, intense pruritus and systemic symptoms such as pyrexia and malaise; this requires urgent medical attention. Pustular psoriasis presents with sterile pustules on erythematous skin, most commonly on the palms and soles or as a generalised disease, often triggered by drugs, infection or abrupt withdrawal of systemic corticosteroids. Psoriasis may also be associated with psoriatic arthritis, causing joint pain, stiffness and swelling in addition to characteristic skin lesions.

Investigations

Diagnosis of psoriasis is usually clinical, based on a detailed history and physical examination, including assessment of lesion morphology, distribution and associated symptoms such as pruritus or joint pain. Skin biopsy is rarely required, except in atypical or unclear cases where the diagnosis is uncertain or to exclude other dermatological conditions. Laboratory tests are generally not necessary for diagnosis, though they may be indicated to assess comorbidities or systemic involvement in severe or erythrodermic forms.

Management

Management of psoriasis is guided by disease severity, type of psoriasis and its impact on the person's quality of life. Patient information giving is essential, including reassurance that psoriasis is chronic but neither infectious nor malignant. Patients should be advised to avoid triggers such as trauma, stress, certain medications, smoking and excessive alcohol. Regular emollient use helps reduce scaling, dryness and pruritus.

Cutaneous management begins with first-line therapy, including topical corticosteroids, vitamin D analogues and emollients, with dithranol or tar preparations used under supervision in selected cases. Second-line therapy includes narrow-band UVB phototherapy and systemic non-biologic agents such as methotrexate, acitretin or ciclosporin. Third-line therapy comprises biologic agents targeting specific immune pathways for patients with severe or treatment-resistant disease.

Psoriatic arthritis requires control of inflammation, preservation of joint function and prevention of structural damage. Symptom relief is achieved with NSAIDs for pain and stiffness and intra-articular corticosteroids for local flares. DMARDs such as methotrexate, sulfasalazine or leflunomide suppress joint inflammation, while gentle activity, splints, appropriate footwear and physiotherapy support joint mobility. Biologic therapies are indicated for refractory arthritis, and surgical intervention, including joint replacement, may be necessary in cases of severe joint destruction.

Clinical considerations

Psoriasis can have a significant psychosocial impact, often causing anxiety, depression and reduced self-esteem due to the visibility of skin lesions. Many individuals experience social stigma, including embarrassment, social withdrawal and discrimination, which can affect work, education and personal relationships. Chronic symptoms such as pruritus and discomfort, along with frequent treatment regimens, may interfere with sleep, daily activities and leisure. Recognising the psychological burden of psoriasis also supports treatment adherence and engagement with care, ultimately improving quality of life.

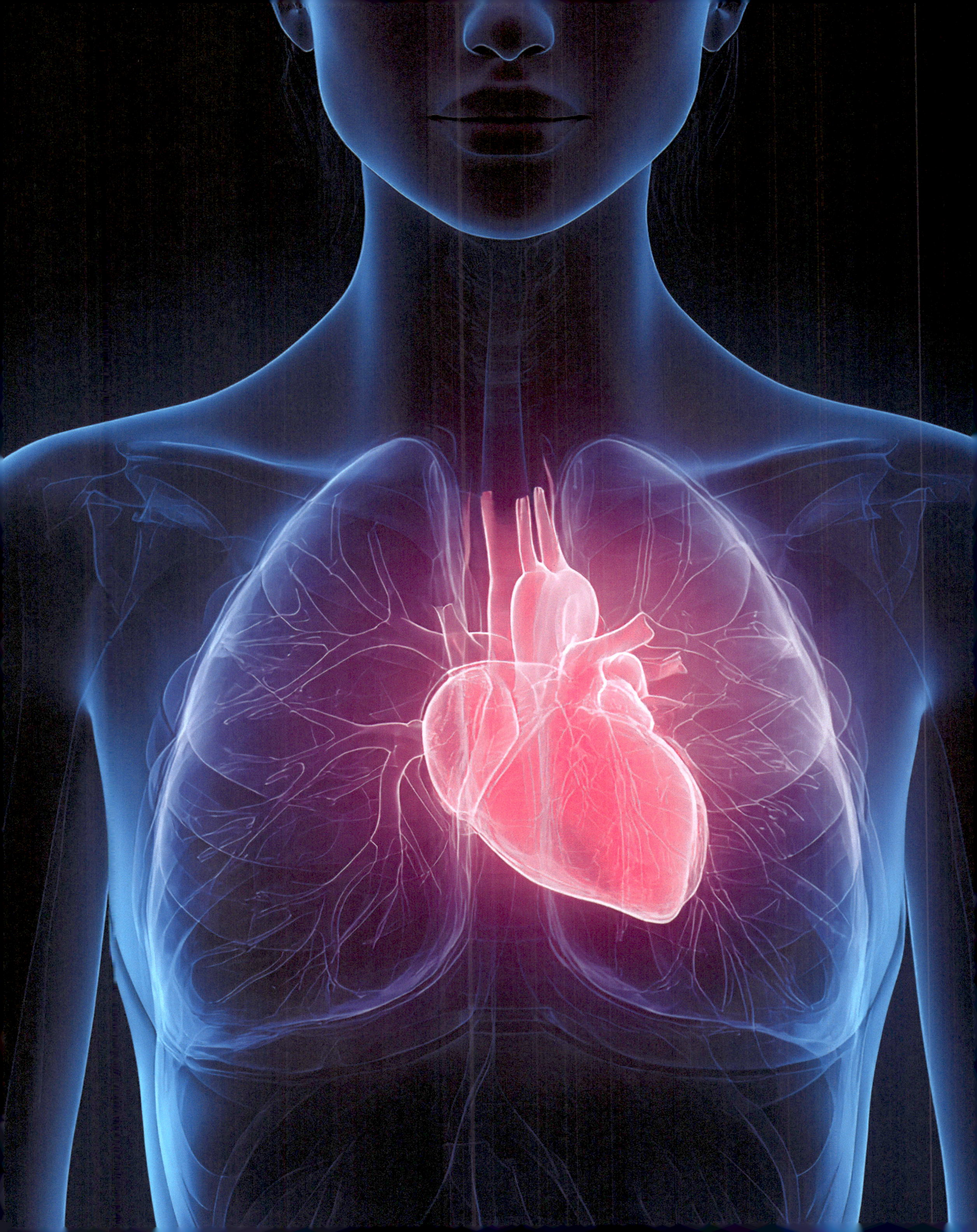

62 Acne vulgaris

Figure 62.1   A pilosebaceous unit.

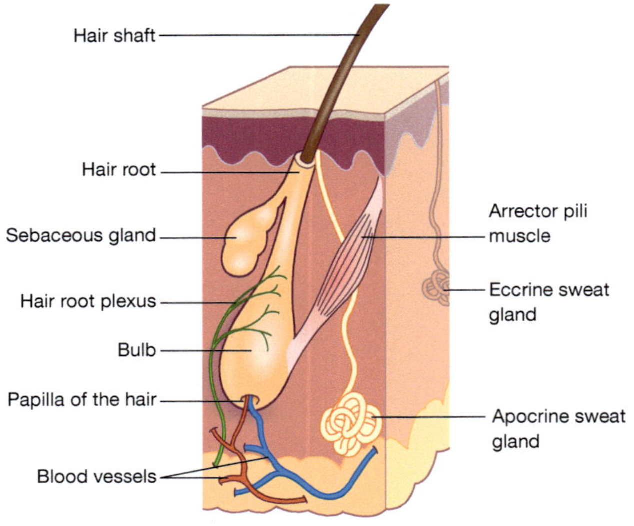

Source:
Peate, Wild & Nair, *Nursing Practice: Knowledge and Care,* 2014

Figure 62.2   The pathogenesis of acne.

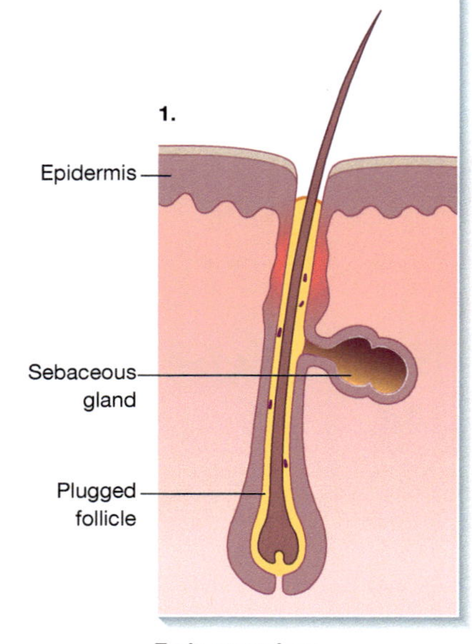

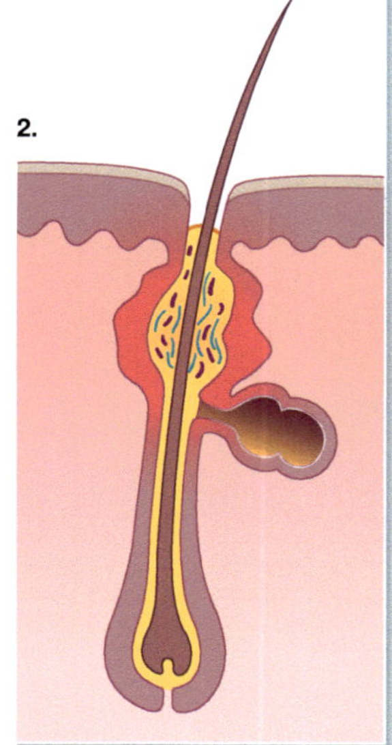

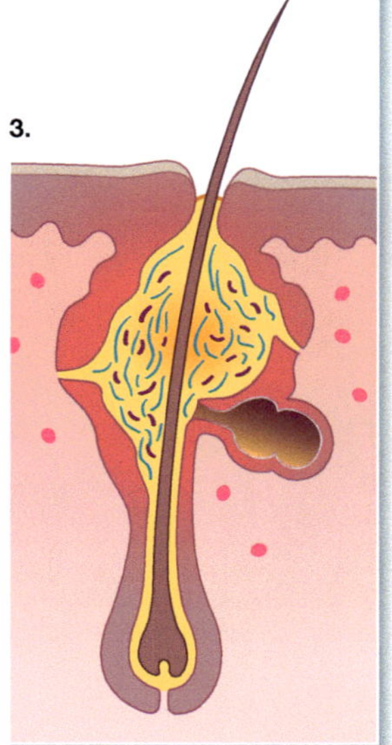

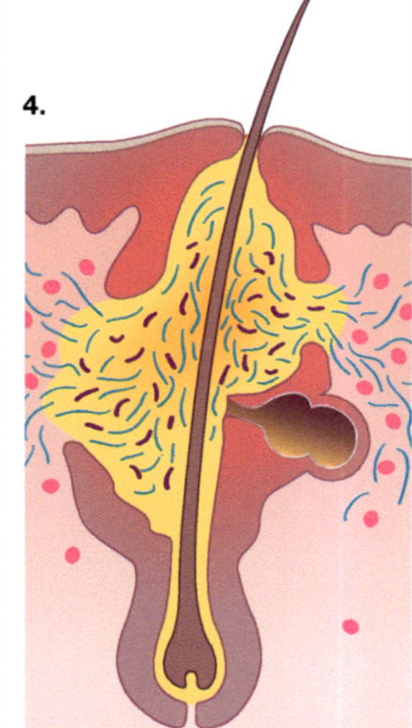

Early comedone
- Accumulation of epithelial cells and keratin

Later comedone
- Accumulation of shed keratin and sebum

Inflammatory papule/pustule
- Propionibacterium acnes proliferation
- Mild inflammation

Nodule cyst
- Marked inflammation
- Scarring

Acne vulgaris

Acne vulgaris is a common skin condition affecting most people in the UK at some stage of their lives. It is a disorder of the pilosebaceous follicles, which are most densely populated on the face, upper chest and back (see Figure 62.1). Acne develops when follicles become blocked with sebum and dead skin cells, which may then become colonised by *Cutibacterium acnes* (*C. acnes*) (a bacterium), triggering an inflammatory response.

During puberty, increased androgen levels stimulate sebum production from enlarged sebaceous glands. Blocked follicles may form comedones, which are classified as open (blackheads) or closed (whiteheads). Inflammation can progress to papules, pustules and nodules, which may be painful or cosmetically distressing.

The condition is more common in boys, although girls are also affected, often experiencing flares in the premenstrual phase. In some cases, acne may be associated with polycystic ovary syndrome or other causes of androgen excess, including exogenous testosterone therapy, anabolic steroid misuse, Cushing's disease or virilising tumours such as Sertoli–Leydig cell tumours.

Most teenagers experience some degree of acne during adolescence, and although many cases are mild, approximately 10–25% develop severe forms. Severe acne can have significant psychological consequences, including low self-esteem, anxiety and social withdrawal, particularly at a time when individuals are navigating major developmental and social changes. Understanding the multifactorial pathogenesis of acne is crucial for appropriate management, which may involve topical or systemic therapies, lifestyle advice and psychosocial support.

Pathophysiology

Acne vulgaris is a multifactorial disorder of the pilosebaceous unit, influenced by genetic, hormonal, microbial and inflammatory factors. Its pathogenesis is commonly described through four interrelated mechanisms: follicular hyperkeratinisation, excess sebum production, colonisation by *C. acnes* and inflammation.

The initial event in acne development is retention hyperkeratosis, in which abnormal proliferation and incomplete desquamation of keratinocytes lead to follicular plugging. These plugged follicles manifest clinically as comedones, which may be open (blackheads) or closed (whiteheads). Genetic predisposition plays a significant role, as evidenced by familial clustering and concordance among twins.

Androgen hormones are key regulators of sebaceous gland activity. Testosterone and its derivatives, including dihydrotestosterone, bind to androgen receptors within sebaceous glands; this leads to the stimulation of sebum production. Circulating androgen levels may be normal in many individuals with acne, highlighting the importance of local androgen metabolism and receptor sensitivity. Other hormonal and metabolic factors, such as growth hormone and insulin-like growth factor-1 (IGF-1), also enhance sebaceous gland activity and contribute to acne development.

The commensal bacterium *C. acnes* colonises the obstructed follicle and plays a critical role in triggering the inflammatory response. *C. acnes* activates monocytes and neutrophils, leading to the release of pro-inflammatory cytokines, including interleukins-8 and -12, and tumour necrosis factor-alpha. This inflammatory cascade will then contribute to the formation of papules, pustules and nodules. Individual susceptibility to inflammation may vary, explaining why there are some people who develop predominantly comedonal acne while others develop more severe inflammatory lesions.

Overall, acne vulgaris results from a dynamic interaction between follicular obstruction, microbial proliferation, sebum overproduction and immune-mediated inflammation, modulated by genetic and hormonal influences. Figure 62.2 illustrates the pathogenesis of acne. Understanding these mechanisms is essential for guiding targeted therapeutic interventions, including topical and systemic agents that can help to reduce sebum production, modulate follicular keratinisation and suppress inflammation or bacterial proliferation.

Signs and symptoms

Acne vulgaris is characterised by non-inflammatory lesions, open and closed comedones and inflammatory lesions, including papules, pustules and nodules. Affected individuals often have oily skin. Local symptoms may include tenderness or pain, particularly over nodules and cysts. Typically, acne vulgaris does not produce systemic symptoms.

Severe acne may present in different forms. Acne fulminans is an acute, severe variant that usually occurs in adolescent males, with painful ulcerative nodules accompanied by systemic symptoms such as pyrexia, malaise and arthralgia. Acne conglobata is a chronic severe form that is characterised by multiple comedones, papules, pustules and nodules, but without any systemic involvement. Acne conglobata can frequently result in disfiguring scarring.

Investigations

The diagnosis of acne vulgaris is usually clinical, based on the patient's history and physical examination. Routine laboratory or imaging investigations are not required in typical cases.

Investigations may be indicated in selected patients to identify an underlying cause, such as androgen excess or a virilising tumour, particularly in females with severe or sudden-onset acne, hirsutism, or menstrual irregularities. Hormonal assays, including testosterone, DHEA-S and 17-hydroxyprogesterone, may be performed, and imaging studies may be considered if a tumour is suspected.

In cases of treatment-resistant or atypical acne, a skin lesion culture may be performed to exclude Gram-negative folliculitis. This is uncommon and it is usually reserved for patients who are not responding to conventional therapies.

Management

The management of acne vulgaris depends on the severity, lesion type and impact on quality of life. Mild acne is often self-limiting, whereas moderate-to-severe acne may require systemic therapy and close follow-up.

General measures include gentle cleansing of affected areas twice daily with a mild, non-comedogenic cleanser. Patients should be advised not to pick or squeeze lesions, which increases the risk of scarring. Adjunctive therapies such as blue light phototherapy or fractional lasers may provide additional benefit in some cases but are not first-line treatments.

Topical therapy is the cornerstone for mild-to-moderate acne. Benzoyl peroxide reduces *C. acnes* colonisation, comedone formation and inflammation. Topical retinoids normalise follicular keratinisation and have anti-inflammatory effects. Topical antibiotics are effective when combined with benzoyl peroxide or a retinoid to reduce the risk of antibiotic resistance. Treatments should be applied to all affected areas, not just visible lesions and continued consistently for several weeks to months for maximum benefit.

Systemic therapy is indicated for moderate-to-severe or treatment-resistant acne. Oral antibiotics are typically prescribed for 6–12 weeks, often combined with topical therapy. Oral isotretinoin is reserved for severe, scarring or refractory acne; it targets all four pathophysiological mechanisms – sebum production, follicular hyperkeratinisation, bacterial proliferation and inflammation – and requires careful monitoring for adverse effects.

Hormonal therapy is particularly effective in females with hormonally driven acne. Combined oral contraceptives containing oestrogen and anti-androgenic progestins can reduce sebum production. Spironolactone may also be used to block androgen receptors in the sebaceous glands.

Management of acne scarring includes procedural interventions. Laser resurfacing, chemical peels and dermabrasion are used for moderate-to-severe scarring. Microdermabrasion, an outpatient procedure using abrasive crystals, is primarily effective for superficial scars.

Successful management combines patient information giving, concordance to topical/systemic therapy, lifestyle guidance and procedural interventions when required, tailored to disease severity and individual patient needs.

Clinical considerations

Acne vulgaris is common and can significantly affect psychological well-being, including self-esteem, body image and social confidence. Acne is not caused by poor hygiene; treatments may take several weeks to show effect. Gentle cleansing twice daily with non-comedogenic products is recommended, and lesions should not be picked or squeezed. Topical treatments should cover all affected areas, and combination therapies (e.g. benzoyl peroxide with topical antibiotics) help reduce bacterial resistance. Lifestyle measures, including a balanced diet and avoidance of exogenous androgens, may be beneficial. Follow-up is essential to monitor treatment response and psychological impact. Patients experiencing low self-esteem, anxiety or social withdrawal, or those with severe, scarring or treatment-resistant acne, are considered for referral, where appropriate, for psychological support.

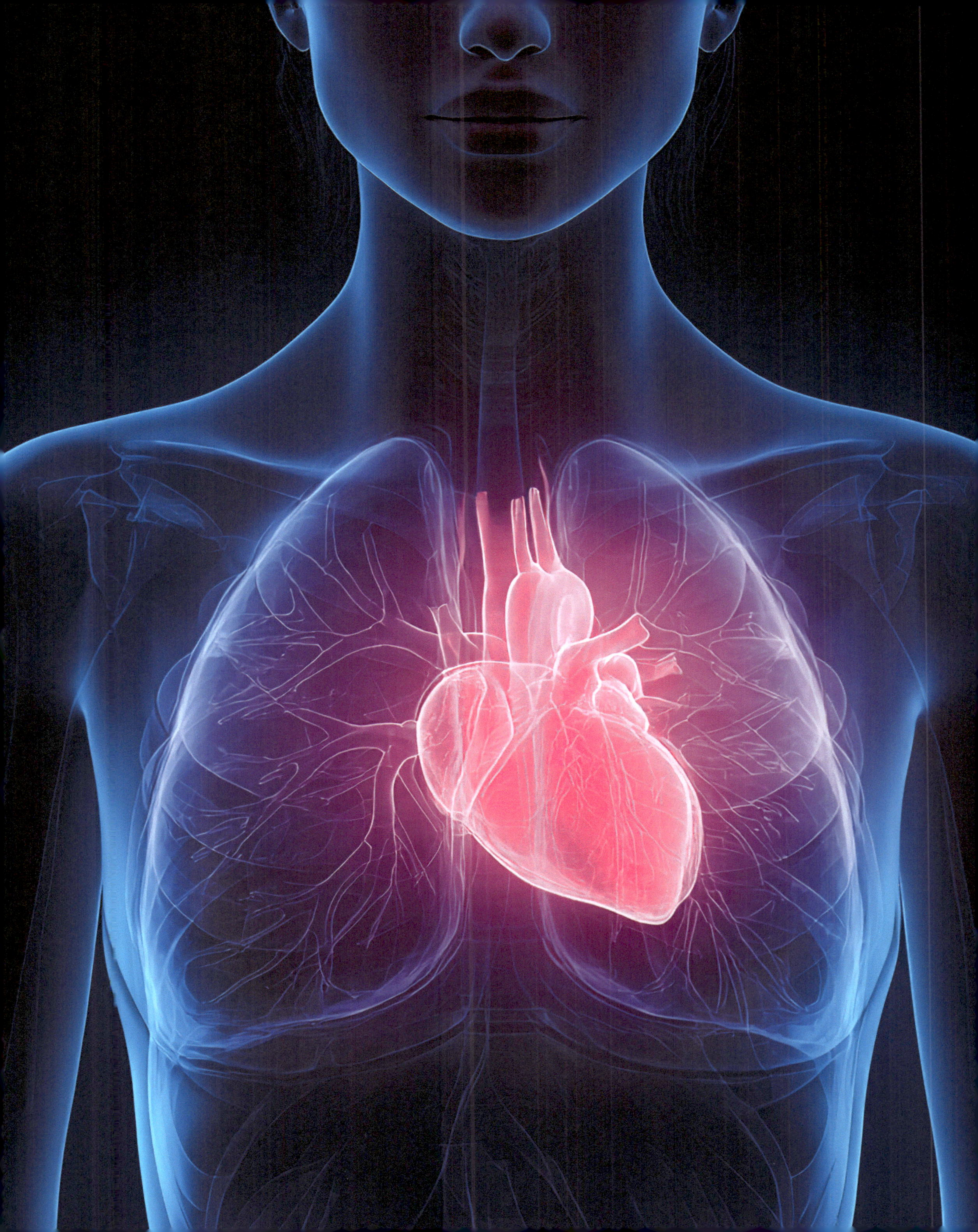

63 Malignant melanoma

Figure 63.1   The location of a melanocyte.

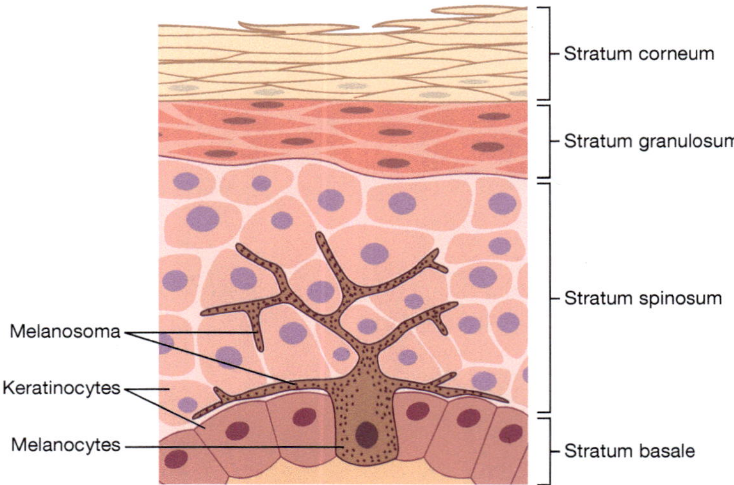

Figure 63.2   Melanocytes and exposure to UV radiation.

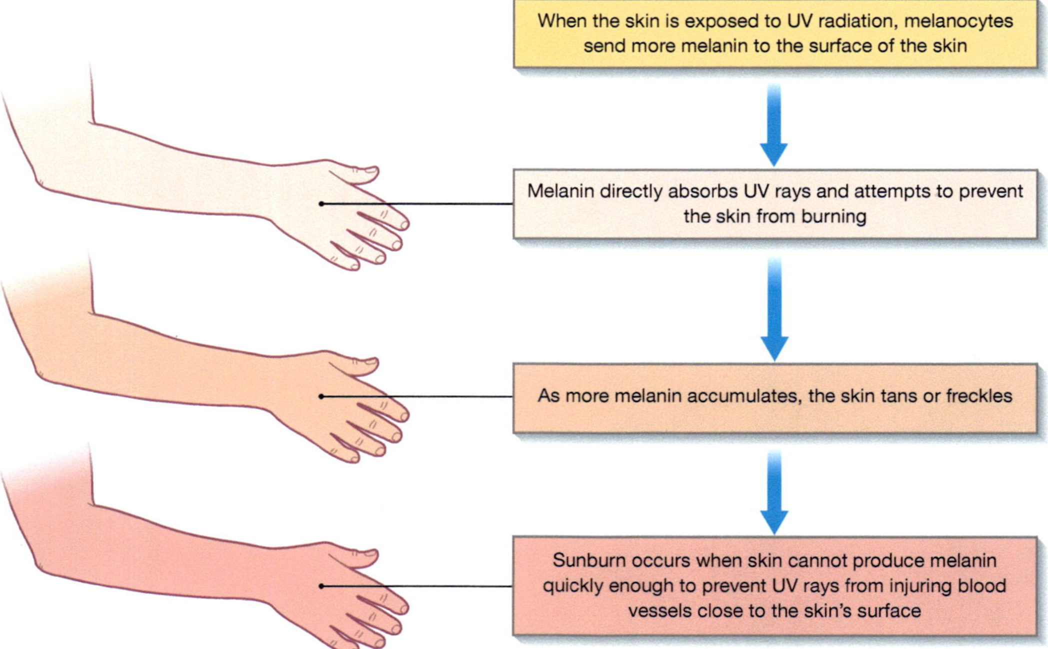

Table 63.1   The ABCDE'S for differentiating early melanoma from benign naevi.

A	Asymmetry: This refers to the shape of the mole or abnormal patch of skin.
B	Borader irregularity: This refers to the edges of the mole or abnormal patch of skin.
C	Colour: This refers to the colour of the mole or abnormal patch of skin.
D	Diameter: This refers to how wide the mole or abnormal patch of skin is.
E	Evolving: Melanomas might change in size, shape or colour.

Melanocytes

Melanocytes are found in the basal layer of the epidermis, the stratum basale and extend branching processes between the keratinocytes in the suprabasal layers. Approximately 5–10% of the cells in the epidermis are melanocytes (Figure 63.1). They are present in similar numbers in both black and white skin, but melanocytes in darker skin types produce more melanin. Differences in skin colour are therefore due to variations in the amount of melanin produced and the size and distribution of the melanin 'packets' (melanosomes) within keratinocytes. People with dark brown or black skin are much less likely to experience damage from ultraviolet (UV) radiation than those with lighter skin.

Non-cancerous growths of melanocytes result in moles (benign melanocytic naevi) and freckles (ephelides and lentigines). Melanin protects the skin from the harmful effects of UV radiation (Figure 63.2).

A mole is a cluster of melanocytes that appears as a pigmented spot on the skin. Moles can be flat or raised and round or oval. They are generally benign and unchanging, but occasionally they can become cancerous. The first sign of melanoma is often a change in the size, shape or colour of an existing mole, or the appearance of a new mole in adulthood.

Skin cancer

Skin cancer is the most common form of cancer in the United Kingdom. The incidence of skin cancer varies geographically, with higher rates observed in regions with greater sun exposure and at higher altitudes. Although skin cancer is more common in people with light skin than in those with dark skin, all skin types are at risk.

Malignant melanoma

Malignant melanoma is a neoplasm of melanocytes, or of cells derived from melanocytes. Once considered uncommon, the annual incidence of this malignancy has increased considerably over the past two decades. One factor contributing to this rise is the increase in intermittent sun exposure associated with outdoor recreational activities and the use of tanning devices. Cancerous growth of melanocytes results in melanoma; most melanomas arise in the skin, although malignant melanomas have been reported in almost every organ of the body.

Surgical excision remains the definitive treatment for early stage melanoma, with histopathological assessment guiding prognosis. Medical management, including immunotherapy and targeted therapy, is used as adjuvant or systemic treatment for advanced disease. Recent advances in these therapies have substantially improved survival outcomes. Prevention through sun protection and early detection remains the most effective strategy for reducing melanoma-related mortality.

Pathophysiology

Most cutaneous melanomas initially spread laterally within the epidermis, known as radial growth. When all malignant cells are confined to the epidermis, the lesion is termed melanoma in situ, which has no metastatic potential and can be effectively treated by local excision. Once malignant cells breach the basement membrane and invade the dermis, the tumour is classified as invasive melanoma, acquiring the potential to metastasise. It is important to note that some aggressive subtypes, such as nodular melanoma, may bypass a prolonged radial growth phase and present primarily with vertical growth.

Four principal clinical subtypes of cutaneous melanoma are recognised: lentigo maligna melanoma, superficial spreading melanoma, nodular melanoma and acral lentiginous melanoma. Nodular melanoma is typically the most aggressive, presenting as a rapidly enlarging, often pigmented nodule that may ulcerate or bleed. Other rarer forms include desmoplastic, mucosal and uveal melanomas, which can arise outside the skin but share similar pathogenic mechanisms.

Invasive melanoma cells can disseminate through the lymphatic system to regional lymph nodes or via the bloodstream to distant organs. Metastases may occur in almost any tissue, most commonly the lymph nodes, liver, lungs, bones and brain. In-transit metastases are tumour deposits found along dermal or subcutaneous lymphatic channels between the primary tumour and regional lymph nodes.

Melanomas progress through two growth phases: radial and vertical. During the radial growth phase, malignant cells proliferate laterally within the epidermis and superficial dermis. The vertical growth phase is characterised by downward invasion into the dermis and acquisition of metastatic potential. Prognostically, tumour thickness (Breslow depth) is a key determinant: lesions are considered thin (same as or less than 1 mm), intermediate (1–4 mm) or thick (more than 4 mm).

UV radiation plays a central role in melanoma development, inducing DNA damage in melanocytes and causing local immunosuppression, including impaired function of epidermal Langerhans cells. This combination reduces the skin's ability to recognise and repair DNA damage, increasing the likelihood of malignant transformation.

Signs and symptoms

Melanoma may present as a multi-coloured or uniformly pigmented lesion that can grow vertically, laterally or irregularly. Lesions are typically asymmetrical, with irregular borders, and may ulcerate, bleed or crust. While melanomas most commonly occur on sun-exposed areas in lighter-skinned individuals, in people with darker skin, they often arise in non-sun-exposed sites, including the palms, soles, nail beds (subungual) and mucosal surfaces such as the oral, genital or vaginal mucosa. Lesions in darker skin may also be less pigmented or amelanotic.

A total body skin examination is essential for patients with suspicious lesions, including assessment of all naevi and high-risk sites. The ABCDE criteria (Asymmetry, Border irregularity, Colour variation, Diameter greater than 6 mm, Evolution) are widely used to help differentiate early melanomas from benign naevi (see Table 63.1). In darker-skinned populations, particular emphasis should be placed on the E (evolution/change) criterion, as colour and diameter may be less reliable indicators. Clinicians should maintain a high index of suspicion for any new or changing lesion, especially on acral (e.g. hands and feet) and mucosal surfaces, to ensure early diagnosis and improved outcomes.

Investigations

Initial investigation of a suspected melanoma is mostly by visual inspection and biopsy for histological confirmation. The recommended approach is a full-thickness excisional biopsy with narrow margins, whenever reasonable. A dermatoscope is used to enhance the assessment of suspicious skin lesions.

For staging and prognostic evaluation, a sentinel lymph node biopsy (SLNB) may be undertaken. This involves identifying and then removing the lymph node(s) that directly drain the area of the primary tumour for histological analysis. SLNB provides important prognostic information and contributes to pathological staging.

Additional investigations to assess for metastases can include imaging studies such as chest X-rays, liver ultrasounds or CT scans of the chest, abdomen and pelvis. Blood tests usually include a full blood count and liver function tests. A bone scan is reserved for those patients with evidence suggestive of bone involvement.

Staging of primary melanoma is based on the histological features of the lesion, including Breslow thickness, ulceration, mitotic rate and lymph node involvement.

Management

Primary treatment for localised malignant melanoma is wide local excision with margins determined by tumour thickness. For advanced or metastatic melanoma, traditional chemotherapy has limited efficacy and is rarely used. Contemporary first-line treatments either boost the immune system or block cancer-specific mutations. Both approaches help patients with advanced melanoma live longer.

Radiotherapy has a limited role but may be used for lentigo maligna in selected cases or palliative treatment of symptomatic metastases, particularly in the brain or bone. For advanced disease, management is palliative.

Clinical considerations

Health promotion for melanoma focuses on sun safety, skin awareness and early detection. Encourage the use of broad-spectrum sunscreen, wear protective clothing and hats, and avoid peak ultraviolet. The use of tanning devices should be avoided due to their association with increased melanoma risk. Perform regular self-examinations, including areas often overlooked, such as the palms, soles, nail beds and mucosal surfaces. Health promotion should target high-risk groups, including those with fair skin, multiple or atypical naevi, a family history of melanoma or a history of severe sunburns. Patients should be advised to seek prompt medical review for any new or changing lesions.

Ear, nose and throat

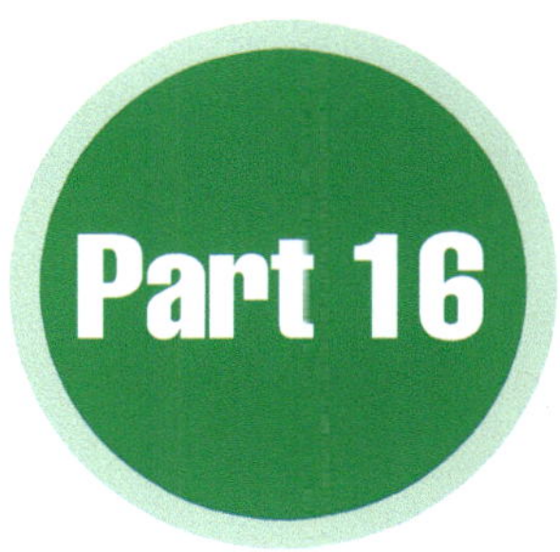

Chapters

64 Otitis media

Figure 64.1 The ear.

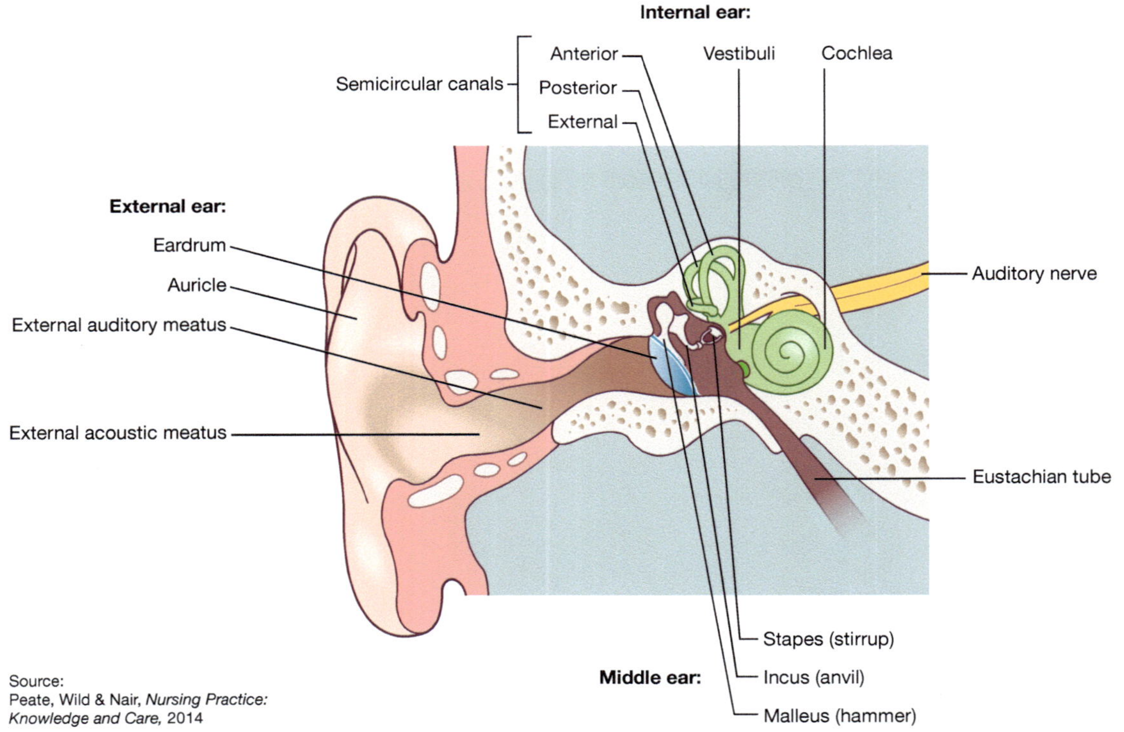

Source:
Peate, Wild & Nair, *Nursing Practice: Knowledge and Care,* 2014

Figure 64.2 Otitis media.

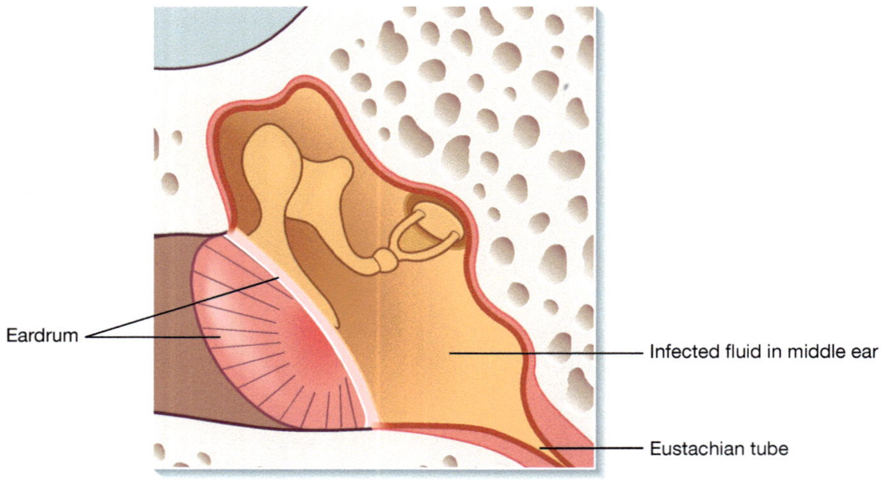

Overview

'Otitis' refers to inflammation of the ear (Figure 64.1). This inflammation can affect the external ear (otitis externa) or the middle ear (otitis media). Otitis media is further classified into acute otitis media (AOM) and otitis media with effusion. Both conditions occur predominantly in children, although they can also affect adults, and may result from bacterial or viral infections.

Otitis media is a common condition frequently encountered in general practice. Most children experience a self-limiting illness; however, some may develop recurrent or chronic problems and require treatment.

In young children, the Eustachian tube is shorter, more horizontal and narrower than in adults. This anatomy makes it easier for infected secretions from the nasopharynx to pass into the middle ear, predisposing them to infection. As children grow, the Eustachian tube becomes longer, more vertical and more angled, improving drainage. Coughing or sneezing in older children and adults tends to promote clearance rather than obstruction.

Pathophysiology

AOM is predominantly a childhood illness, affecting more than two-thirds of children in the UK by the age of three, with approximately half experiencing three or more episodes. The peak incidence occurs between 6 and 24 months, after which the risk declines sharply. AOM is relatively uncommon in adults, and when it does occur, it is often associated with Eustachian tube dysfunction, recent upper respiratory tract infection, sinusitis or immunosuppression. Adults may also develop AOM secondary to structural abnormalities, allergies or following barotrauma (e.g. air travel or diving).

Episodes are more frequent during the winter months, often following a viral upper respiratory tract infection. Several risk factors increase susceptibility, including male sex, exposure to older siblings in school or nursery settings, pacifier use and parental smoking.

The central event in the development of AOM is Eustachian tube dysfunction, which impairs ventilation of the middle ear. In young children, the Eustachian tube is shorter, narrower and more horizontal than in adults, which facilitates the reflux of nasopharyngeal secretions into the middle ear. Inflammation of the nasopharynx, commonly following a viral upper respiratory tract infection, can extend to the medial end of the Eustachian tube, causing swelling, obstruction and fluid stasis. This results in altered middle ear pressures, often negative relative to ambient pressure, which promotes the accumulation of sterile or infected fluid (see Figure 64.2). Allergic inflammation or structural abnormalities, such as craniofacial malformations or neuromuscular disorders, may produce similar dysfunction.

Bacterial colonisation of the middle ear usually follows the establishment of fluid stasis. The most frequent bacterial pathogens are *Streptococcus pneumoniae*, *Haemophilus influenzae* and *Moraxella catarrhalis*, which colonise the nasopharynx and may gain access to the middle ear via reflux or aspiration through the dysfunctional Eustachian tube. Successful colonisation requires bacterial adherence to the mucosal epithelium, which is facilitated by prior viral damage to the respiratory mucosa. Although viruses often trigger AOM, they rarely appear as the primary pathogen in the middle ear fluid.

Once bacteria reach the middle ear, an acute inflammatory response ensues. This is characterised by vasodilatation, increased vascular permeability, exudation, leukocyte infiltration and local immune activation. These processes lead to the classical clinical features of AOM, including ear pain, fever and impaired hearing. In children with recurrent or chronic disease, Eustachian tube dysfunction may be persistent, or the tube may be patulous or hypotonic, further predisposing them to repeated infections.

Immunological factors play a significant role in both susceptibility and resolution of AOM. The nasopharyngeal lymphoid tissue, including adenoids, contributes to local defence by limiting bacterial adherence to the mucosa. Variations in mucosal and systemic immunity may explain why some children experience recurrent episodes while others recover rapidly.

In summary, AOM arises from a complex interplay between anatomical predisposition, viral infection, bacterial colonisation and host immune response. Understanding these mechanisms highlights why AOM is particularly common in young children and provides the rationale for preventive and therapeutic strategies, including immunisation, minimising exposure to respiratory pathogens and judicious use of antibiotics.

Signs and symptoms

Inflammation of the middle ear often occurs in association with an upper respiratory tract infection. Typical symptoms include otalgia (ear pain), irritability, malaise, fever and occasionally vomiting. In some children, pyrexia may trigger febrile convulsions.

On examination, the tympanic membrane may appear red, inflamed and bulging. In some cases, the outer ear may appear erythematous. Hearing loss is commonly reported due to fluid accumulation in the middle ear. If the tympanic membrane ruptures, otorrhoea (discharge from the ear) may be observed.

Investigations

In most cases, no investigations are required, as the diagnosis is primarily clinical. Otoscopy is the main diagnostic tool, allowing assessment of the tympanic membrane for redness, bulging or perforation.

Microbiological culture of ear discharge may be indicated in cases of chronic or recurrent tympanic membrane perforation or when grommets (ventilation tubes) are present, to guide antibiotic therapy.

Audiometry is not routinely performed during the acute phase but should be considered if chronic hearing loss is suspected. Imaging with CT or MRI is reserved for cases where complications are suspected, such as mastoiditis, intracranial spread or atypical presentations.

Management

Most cases of AOM resolve spontaneously, and routine antibiotic therapy is not required. Management is therefore primarily symptomatic, with adequate analgesia and antipyretics prescribed to relieve pain and fever in all patients. In mild to moderate cases, a watchful waiting approach is recommended, with antibiotics reserved for specific situations.

Antibiotic therapy should be considered in children under 2 years with bilateral AOM or a bulging tympanic membrane accompanied by multiple symptoms, in any patient whose symptoms persist for more than 2 to 3 days, and in those with otorrhoea. Children or adults at high risk of complications, including those with significant cardiac, pulmonary, renal, hepatic or neuromuscular disease, immunosuppression, cystic fibrosis or a history of prematurity, should also receive antibiotics promptly.

When indicated, antibiotics remain the only medications with proven efficacy in modifying the course of AOM. Most agents can be administered once or twice daily, improving compliance and reducing the need for school- or daycare-based dosing. The overall approach emphasises targeted antibiotic use, minimising unnecessary exposure while ensuring that patients at higher risk of complications receive appropriate therapy.

Clinical considerations

Patients with acute otitis media should avoid swimming until the infection has resolved and the tympanic membrane is intact, as water exposure may worsen the infection or introduce new pathogens into the middle ear. Similarly, air travel during an active episode can exacerbate ear pain and discomfort due to pressure changes in the middle ear from Eustachian tube dysfunction. If flying is unavoidable, techniques such as chewing gum, swallowing or gentle autoinflation may help to equalise pressure, though these measures are often less effective during acute infection. Swimming and flying can generally be resumed once symptoms have resolved and the tympanic membrane is no longer inflamed or perforated.

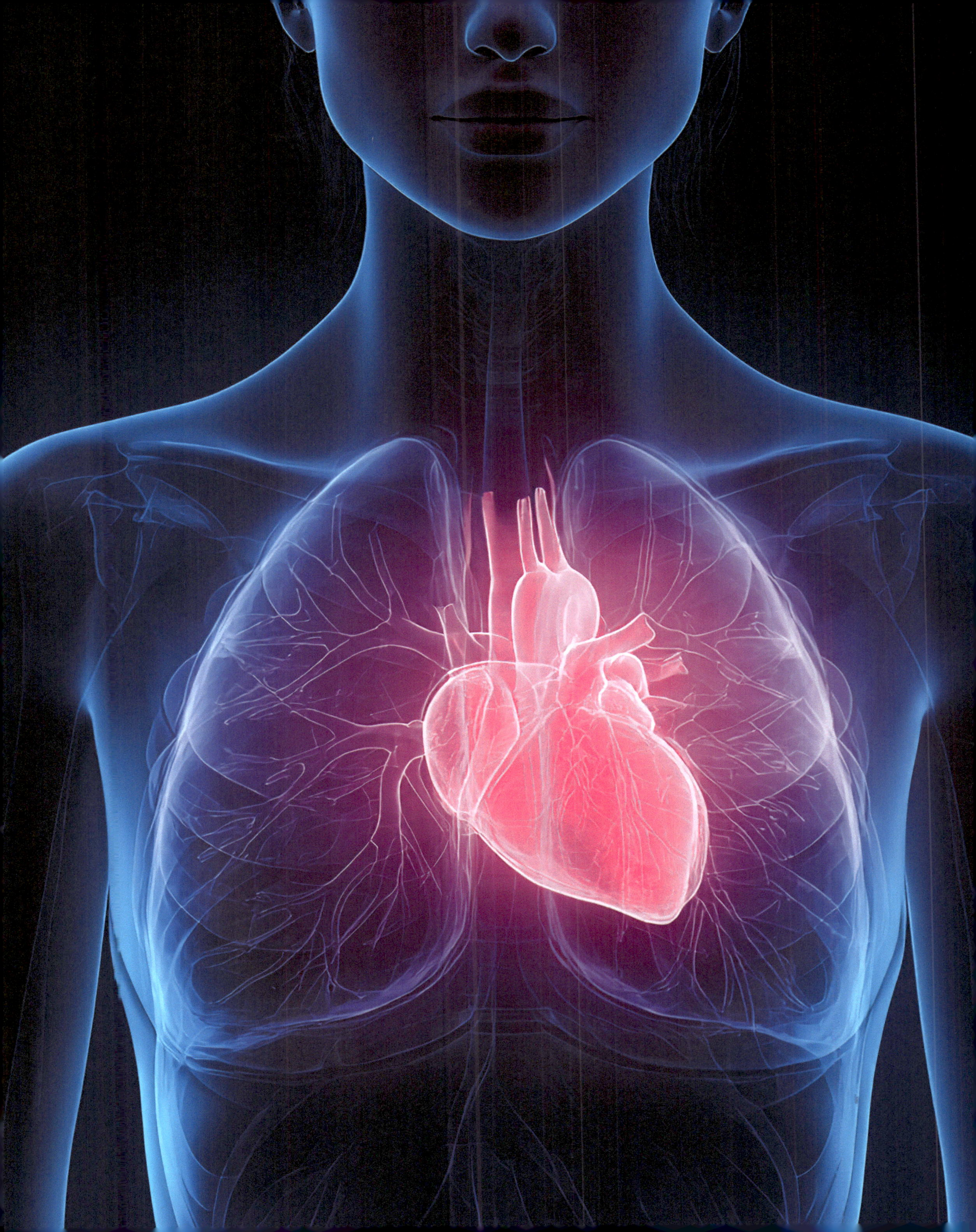

65 Ménière's disease

Figure 65.1 (a) Normal membranous labyrinth and (b) dilated membranous labyrinth in Ménière's disease.

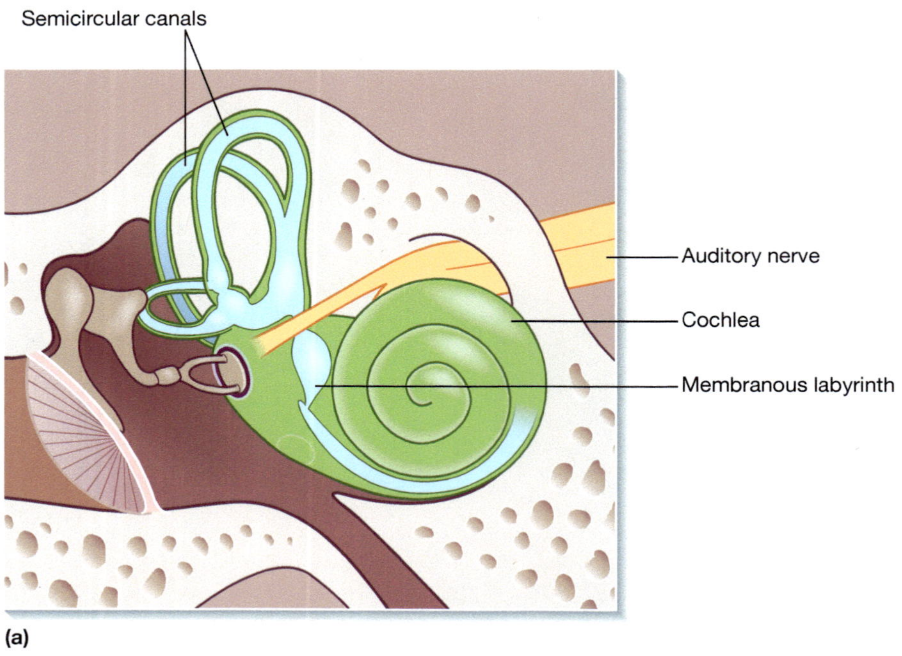

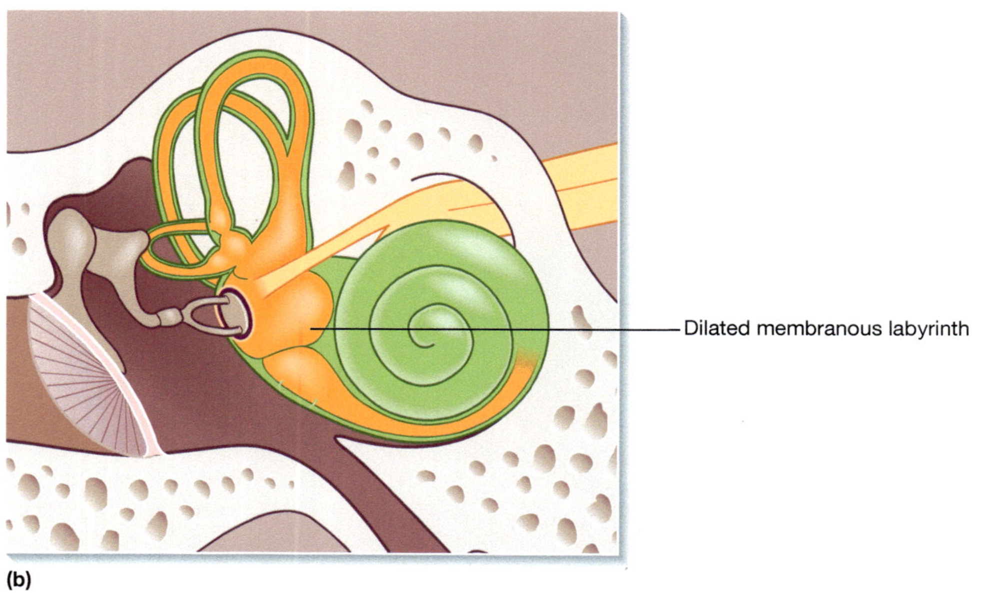

Overview

Ménière's disease is a disorder of the inner ear caused by abnormal fluid dynamics within the membranous labyrinth. The inner ear comprises the cochlea, responsible for hearing and the vestibular apparatus, responsible for balance. The vestibular apparatus includes the semicircular canals, utricle and saccule, all of which are enclosed within the membranous labyrinth, containing a fluid called endolymph. In Ménière's disease, there is a progressive distension of the membranous labyrinth, a condition known as endolymphatic hydrops (see Figure 65.1a and b). This distension can damage the vestibular system, resulting in vertigo or the cochlea nerve, causing hearing loss. Endolymphatic hydrops refers to increased hydraulic pressure within the endolymphatic system of the inner ear.

The reported prevalence of Ménière's disease varies. Bilateral involvement is observed in approximately 10% of patients at initial diagnosis, increasing to over 40% as the disease progresses. Familial predisposition may play a role, with up to half of patients reporting a significant family history. Ménière's disease can occur at almost any age, with cases documented in children as young as four and in elderly adults over 90 years. Onset typically occurs in early to middle adulthood, with peak incidence between 40 and 60 years. Slight female predominance has been reported, and historically, the disease has been noted more frequently in white populations, although it can occur in individuals of any ethnicity.

Ménière's disease is considered idiopathic, and if a specific cause is identified, the condition is classified as secondary endolymphatic hydrops rather than Ménière's disease. Nevertheless, several factors can lead to elevated endolymphatic pressure, including metabolic disturbances, hormonal imbalances, trauma, infections, autoimmune conditions such as lupus or rheumatoid arthritis, allergies and dietary triggers. Identifying and managing these contributing factors is important in differentiating Ménière's disease from other causes of endolymphatic hydrops.

Pathophysiology

The exact pathophysiology of Ménière's disease remains incompletely understood. The endolymph and perilymph, the fluids within the inner ear, are separated by delicate membranes that house the neural apparatus of hearing and balance. Changes in fluid pressure place stress on these membranes, resulting in hearing disturbance, tinnitus, vertigo, imbalance and aural fullness.

In some cases, increased endolymphatic pressure may lead to rupture of Reissner's membrane, allowing endolymph and perilymph to mix. This sudden change in the ionic environment can trigger abrupt alterations in vestibular nerve firing, producing acute vertigo attacks. The distension of the membranous labyrinth also causes mechanical disruption of the auditory and vestibular organs. Stretching of the utricle and saccule may produce non-rotational vestibular symptoms, such as imbalance or light-headedness.

Similarly, distortion of the organ of Corti and its inner and outer hair cells can lead to sensorineural hearing loss and tinnitus. These pathophysiological changes underlie the characteristic episodic nature of Ménière's disease symptoms.

Signs and symptoms

Ménière's disease is characterised by a classic tetrad (four) of symptoms: episodic vertigo, tinnitus, fluctuating sensorineural hearing loss and a sensation of aural fullness or pressure. These features arise in a fluctuating and episodic pattern, which is the hallmark of the condition. Acute attacks of vertigo typically last from several minutes to a few hours, most commonly around 2 to 3 hours

and may occur in clusters of several episodes each year. Periods of remission, in which symptoms may completely resolve, can last for weeks or months. In the majority of cases, the disease initially affects one ear, although bilateral involvement may develop gradually over many years.

In addition to the classic symptoms, some patients experience 'drop attacks', also known as Tumarkin's otolithic crisis, in which sudden falls occur without loss of consciousness or associated vertigo. Imbalance is another frequent complaint, often persisting between acute attacks or emerging as vertigo episodes become less prominent over time.

The clinical course of Ménière's disease can be described in three stages, though not all patients progress through each of these. In the early stage, symptoms are dominated by sudden, unpredictable attacks of vertigo accompanied by fluctuating hearing loss and worsening tinnitus. During the middle stage, vertigo episodes continue and patients may report unsteadiness or light-headedness both before and after attacks. Hearing loss becomes more evident and typically sensorineural in nature, while tinnitus tends to intensify. In the late stage, hearing loss often becomes permanent, vertigo attacks lessen in frequency or cease altogether, and persistent imbalance may develop. Tinnitus usually remains a constant feature throughout.

Investigations

A diagnosis of Ménière's disease is clinical and based on the characteristic symptom complex of recurrent vertigo, fluctuating sensorineural hearing loss, tinnitus and aural fullness. Ménière's disease is defined by two or more spontaneous episodes of vertigo lasting 20 minutes to 12 hours, documented low- to mid-frequency sensorineural hearing loss and associated tinnitus or aural pressure in the affected ear. There are no specific diagnostic signs on examination between attacks.

Because these symptoms may occur in many other conditions, clinicians should perform a thorough assessment to exclude alternative causes. Other ear, nose and throat conditions that may present with similar features include vestibular schwannoma (acoustic neuroma), particularly in patients with unilateral hearing loss, tinnitus or facial nerve involvement, as well as otitis media, impacted cerumen and ototoxicity from certain medications. Clinicians should also consider neurological and intracranial causes of vertigo and hearing loss.

Audiometry is the cornerstone of investigation and typically reveals a fluctuating sensorineural hearing loss, initially affecting low frequencies. Specialised vestibular and auditory tests can support the diagnosis of Ménière's disease and help exclude other causes of vertigo or hearing loss. These include video nystagmography or electronystagmography, often combined with bithermal caloric testing to assess vestibular function; electrocochleography to detect elevated endolymphatic pressure; and brainstem auditory evoked potentials to evaluate the integrity of the auditory nerve and brainstem pathways.

In unilateral cases, MRI of the brain and internal auditory canals with contrast is recommended to rule out vestibular schwannoma and other intracranial lesions.

Further investigations may be undertaken as indicated to exclude systemic causes. These may include thyroid function tests, fasting glucose, autoimmune and syphilis screening, and renal function tests.

Management

The aim of treatment in Ménière's disease is to alleviate acute attacks, reduce the frequency and severity of episodes, preserve hearing and minimise the impact of tinnitus.

Acute attacks of vertigo and associated nausea can be managed with medications such as prochlorperazine, cinnarizine or cyclizine. These may be administered orally, buccally or intramuscularly if vomiting prevents oral intake. In selected cases, short courses of oral steroids or intratympanic steroid injections may be considered.

Patients are advised to follow a low-salt diet and limit alcohol intake. Some clinicians also recommend avoiding caffeine, chocolate and tobacco, although evidence for these triggers is less robust.

Surgical interventions may be considered, such as endolymphatic sac decompression, vestibular nerve section or labyrinthectomy. Patients must be informed of potential risks, including hearing loss and persistent imbalance.

In the UK, patients experiencing vertigo from any cause are required to notify the Driver and Vehicle Licensing Agency (DVLA), as it may affect their ability to drive safely.

Clinical considerations

Patients with Ménière's disease are at increased risk of falls. It is essential to ensure that their environment is safe, with hazards such as loose rugs, clutter or uneven flooring minimised. Patients should be encouraged to use supportive aids, such as handrails and stable furniture, and to move cautiously during acute episodes, sitting or lying down at the onset of vertigo.

Driving during vertigo episodes should be avoided, and patients must comply with reporting requirements to the Driver and Vehicle Licensing Agency (DVLA) in the UK.

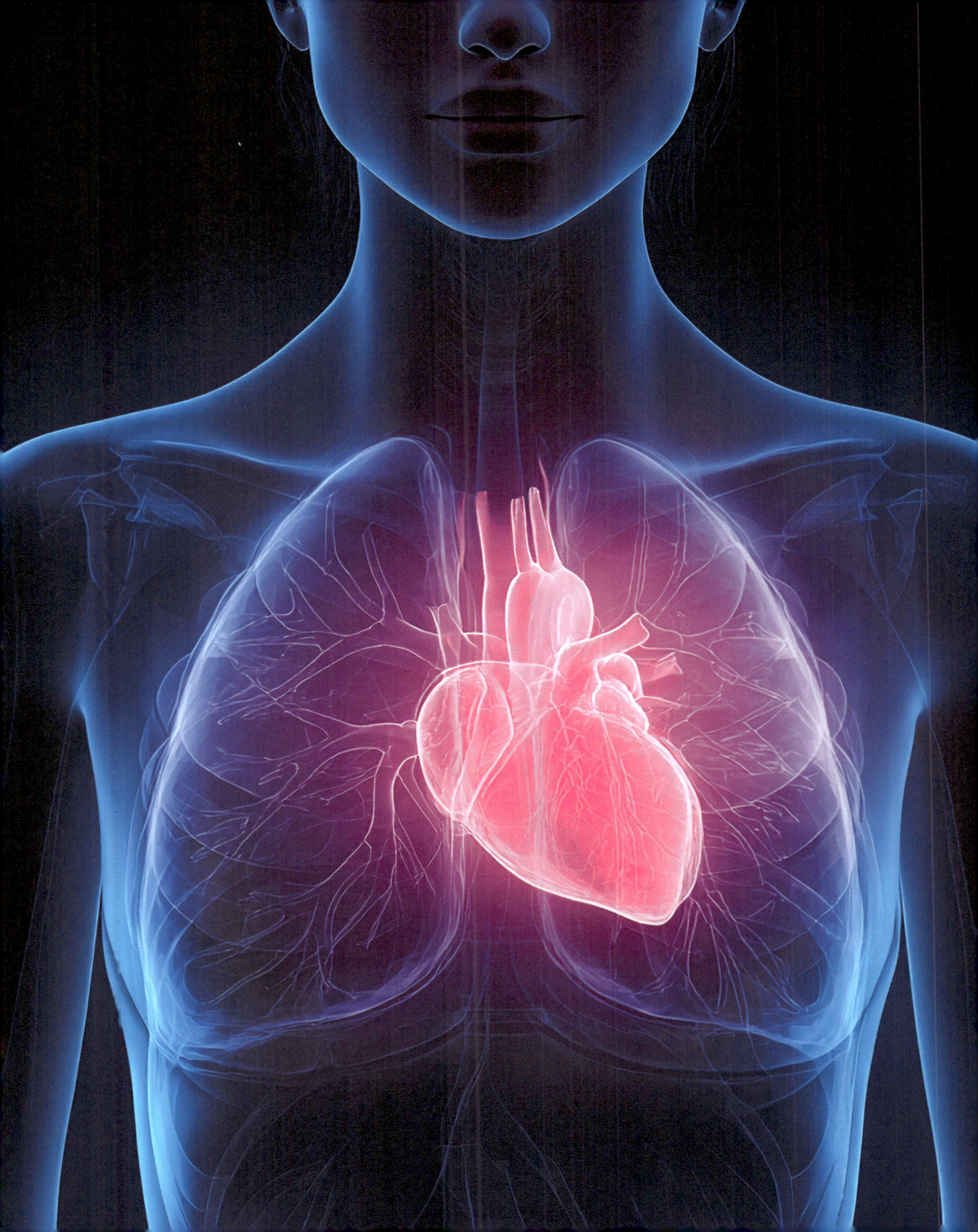

66 Pharyngitis

Figure 66.1 Normal and infected throat.

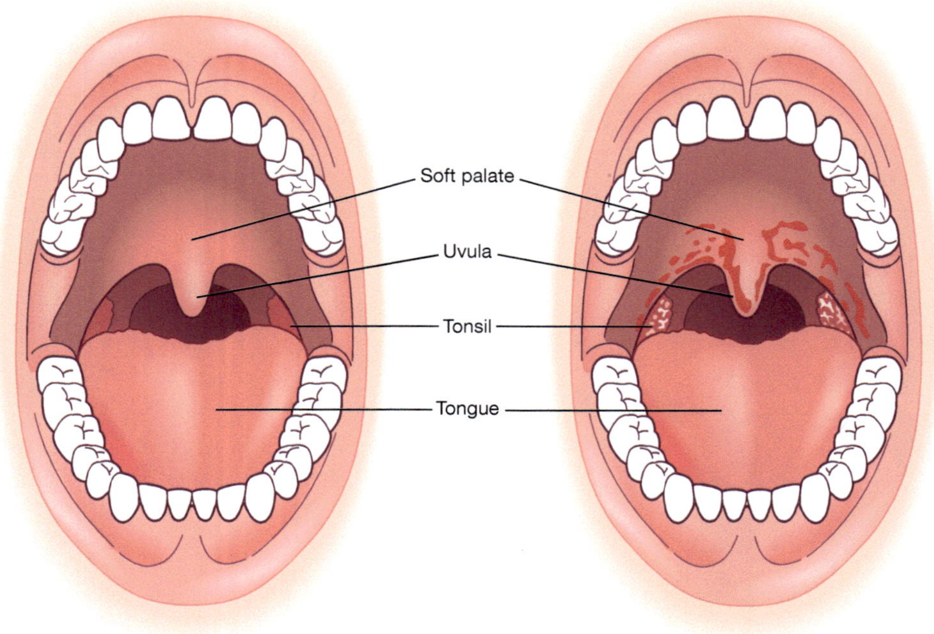

Figure 66.2 Taking a throat swab.

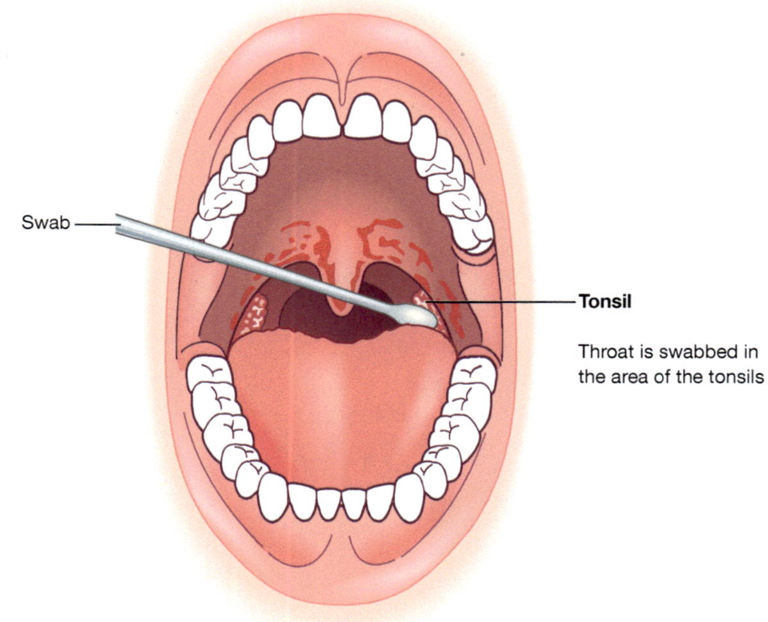

Pharyngitis

Pharyngitis is an inflammation or infection of the pharynx and/or tonsils. The majority of cases are viral in origin and are most commonly caused by rhinovirus, adenovirus, influenza, parainfluenza and Epstein–Barr virus; the condition is usually self-limiting, resolving without specific treatment. Bacterial pharyngitis, most frequently caused by group A beta-haemolytic streptococcus (GABHS), is less common but clinically significant due to the potential for suppurative (complications from pus formation) and non-suppurative complications. Other causes include allergic reactions, trauma, exposure to toxins and neoplasia (Figure 66.1).

Pharyngitis is common but often under-reported because of its self-limiting nature. It occurs more frequently in children, with peak incidence of GABHS and viral pharyngitis in school-aged children (approximately 5–15 years). Pharyngitis is rare in children younger than 3 years. Mortality is uncommon but may occur as a result of complications such as airway obstruction, peritonsillar abscess, toxic shock syndrome or rheumatic carditis. Other sequelae of streptococcal infection include acute glomerulonephritis.

Pathophysiology

In viral pharyngitis, viruses may directly infect the pharyngeal mucosa, causing local inflammation. In some cases, irritation of the pharynx is secondary to post-nasal secretions, as seen with rhinovirus and coronavirus infections.

In bacterial pharyngitis, particularly infections caused by GABHS, the bacteria invade the pharyngeal mucosa and release extracellular toxins and proteases, which contribute to tissue inflammation and local symptoms. Certain strains of GABHS produce M protein, a virulence factor that helps the bacteria evade the immune system. Because the M protein resembles proteins that are in the heart muscle, the immune response against the bacteria can mistakenly attack the heart; this can lead to rheumatic fever and potential heart valve damage.

The prevalence of rheumatogenic GABHS strains has declined in many countries, contributing to a reduction in rheumatic fever incidence.

Signs and symptoms

The causes of viral and bacterial pharyngitis are similar, and differentiation based solely on history and physical examination can often be difficult. Signs and symptoms alone cannot reliably confirm or exclude a GABHS infection.

Certain features increase the likelihood of bacterial (GABHS) pharyngitis, including:

- Sudden onset of sore throat
- Pyrexia
- Headache
- Vomiting (particularly in children)
- Tonsillar exudates (these are white or yellow patches or coatings on the tonsils)
- Anterior cervical lymphadenopathy
- Recent contact with individuals diagnosed with streptococcal pharyngitis or rheumatic fever.

A recent history of orogenital contact raises the possibility of gonococcal pharyngitis. A past history of rheumatic fever is important to consider when planning management.

Symptoms more suggestive of viral pharyngitis include:

- Gradual onset
- Associated cough
- Rhinorrhoea (runny nose)
- Hoarseness
- Other features of upper respiratory tract infection such as malaise and rhinitis.
- Odynophagia (pain on swallowing) may be present in both viral and bacterial infections.

During assessment, the practitioner should explore the duration and severity of symptoms, any self-medication, relevant past medical history and comorbidities, presence of trismus (restricted opening of the mouth), dysphagia, stridor, systemic illness and rash, which may indicate complications or alternative diagnoses.

Investigations

In primary care, investigations for pharyngitis are generally not required, as most cases are viral and self-limiting. Clinical assessment alone is usually sufficient, and most patients improve without intervention. Investigation should be considered when symptoms are prolonged, severe or atypical, or when there is suspicion of complications or underlying systemic illness.

A throat swab may be useful when bacterial infection is suspected, particularly in the presence of tonsillar exudates, marked erythema, or tender anterior cervical lymphadenopathy (see Figure 66.2). Rapid antigen detection tests or culture can confirm GABHS infection and guide the use of antibiotic therapy. Full blood count and glandular fever screening tests are indicated if infectious mononucleosis is suspected, as this may present with atypical lymphocytosis and prolonged symptoms. Antistreptolysin O (ASO) titres (this is an antibody produced by the body in response to infection with GABHS) can help identify recent streptococcal infection in patients who are systemically unwell or have persistent symptoms, although they are not useful for acute diagnosis. Gonococcal culture should be performed if the patient's history indicates potential orogenital exposure.

Examination caution is essential: a throat examination using a tongue depressor must never be attempted in patients with stridor, drooling or difficulty breathing, as this may indicate epiglottitis and could provoke laryngeal spasm, a life-threatening emergency. Typical examination findings in pharyngitis include pharyngeal and tonsillar erythema, tonsillar enlargement, exudate and tender anterior cervical lymphadenopathy. Careful documentation of symptom duration, severity, systemic features and red-flag signs is important to identify patients requiring further investigation or urgent referral.

Management

Efforts should be made to make an accurate diagnosis before initiating treatment, as pharyngitis is a symptom of an underlying condition. National guidelines for the assessment of patients presenting with sore throats are available to aid clinical decision-making. Most cases are self-limiting, with natural resolution within about 1 week. Patients should be advised to rest, maintain hydration and practise good hygiene to reduce the risk of transmission.

Symptomatic relief can be provided with antipyretic analgesics, such as paracetamol or ibuprofen. Antibiotic therapy may be considered depending on the likelihood of bacterial infection:

1 No antibiotics – for most viral cases.
2 Delayed prescription – for mild or uncertain bacterial infection.
3 Immediate prescription – for high likelihood of bacterial infection, particularly GABHS, to prevent complications.

In rare cases with airway compromise or severe inflammation, short-term systemic steroids may be considered under specialist guidance, but they are not part of routine management.

Clinical considerations

Most cases of pharyngitis are caused by viruses, and antibiotics are rarely required. Local protocols are used to guide the need for testing or antibiotic therapy. When bacterial infection is possible but uncertain, a delayed prescription or 'watchful waiting' approach may be appropriate. Antibiotics should be prescribed only for confirmed or highly suspected group A streptococcal infection, primarily to prevent serious complications such as rheumatic fever. Patients should be informed that antibiotics do not relieve viral symptoms, and overuse contributes to antimicrobial resistance.

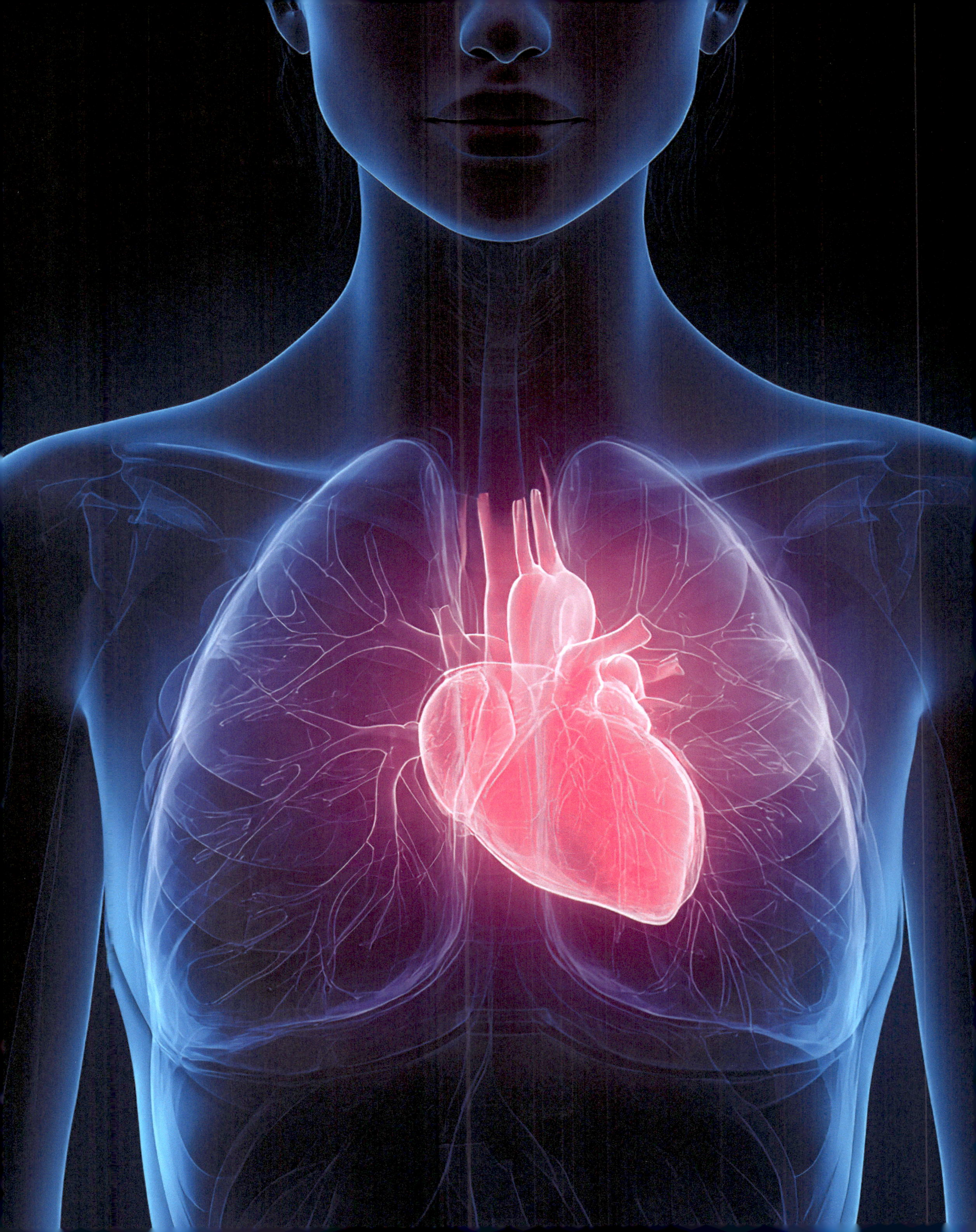

67 Rhinosinusitis

Figure 67.1 The nasal cavity.

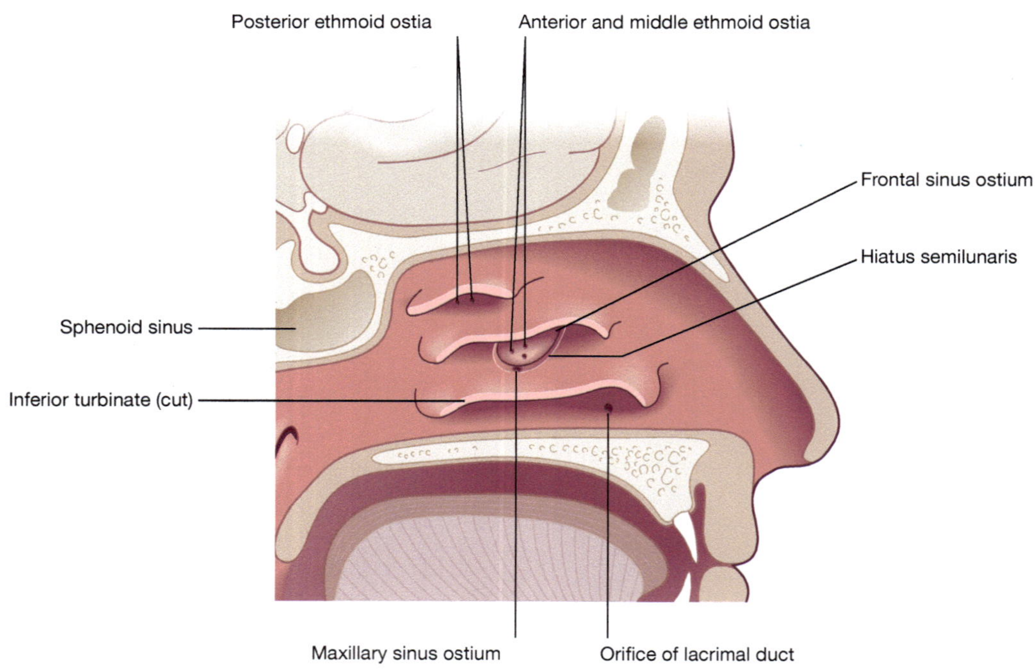

Figure 67.2 Symptoms of rhinosinusitis.

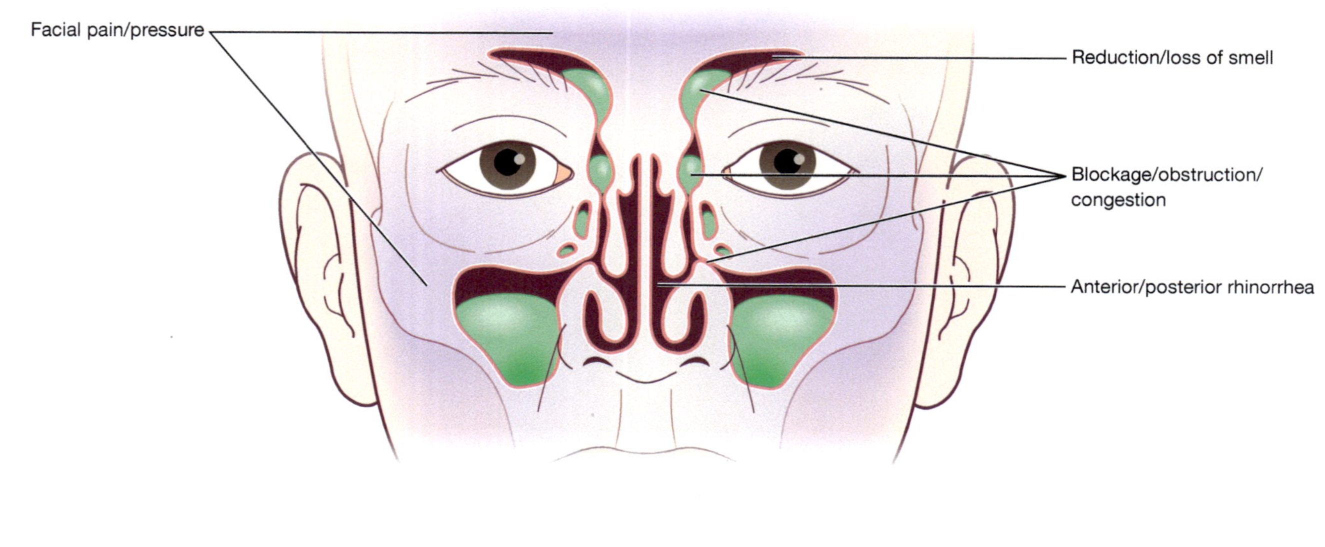

Rhinosinusitis

The nasal cavity is illustrated in Figure 67.1. Sinusitis, more accurately referred to as rhinosinusitis, is characterised by inflammation of the paranasal sinuses and the nasal mucosa, as sinus involvement rarely occurs in isolation. The paranasal sinuses comprise the frontal, maxillary, sphenoidal and ethmoidal sinuses. They develop as diverticula from the nasal mucosa, being rudimentary or absent at birth, with rapid expansion during the eruption of permanent teeth and again at puberty.

The presentation of sinus pathology may be complicated by referred pain. The maxillary sinus receives innervation from the infraorbital nerve and the anterior, middle and posterior superior alveolar nerves. Consequently, pathology within the maxillary sinus may manifest as upper jaw pain, toothache or discomfort in the overlying skin of the cheek, potentially complicating diagnosis.

Rhinosinusitis is a common condition, affecting approximately 15% of the population in Western countries, and exhibits seasonal variation, with a higher prevalence during winter. Children typically experience six to eight upper respiratory tract infections annually, some of which may be complicated by the development of acute bacterial sinusitis. Infective sinusitis is observed more frequently in women than in men, which may reflect closer contact with young children and increased exposure to pathogens.

Understanding the anatomical development, innervation and epidemiology of the paranasal sinuses is essential for accurate diagnosis and management of rhinosinusitis. Awareness of referred pain patterns and patient demographics can aid clinicians in differentiating sinus pathology from other causes of facial or dental discomfort.

Pathophysiology

The paranasal sinuses are normally sterile cavities lined by respiratory epithelium with ciliated cells that propel mucus toward the sinus ostia, ensuring unidirectional flow into the nasal cavity and preventing microbial contamination. The maxillary sinus typically has a single ostium positioned high on the medial wall, which may predispose to impaired drainage in a non-dependent position.

Acute rhinosinusitis usually begins with mucosal inflammation, often triggered by viral upper respiratory tract infections, allergy or chemical irritation. Inflammation and oedema of the sinus ostia obstruct mucus flow, creating stasis and negative pressure within the sinus, which can rarely allow bacterial superinfection. While most acute episodes are viral (90–98%), bacterial infection may be suspected when symptoms worsen after 5 days or persist beyond 10 days. Impairment of mucociliary clearance, whether from host factors such as smoking, anatomical variants or immunodeficiency, can increase the risk of infection.

Chronic rhinosinusitis is defined as symptoms persisting for more than 12 weeks and is associated with ongoing inflammation rather than repeated acute infections alone. It can be classified into phenotypes with or without nasal polyps and may involve irreversible changes in the mucosa, often compounded by host or environmental factors.

Temporal classification of rhinosinusitis includes:

- Acute: 7–30 days
- Subacute: 4–12 weeks
- Recurrent: 3 or more significant acute episodes per year, each lasting 10 or more days
- Chronic: More than 12 weeks, with or without acute exacerbations

Understanding sinus anatomy, mucociliary function and host susceptibility is essential for recognising the mechanisms underlying both acute and chronic rhinosinusitis and for guiding appropriate management.

Signs and symptoms

There is no single clinical sign or symptom that is sufficiently sensitive or specific to diagnose acute sinusitis; therefore, management is guided by the overall clinical impression. Acute sinusitis typically follows an upper respiratory tract infection and is identified by nasal obstruction or congestion, anterior or posterior nasal discharge, facial pain or pressure, and/or reduced or lost sense of smell.

Nasal discharge that is thick, purulent (containing or producing pus) or green may raise suspicion of bacterial involvement, although colour alone is not definitive. Nasal blockage is often bilateral and may result from underlying rhinitis. Facial pain or pressure is usually localised over the affected sinus but may be referred to the upper jaw, teeth, forehead or orbit. Isolated facial pain without accompanying nasal symptoms is unlikely to indicate sinusitis. Figure 67.2 depicts the paranasal sinuses and common sites of referred facial pain.

Investigations

Investigations are generally not required to diagnose acute sinusitis, although this remains a matter of clinical debate. Physical examination has limited sensitivity, but this may reveal purulent nasal discharge, mucosal swelling and tenderness over the affected sinuses.

Anterior rhinoscopy, with or without a topical decongestant, is useful to assess the nasal mucosa, the presence and colour of discharge, and any predisposing anatomical variations. Nasal endoscopy can provide additional information in selected cases, such as recurrent, complicated or chronic sinusitis, by identifying the origin of purulent discharge and evaluating ostiomeatal obstruction.

Management

Acute rhinosinusitis

Diagnosis is primarily clinical, based on history and presenting signs and symptoms. Most cases are viral, and patients should be reassured that the illness is self-limiting, similar to a prolonged cold.

Symptomatic measures include:

- Analgesics such as paracetamol or ibuprofen for pain or fever
- Short-term intranasal decongestants (maximum 7 days)
- Nasal irrigation with warm saline solution
- Warm face packs for localised pain relief

Antibiotics are reserved for patients with severe symptoms, persistent illness beyond 10 days or worsening symptoms after initial improvement. First-line agents typically include amoxicillin, guided by local protocols.

Patients who deteriorate or develop complications (such as orbital or intracranial involvement) may require hospital assessment. In such cases, management can include microbiological investigations, intravenous antibiotics and, rarely, surgical intervention to restore sinus ventilation and mucociliary function.

Chronic rhinosinusitis

Chronic rhinosinusitis is less common than acute rhinosinusitis and is defined by the presence of nasal and sinus symptoms persisting for more than 12 weeks. Chronic rhinosinusitis is classified into chronic rhinosinusitis without nasal polyps (CRSsNP) and chronic rhinosinusitis with nasal polyps (CRSwNP). Rare forms include allergic or invasive fungal sinusitis.

Symptoms are generally less acute than in acute sinusitis and include nasal obstruction or congestion, nasal discharge, post-nasal drip and reduced sense of smell. Facial pain may occur but is usually mild. Examination may reveal nasal mucosal inflammation, polyps and purulent discharge in some cases.

Diagnosis is primarily clinical. Investigations are not usually required, but imaging (CT scan) may be indicated if the diagnosis is uncertain or if surgery is being considered.

Management is initially medical and aims to restore sinus ventilation and reduce inflammation. First-line therapy includes:

- Intranasal corticosteroids
- Saline nasal irrigation for symptomatic relief

Antibiotics are reserved for acute bacterial exacerbations. Surgical intervention, such as functional endoscopic sinus surgery, may be considered if symptoms persist despite maximal medical therapy, particularly in CRSwNP.

Clinical considerations

Acute rhinosinusitis is usually viral, and purulent discharge alone does not indicate bacterial infection. Bacterial involvement is more likely when symptoms persist beyond 10 days or worsen after initial improvement. Red flags such as severe headache, periorbital swelling, visual changes or neurological signs require urgent assessment.

Chronic rhinosinusitis lasts more than 12 weeks, with nasal obstruction and reduced sense of smell often more prominent than pain. Examination may reveal mucosal inflammation, polyps or anatomical factors affecting sinus drainage.

Management is primarily supportive, including analgesics, saline irrigation, and short-term decongestants. Intranasal corticosteroids are used for persistent inflammation, antibiotics are reserved for severe or prolonged bacterial cases, and surgery is considered only when medical therapy fails or complications arise.

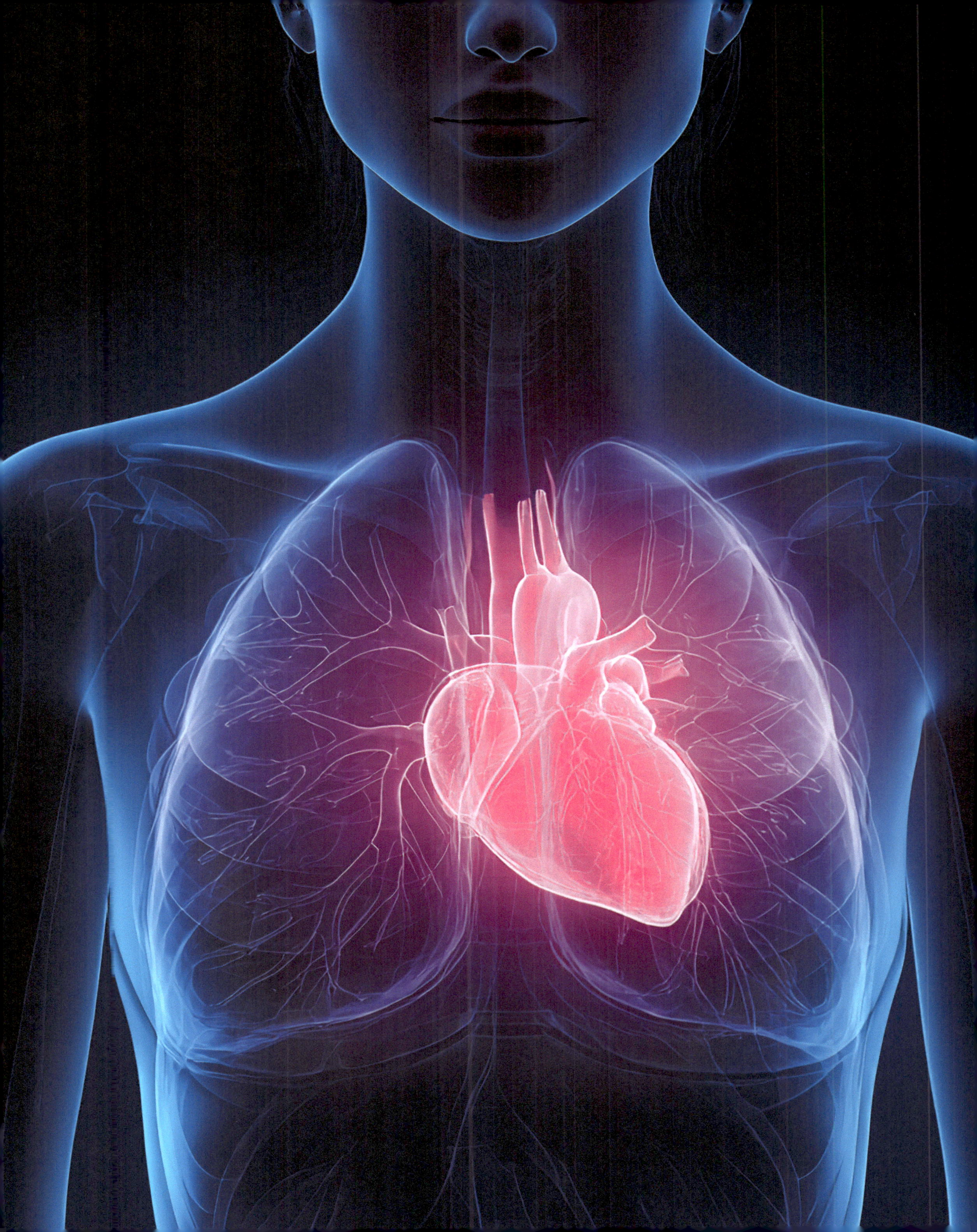

68 Epistaxis

Figure 68.1 Cross-section of the nasal cavity and vasculature.

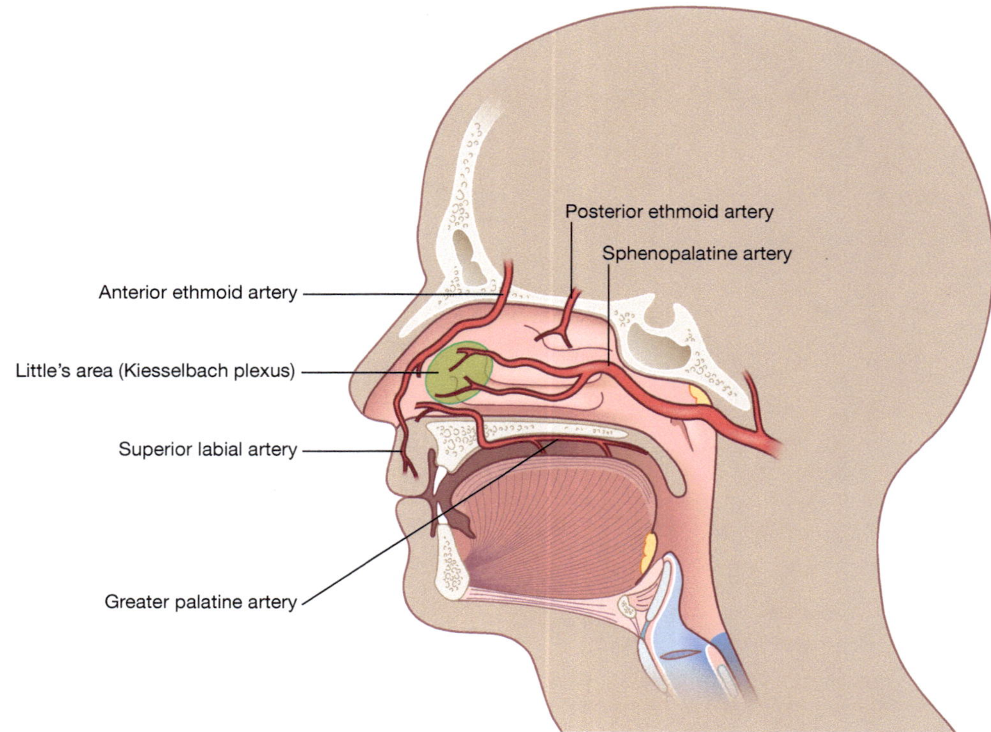

Box 68.1 First aid for a nosebleed.

1.	Reassure the patient and remain calm. Anxiety can worsen bleeding.
2.	Positioning: ask the patient to sit down and lean slightly forward. This prevents blood from flowing down the throat, which could cause nausea or compromise the airway.
3.	Maintain airway: ensure the patient's airway remains clear at all times.
4.	Pinch the nose: using the thumb and index finger, pinch the soft part of the nose (just below the nasal bone) firmly for 10 minutes without checking too early.
5.	Provide support: give tissues to catch blood and a bowl if necessary. Avoid tilting the head back.
6.	After 10 minutes: release the pressure slowly to check if bleeding has stopped.
7.	If bleeding continues: reapply pressure for another 10 minutes. You may repeat once more if necessary.
8.	Seek urgent medical help if bleeding persists after 30 minutes or if the patient has recurrent nosebleeds, is on anticoagulants or experiences dizziness, weakness or heavy bleeding.

•	Using a cold compress or ice on the bridge of the nose can help constrict vessels.
•	Avoiding nose blowing, picking or heavy exertion for several hours afterwards.
•	Being aware of risk factors (anticoagulants, hypertension and repeated bleeds) that may necessitate earlier medical review.

Epistaxis

Epistaxis (nosebleed) is usually self-limiting and harmless, and in most cases, the underlying cause of vascular damage is not identified. Rarely, epistaxis can be life-threatening, but it often causes significant concern, particularly for parents of young children. Most epistaxis originates from Little's area on the anterior nasal septum, which contains the Kiesselbach plexus of vessels (see Figure 68.1). Less commonly, bleeding arises from branches of the sphenopalatine artery in the posterior nasal cavity.

Over half of the population experiences at least one episode of epistaxis, although the true prevalence is uncertain because most episodes are self-limited and unreported. The incidence varies with age, peaking in children under ten years and adults over 45 years. Epistaxis is unusual in children under 2 years, and when it occurs, it may indicate injury or a more serious illness. In older adults, posterior epistaxis is relatively more common than in younger individuals.

Pathophysiology

Nosebleeds can arise from a wide range of causes, which are conventionally divided into local, systemic and idiopathic factors.

Local trauma

Epistaxis is most commonly caused by local trauma. Self-induced injury, such as nasal picking, frequently affects young children and can result in anterior septal mucosal ulceration and bleeding. Facial trauma, nasal fractures and foreign bodies, including nasogastric or nasotracheal tubes, can also precipitate nosebleeds. Bleeding may range from minor and self-limiting to severe haemorrhage in the context of extensive injury, sometimes requiring nasal packing. Iatrogenic causes, including nasal or sinus surgery, can result in minor mucosal lacerations or, less commonly, significant bleeding due to transection of major vessels.

Mucosal irritation

Mucosal irritation is another frequent contributor to epistaxis. Dry climates, cold weather and home heating systems can dehydrate the nasal mucosa, increasing susceptibility to bleeding. Topical nasal medications, including corticosteroids and antihistamines, as well as systemic agents such as non-steroidal anti-inflammatory drugs, may further predispose patients to minor epistaxis.

Structural abnormalities

Structural changes in the nasal septum, including deviations, spurs and perforations, can disrupt airflow, induce mucosal dryness and contribute to epistaxis. Bleeding often occurs anterior to the site of abnormality, and crusting at the edges of septal perforations is a common locus for recurrent bleeding.

Inflammatory diseases

Inflammatory conditions, such as bacterial, viral or allergic rhinosinusitis, may inflame the nasal mucosa, causing minor blood-streaked discharge. Granulomatous diseases, including sarcoidosis, granulomatosis with polyangiitis, tuberculosis, syphilis and rhinoscleroma, can result in friable mucosa and recurrent epistaxis.

Neoplasms

Benign and malignant tumours of the nasal cavity may also present with epistaxis, often accompanied by unilateral obstruction or symptoms resembling rhinosinusitis. Recognition of neoplasms is essential to ensure timely diagnosis and management.

Systemic causes

Systemic factors include congenital and acquired coagulopathies (these are disorders that affect the blood's ability to clot properly). Congenital bleeding disorders, such as haemophilia and von Willebrand disease, should be considered in patients with a positive family history, easy bruising or prolonged bleeding. Acquired coagulopathies, including thrombocytopaenia or liver disease, and the use of oral anticoagulants increase the risk of epistaxis. Substance use, particularly intranasal cocaine, can lead to severe vasoconstriction, septal necrosis and bleeding. Age-related vascular fragility due to arteriosclerosis contributes to the higher prevalence of epistaxis in older adults. Although hypertension is frequently observed in patients with nosebleeds, it is rarely a direct cause; elevated blood pressure is usually reactive due to stress and anxiety.

Idiopathic epistaxis

In many cases, despite careful evaluation, no definitive cause is identified. These episodes are classified as idiopathic and are often self-limiting.

Signs and symptoms

Determine the site of bleeding. Bleeding from a single nostril is usually anterior in origin, whereas blood from both nostrils or flowing into the throat typically indicates a posterior source, which may be more serious. History explores any recent trauma, including nose picking, facial injuries or prior nasal surgery – common triggers of bleeding. Review the patient's family and personal history for bleeding or clotting disorders, hypertension and previous episodes of epistaxis. Medications should be assessed, particularly anticoagulants, non-steroidal anti-inflammatory drugs and topical nasal therapies, as these can increase the risk of prolonged bleeding. Additional associated symptoms, such as facial pain, earache, dizziness or other systemic signs, should be noted, as they may indicate local complications or more extensive blood loss.

Investigations

Routine laboratory investigations are generally not required in patients with a first-time nosebleed or infrequent episodes when there is a clear history of trauma, nose picking or other minor local causes. Laboratory studies should be considered if the bleeding is severe, recurrent or unexplained, or if a coagulopathy is suspected. Appropriate investigations may include a full blood count, coagulation profile and liver function tests, depending on the clinical context.

Management

Medical attention is typically needed when epistaxis is recurrent, severe or unresponsive to initial first-aid measures. Management depends on the location and severity of bleeding. Localised anterior bleeding often responds to chemical or electrical cauterisation; persistent bleeding, particularly from posterior sites, may require nasal packing. In recurrent or severe epistaxis not responding to medical therapy, surgical options such as arterial ligation or endovascular embolisation are available.

Following intervention, patients should be closely monitored for rebleeding or complications, and adequate pain control should be provided, particularly in cases involving posterior packing. Antibiotic prophylaxis may be indicated for patients with nasal packing at risk of rhinosinusitis or toxic shock syndrome but it is not routinely required for all patients. Patients should avoid aspirin and other non-steroidal anti-inflammatory drugs, which can exacerbate bleeding. In addition, any underlying medical conditions, such as hypertension, coagulopathies or vitamin K deficiency, should be optimally managed in collaboration with appropriate specialists. Box 68.1 outlines first aid treatment.

Clinical considerations

Most nosebleeds are minor; certain features indicate the need for urgent assessment. Red flags include bleeding longer than 20–30 minutes despite first aid, posterior bleeding with blood flowing into the throat or from both nostrils, recurrent or severe epistaxis, especially in patients on anticoagulants or with known bleeding disorders and signs of haemodynamic compromise. Unexplained unilateral nasal obstruction or the presence of a mass should also prompt specialist evaluation, as it may indicate an underlying tumour or structural pathology.

Vision

Chapters

69 Cataracts

Figure 69.1   The eye.

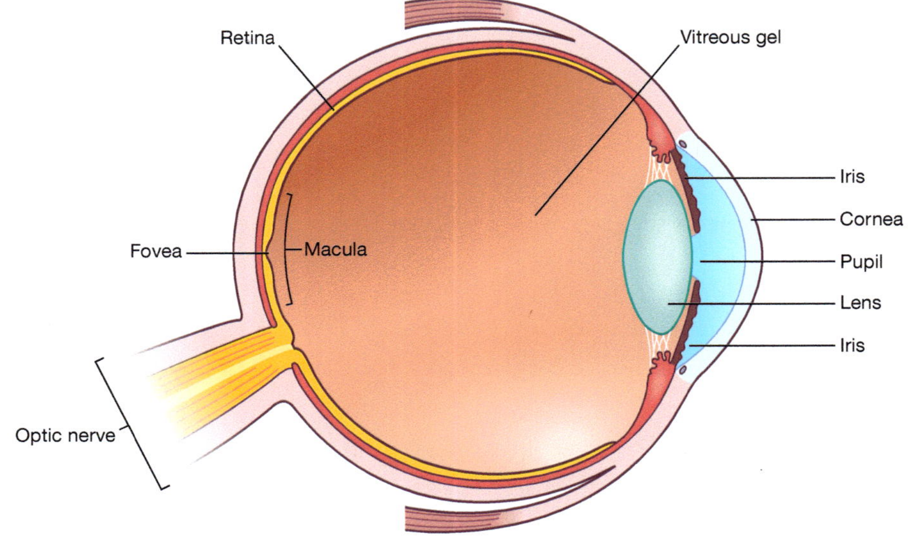

Figure 69.2   Normal lens (a) and lens affected by cataract (b).

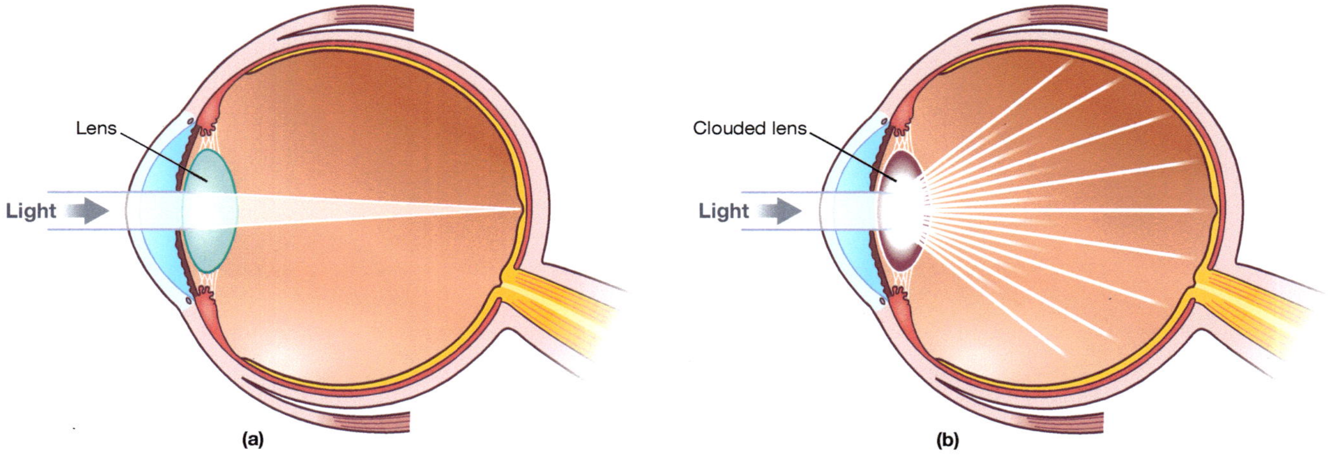

Figure 69.3   Phacoemulsification.

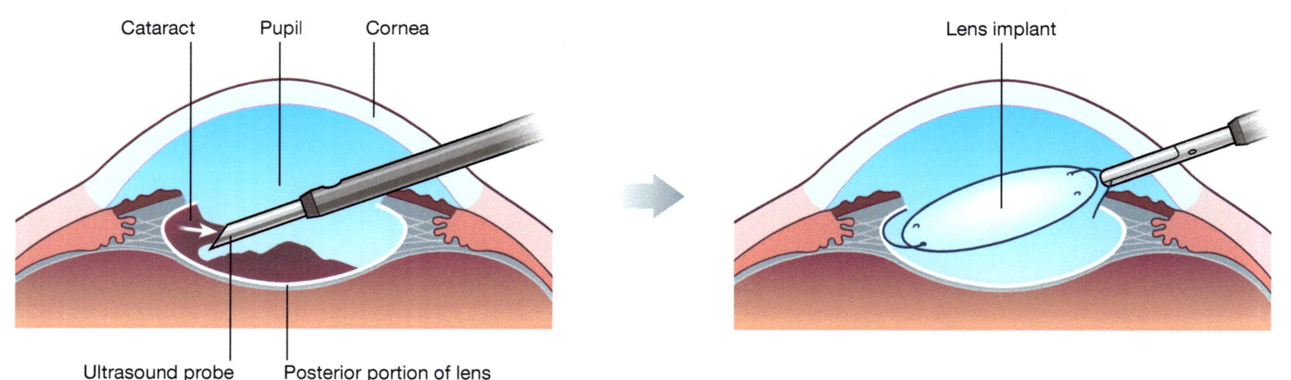

Overview

Cataract is an age-related, vision-impairing condition characterised by gradual opacification of the lens of the eye. Globally, it is one of the leading causes of blindness. Cataracts can vary in severity, ranging from small, subtle opacities to complete lens clouding. While age-related changes are the most common cause, congenital cataracts may also occur.

Age-related cataract is a progressive condition in which the lens of the eye gradually becomes cloudy, leading to blurred or misty vision. Early detection, regular monitoring and timely surgical intervention are essential in its management.

When light passes through the front of the eye, it is focused by the cornea and lens onto the retina (see Figure 69.1). The lens is normally transparent, allowing light to pass directly through and focus precisely on the retina. The retina then converts light into electrical signals, which are transmitted via a network of nerves to the optic nerve and ultimately to the brain. The brain interprets these signals, enabling vision.

Cataracts result from changes in the arrangement of lens proteins and their water content, causing the lens to become opaque rather than clear (see Figure 69.2). This clouding prevents light from passing directly through the lens, leading to visual impairment. A cataract is not a tumour or a growth over the eye; it is simply the lens becoming opaque or 'misty'.

Pathophysiology

Cataract is a progressive opacification of the lens that leads to impaired vision. While age is the most significant risk factor for adult cataracts, cataracts can also occur in children. Congenital or paediatric cataracts may result from genetic mutations, intrauterine infections (e.g. rubella), metabolic disorders, trauma or systemic diseases. These cataracts can be present at birth or develop during childhood and, if untreated, can lead to permanent visual impairment due to amblyopia. Age-related (senile) cataracts, which typically develop in older adults, are primarily caused by biochemical and structural changes in the lens over time, leading to protein aggregation, oxidative stress and progressive lens opacification.

Age is the most significant risk factor in cataracts, but other contributors include diabetes mellitus, prolonged corticosteroid use, ocular trauma, ultraviolet (UV) exposure, uveitis, smoking, excessive alcohol intake, poor nutrition and socioeconomic factors. These factors can accelerate the biochemical and structural changes that compromise lens transparency.

The lens is normally transparent due to the highly organised arrangement of lens fibre cells and the precise structure of crystallin proteins, which maintain clarity and refractive function. With ageing, the lens undergoes structural and biochemical changes: it increases in thickness and weight, while its ability to accommodate declines. New cortical fibres are added in concentric layers, compressing the central nucleus and resulting in nuclear sclerosis. The accumulation of insoluble proteins, oxidative damage and impaired antioxidant mechanisms further reduces transparency.

Lens epithelial cells, responsible for maintaining lens homeostasis and generating new fibre cells, experience age-related alterations, including aberrant differentiation and subtle losses in cell density. These changes, combined with a reduction in water and nutrient transport through the epithelium and cortex, contribute to protein aggregation, lens opacification and decreased refractive quality.

Age-related cataracts are classified into three main types:

1 Nuclear cataract – characterised by central hardening and yellowing of the lens nucleus due to compression from newly formed cortical fibres. Vision loss typically progresses slowly.
2 Cortical cataract – presents as wedge-shaped opacities in the lens cortex, forming 'spokes' that may interfere with vision if they extend into the visual axis or if the cataract becomes mature.
3 Posterior subcapsular cataract – occurs at the back of the lens, often in younger individuals or patients exposed to steroids or radiation. It causes glare and may impair near vision even in the early stages.

The pathogenesis of cataract is therefore multifactorial, involving oxidative stress, protein aggregation, cellular changes and structural alterations, all culminating in progressive lens opacity and visual impairment.

Signs and symptoms

Cataracts can affect one or both eyes. Coexisting ocular conditions, such as glaucoma, age-related macular degeneration, diabetic retinopathy and amblyopia, may be present in individuals requiring cataract surgery.

Typical symptoms include a gradual, painless loss of vision, difficulty reading, trouble recognising faces, problems watching television, increased sensitivity to glare and monocular diplopia.

Lens opacities can often be detected as defects in the red reflex when viewed with an ophthalmoscope held approximately 50–60 cm from the eye. Pupil dilation may aid visualisation. Depending on the type and severity of the cataract, the lens may appear white, yellow or brown when a bright light is shone onto it.

Investigations

After a thorough history, a careful physical examination of the eye should be performed. The examination can reveal abnormalities that may indicate systemic conditions affecting the eye and contributing to cataract development. The diagnosis of cataract is based on the combination of a detailed history and a comprehensive eye examination.

Management

Failure to treat a developing cataract surgically can lead to complications such as lens swelling and intumescence, secondary glaucoma and eventual visual loss. Currently, there is no medical therapy proven to prevent, delay or reverse cataract formation. Surgical removal remains the only effective intervention to restore or maintain vision.

Most cataract surgery is performed in older adults, with the majority of patients over 60 years of age. Phacoemulsification is the most widely used technique and is considered the safest and most effective method (see Figure 69.3). There is no absolute visual acuity threshold for surgery; the impact on the patient's quality of life and daily functioning is the primary deciding factor.

During phacoemulsification, a small corneal incision (approximately 2.2–3 mm) is made, followed by a circular opening (capsulorhexis) in the anterior lens capsule of around 5 mm. The lens nucleus is emulsified using an ultrasonic probe, and cortical material is aspirated. A folded intraocular lens is then inserted into the empty capsular bag, where it unfolds. The incision is self-sealing and rarely requires sutures.

The procedure is usually performed on a day-case basis under local or topical anaesthesia. Postoperative management includes topical antibiotics and corticosteroids, and patients are advised to avoid strenuous activity and eye rubbing for several weeks.

Clinical considerations

After cataract surgery, patient safety is paramount. Advise patients to use all prescribed topical antibiotics and corticosteroids as directed to prevent infection and control inflammation. Avoid strenuous activity, heavy lifting, bending or rubbing the operated eye for 4–6 weeks to reduce the risk of wound complications. Wearing sunglasses outdoors to protect from bright light and trauma. Report any sudden pain, redness, discharge or loss of vision promptly; these may indicate infection or other complications. Follow-up appointments are essential to monitor healing, intraocular pressure and the position of the intraocular lens.

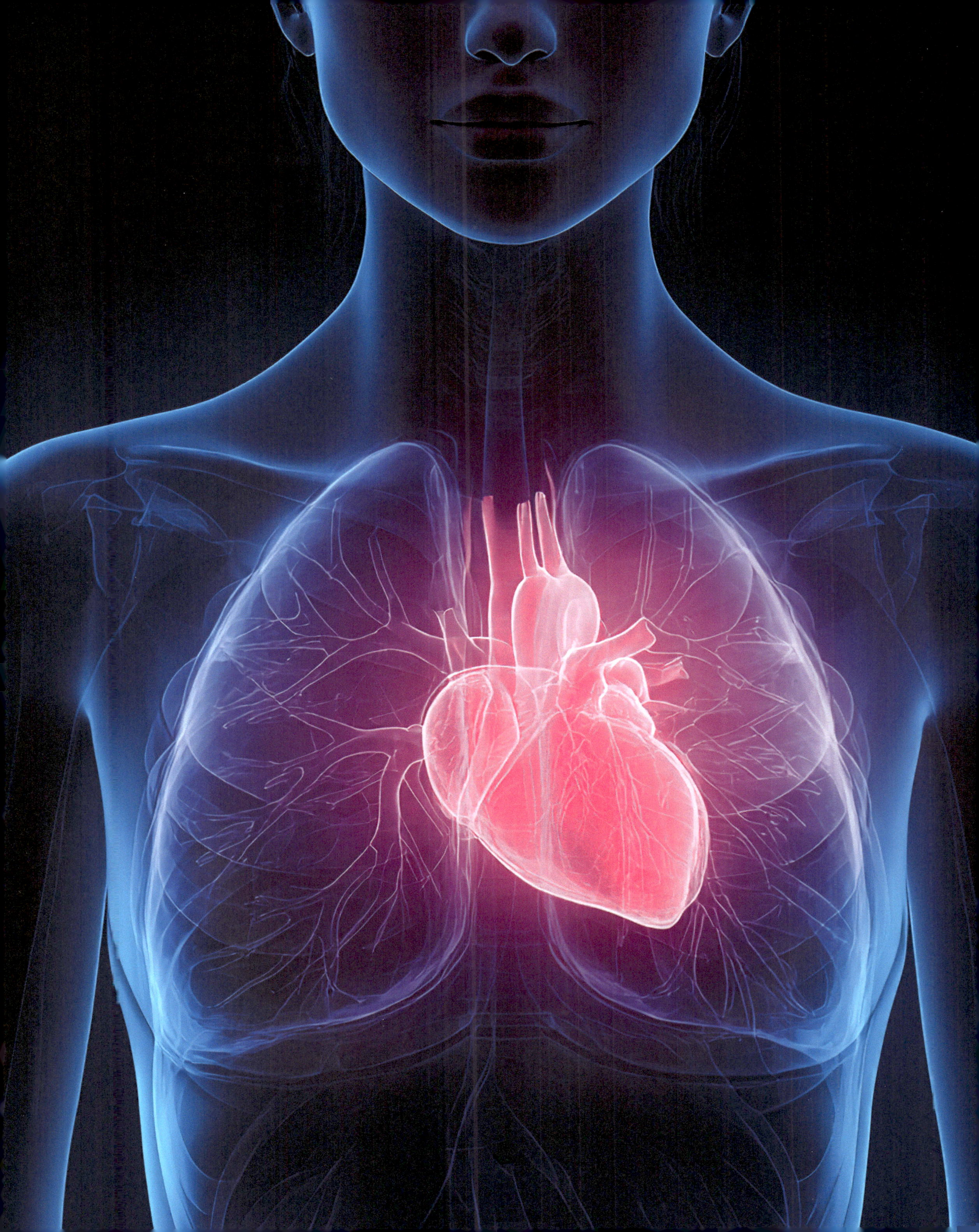

70 Glaucoma

Figure 70.1 Glaucoma.

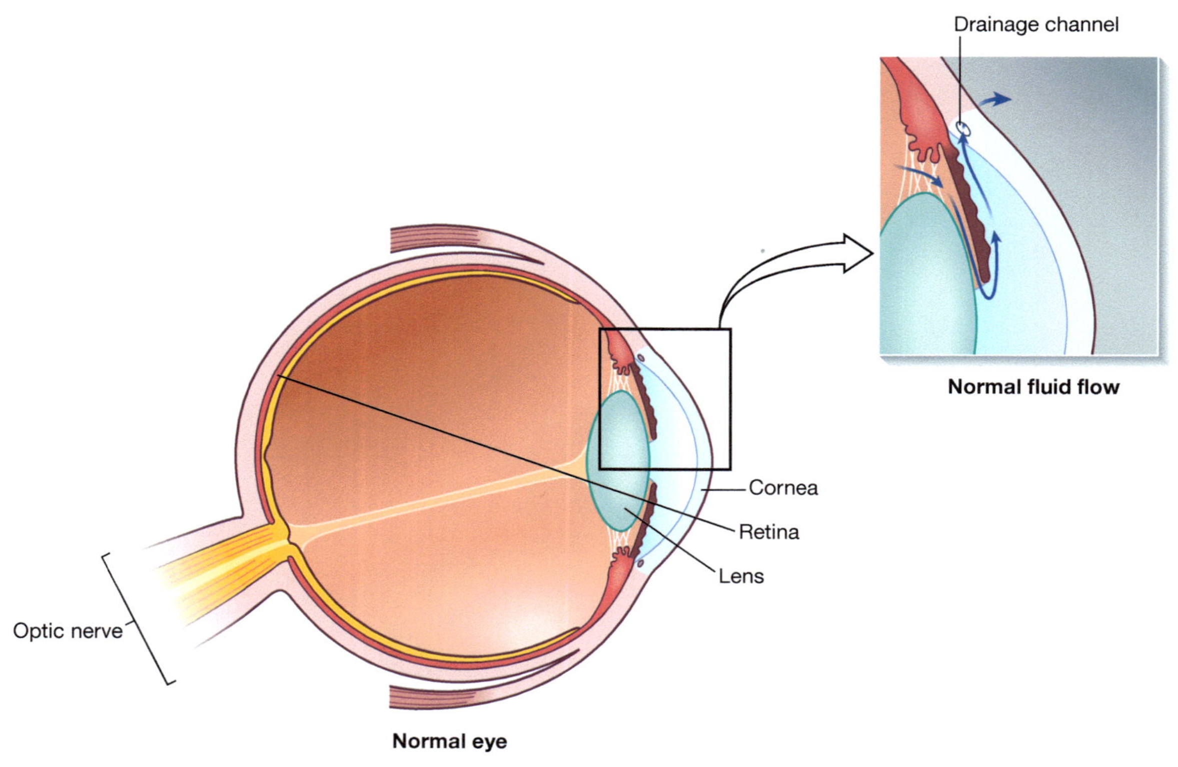

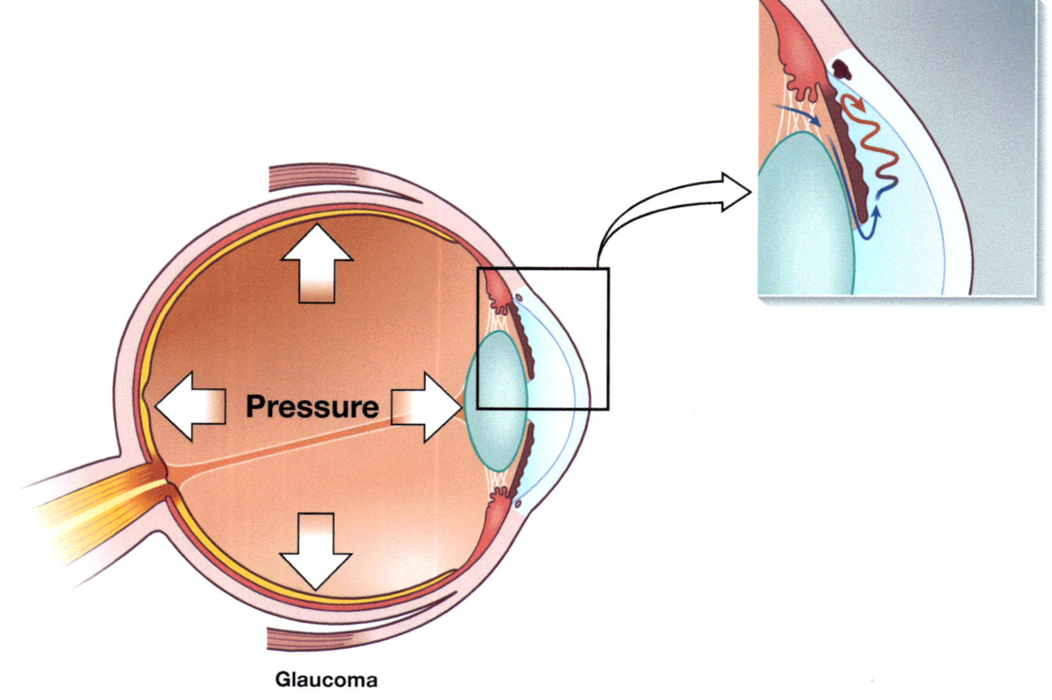

Overview

Glaucoma is a group of eye disorders characterised by progressive optic neuropathy, often associated with increased intraocular pressure (IOP), typically above 21 mmHg, though optic nerve damage can occur at lower pressures in normal-tension glaucoma. Extremely high pressures, sometimes reaching 70–80 mmHg, may occur in rare cases of acute angle-closure glaucoma, causing compression of the optic nerve as it exits the eyeball (see Figure 70.1).

Glaucoma involves structural and functional damage to the optic nerve, resulting in characteristic optic disc changes and progressive visual field defects. Existing optic nerve damage is usually irreversible, but lowering IOP can slow or halt disease progression.

The term 'glaucoma' refers to a family of disorders characterised by optic neuropathy. When the specific type is known, a more precise term should be used.

Glaucoma is classified as congenital or acquired. Acquired glaucoma is further subdivided into primary open-angle or primary angle-closure types, depending on the mechanism of aqueous outflow obstruction, and may be secondary when an identifiable underlying cause is present.

Pathophysiology

The exact mechanisms of glaucoma are not fully understood, but elevated IOP is a major risk factor in most types. Elevated IOP can distort the lamina cribrosa at the optic nerve head, reduce blood flow and interfere with axonal transport, ultimately causing retinal ganglion cells to die. These changes result in the gradual loss of peripheral visual field, a hallmark of the disease.

While optic nerve damage is most commonly associated with elevated IOP, some patients develop normal-tension glaucoma, indicating additional susceptibility factors such as vascular dysregulation.

Glaucoma includes several forms, with the most common being primary open-angle glaucoma (POAG) and angle-closure glaucoma. The pathophysiology differs between these forms: POAG usually develops slowly due to trabecular meshwork dysfunction and impaired aqueous outflow, whereas angle-closure glaucoma results from sudden obstruction of the anterior chamber angle, causing rapid IOP elevation and acute optic nerve injury.

Primary open-angle glaucoma

Signs and symptoms

Open-angle glaucoma is often called 'the sneak thief of sight' because it usually causes no symptoms until significant vision loss has occurred. The condition develops slowly, often over several years and early changes in vision are typically unnoticed. Visual acuity is generally preserved until the late stages of the disease. By the time vision loss becomes apparent to the individual, the glaucoma is usually advanced.

Loss of vision from glaucoma is irreversible, but the disease can be detected during routine eye examinations, where changes in the optic disc, raised IOP or visual field defects may be noted.

Risk factors for open-angle glaucoma include increasing age, family history, Afro-Caribbean ethnicity and, to a lesser extent, diabetes mellitus or cardiovascular disease.

Investigations

A detailed history is taken, and the eye is examined thoroughly for evidence of glaucoma, comorbidities or alternative causes for any clinical findings.

Glaucoma assessment typically includes IOP measurement (tonometry), optic disc evaluation, visual field testing, gonioscopy to assess the anterior chamber angle and measurement of central corneal thickness (pachymetry).

Management

Management of glaucoma varies depending on disease severity and patient factors, and national guidelines (e.g. National Institute for Health and Care Excellence) provide structured recommendations. Treatment may not be started immediately; repeated assessments are usually necessary to confirm the diagnosis and assess progression, unless the disease is advanced and unequivocal, in which case treatment should commence promptly.

First-line treatment is typically medical therapy, often with topical eye drops and may be required for one or both eyes. Prostaglandin analogues are generally preferred due to their efficacy and once-daily dosing. Other medications, such as beta-blockers, carbonic anhydrase inhibitors and sympathomimetics, may be used alone or in combination. Miotics are used less commonly in modern practice.

Laser therapy, such as selective laser trabeculoplasty, may be considered when medications are insufficient or as an alternative first-line treatment in selected cases. Surgical interventions, including trabeculectomy or tube shunt procedures, are reserved for patients whose glaucoma remains uncontrolled despite maximal tolerated medical therapy.

Angle-closure glaucoma

Signs and symptoms

Acute angle-closure glaucoma typically presents with sudden, severe ocular pain that may radiate around the orbit and is often associated with a frontal or generalised headache. Visual symptoms include blurred vision, rapidly progressing visual loss and seeing rainbow-coloured halos around lights. Some patients may report subacute or intermittent attacks with transient blurring of vision and halos prior to a full acute episode. Systemic symptoms such as nausea and vomiting are common, and these may be the main presenting feature.

Investigations

The diagnosis of acute angle-closure glaucoma is primarily based on history and clinical examination. Examination of the affected eye typically reveals a red eye with a hazy cornea, a mid-dilated pupil that is minimally reactive or non-reactive and a firm globe on palpation. Slit-lamp examination can confirm corneal oedema and anterior chamber findings, while tonometry is used to measure the markedly elevated IOP.

Acute attacks are usually unilateral, but predisposing anatomical factors are often present in both eyes. Long-term management frequently includes prophylactic laser peripheral iridotomy of the fellow eye to reduce the risk of a future attack. Urgent recognition and treatment are essential to preserve vision.

Management

The immediate priority, at any time of day, is to reduce IOP to preserve vision. Rapid assessment by an ophthalmologist is essential. Topical therapy may include beta-blockers (e.g. timolol) and apraclonidine. Pilocarpine can be used in phakic eyes once the IOP begins to fall, while phenylephrine may be considered in select pseudophakic patients.

Systemic therapy includes intravenous acetazolamide. If IOP remains elevated, systemic hyperosmotics such as oral glycerol or intravenous mannitol (20% solution, 1–2 g/kg) may be administered. Pain relief and antiemetics should also be provided.

Once the acute attack is partially controlled, definitive treatment is aimed at correcting the underlying mechanism of angle closure, usually by early laser peripheral iridotomy or, in some cases, surgical intervention if laser is not feasible or insufficient.

Clinical considerations

Acute angle-closure glaucoma is an ophthalmic emergency; urgent recognition and treatment are essential to prevent permanent vision loss. Patients typically present with sudden eye pain, blurred vision, halos around lights, headaches and sometimes nausea and vomiting. The priority is to lower IOP as quickly as possible; urgent assessment by an ophthalmologist should be sought, regardless of the time of day. Once controlled, definitive treatment, usually laser peripheral iridotomy, should be instigated promptly. Any delay can result in irreversible optic nerve damage and permanent visual impairment.

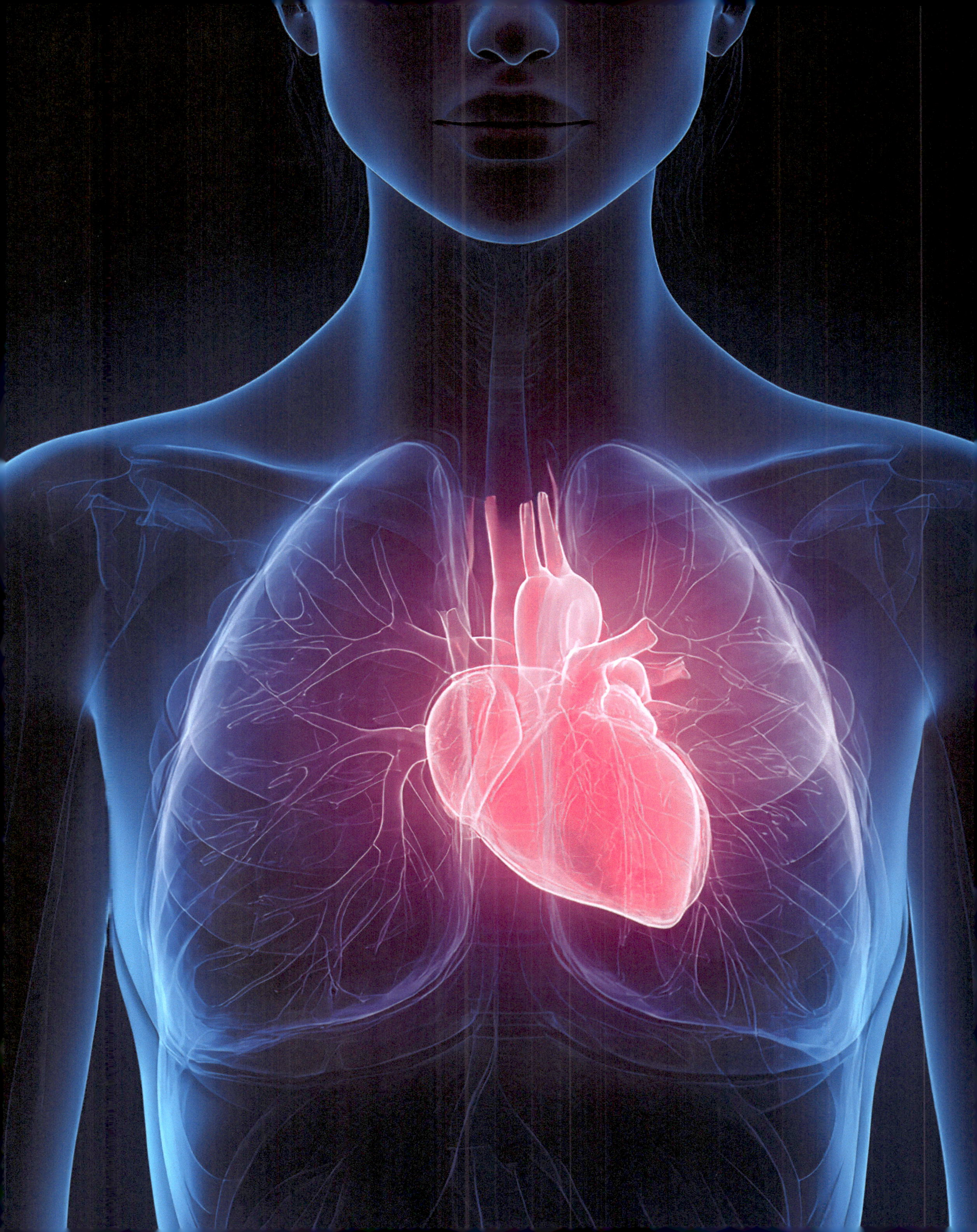

71 Age-related macular degeneration

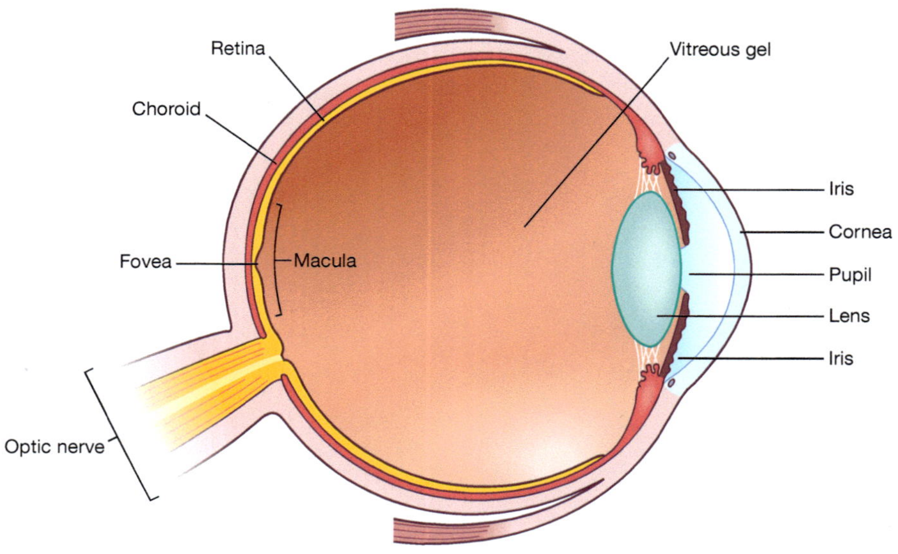

Figure 71.1 The eye showing the position of the macula.

Figure 71.2 Normal macula and degenerated.

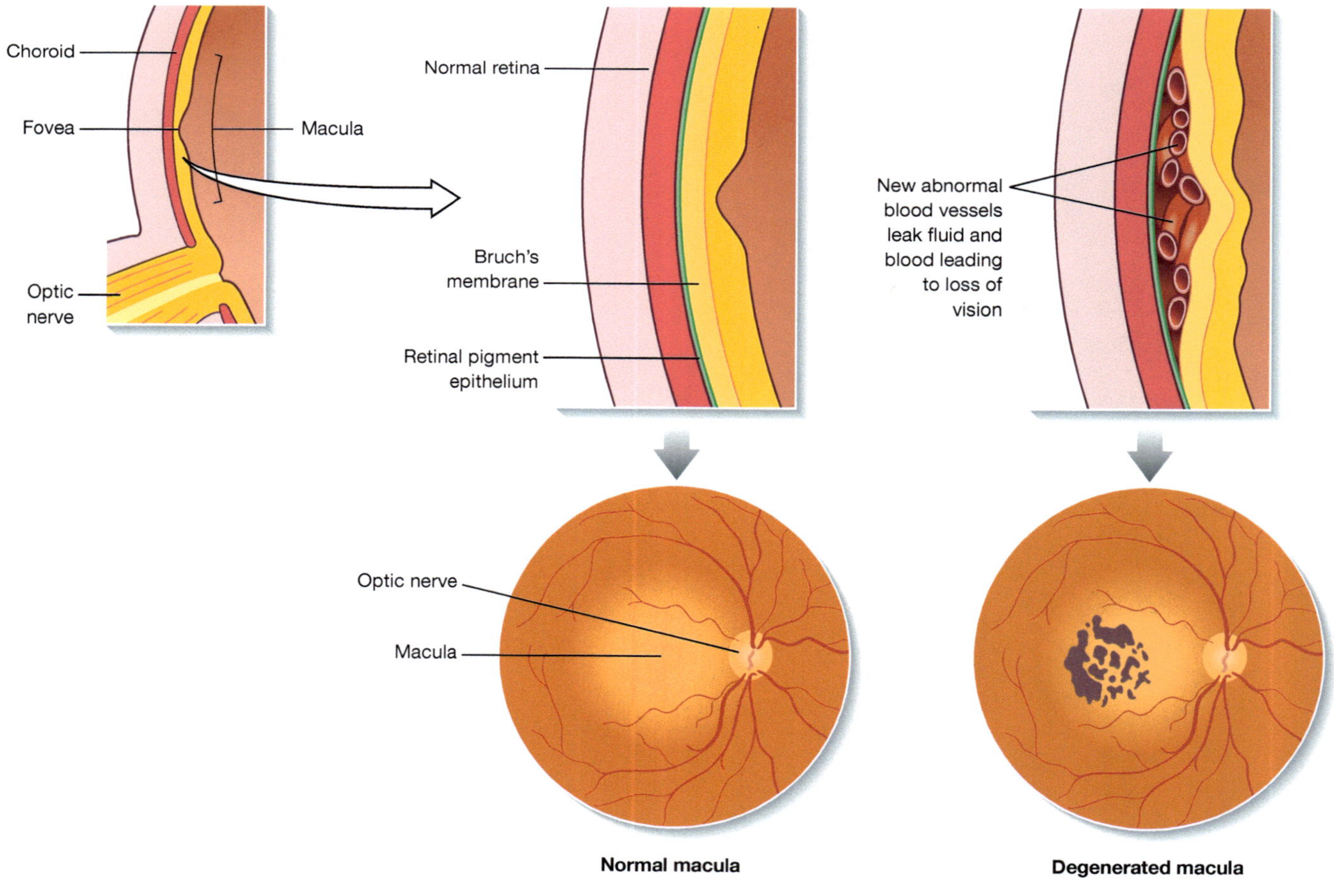

AMD is also known as age-related macular degeneration.

Overview

Age-related macular degeneration (AMD) affects the macula, a small central area of the retina approximately 5 mm in diameter that is critical for seeing fine detail, colour and objects directly in front of the person (see Figure 71.1). When light enters the eye, it is focused onto the retina, which contains multiple layers. Of these, the photoreceptor layer is key for vision, as it contains cells sensitive to light.

The macula is densely packed with cone photoreceptors, which function best in bright light and enable central vision, detailed perception, and colour recognition. In contrast, the peripheral retina contains predominantly rod cells, which are more sensitive in dim light and provide peripheral vision.

Pathophysiology

AMD is the leading cause of irreversible visual loss in people over 50 in the UK, and its prevalence is rising with an ageing population. Ageing and smoking are the most consistent risk factors, while cardiovascular conditions, particularly hypertension and a positive family history, further increase susceptibility. White individuals are more commonly affected by AMD than other ethnic groups.

AMD primarily affects the macula, the central portion of the retina responsible for high-acuity vision and colour perception. Early changes, often asymptomatic, are characterised by the accumulation of small extracellular deposits known as drusen between the retinal pigment epithelium (RPE) and Bruch's membrane. Drusen are composed of lipids, proteins and cellular debris, and their presence indicates age-related maculopathy. Over time, these deposits may interfere with RPE function, leading to photoreceptor stress and degeneration.

Late AMD manifests in two principal forms: atrophic (dry, non-exudative) and exudative (wet, neovascular). Atrophic AMD accounts for approximately 90% of cases and is characterised by progressive atrophy of the RPE, photoreceptors and underlying choriocapillaris, often associated with confluent drusen. This gradual degeneration results in central visual loss while peripheral vision is preserved.

Exudative AMD, present in roughly 10% of patients, involves the growth of abnormal choroidal vessels under or into the retina, forming a neovascular membrane. These vessels are fragile and prone to leakage, causing serous fluid accumulation, haemorrhage and serous retinal detachment. Retinal angiomatous proliferation (RAP), originating from retinal vessels, may also contribute. Chronic exudation and fibrovascular proliferation ultimately lead to scar formation, known as disciform macular degeneration, resulting in severe central vision loss.

Emerging research highlights the role of oxidative stress, complement system dysregulation and RPE dysfunction in AMD pathogenesis, explaining why the disease is strongly age-related. While early AMD may be asymptomatic, the progressive nature of photoreceptor and RPE damage underlies the characteristic central vision loss and difficulty with detailed or colour vision that define this condition (see Figure 71.2).

Signs and symptoms

AMD may be detected incidentally during routine optometrist visits, particularly when only one eye is affected. Patients may report difficulty with tasks requiring detailed central vision, such as reading, driving or recognising faces. In the early stages of geographic atrophy (dry AMD), diagnosis is often secondary to incidental fundus findings. As the disease progresses, central vision gradually declines, and patients may notice distortion of straight lines (metamorphopsia) or, occasionally, visual size distortions (micropsia or macropsia).

Exudative (wet) AMD may present similarly, but sudden deterioration of central vision can occur due to macular haemorrhage. A shower of floaters may occasionally precede bleeding.

Examination may reveal normal or reduced visual acuity. Fundus examination typically shows discrete yellow drusen in the macular area, which may enlarge, coalesce and become paler as AMD progresses. In wet AMD, haemorrhage appears as a dark red, well-defined patch in the macula. Late-stage disease may result in macular scarring, seen as a thick, fibrotic lesion in the central macular region.

Investigations

Slit-lamp biomicroscopy is essential for examining the macula and retinal changes and is typically performed with pupil dilation. Optical coherence tomography (OCT) is widely used to support the initial diagnosis, assess disease severity and monitor response to treatment. OCT provides high-resolution cross-sectional images of the retina and can be performed quickly and painlessly in the clinic.

In patients with suspected choroidal neovascularisation (CNV), fluorescein angiography (FA) is used to confirm and characterise abnormal vessels, which guides treatment decisions. Indocyanine green angiography (ICGA) may be employed selectively to provide additional detail, particularly in atypical cases such as RAP or polypoidal choroidal vasculopathy. Both FA and ICGA require intravenous dye injection.

Management

There are a number of treatments available for wet AMD. Wet AMD (neovascular AMD) is treated to prevent the growth of abnormal blood vessels that can leak, bleed and scar the retina. Early treatment is essential to preserve central vision, as delayed therapy may result in irreversible visual loss.

First-line treatment is intravitreal anti-vascular endothelial growth factor (anti-VEGF) therapy (the medication is injected directly into the vitreous cavity of the eye), which inhibits abnormal CNV and prevents further leakage. The injections are performed under local anaesthetic drops using a sterile technique. Multiple injections are usually required over time to maintain disease control.

Photodynamic therapy (PDT), which combines a light-sensitive drug with a low-energy laser, may be considered in cases where anti-VEGF therapy is ineffective or cannot be tolerated by the patient.

Currently, there is no approved treatment for dry AMD, as this form does not involve neovascularisation; management focuses on monitoring and lifestyle measures, including smoking cessation and nutritional support. Research is on-going, and there are new treatment modalities being developed.

Clinical considerations

AMD may be asymptomatic in its early stages; regular eye examinations are particularly important for individuals over 50 years old or those with risk factors such as smoking, hypertension or a family history of AMD. Patients with dry AMD require ongoing monitoring to detect progression to geographic atrophy or the development of wet AMD. Wet AMD, in particular, requires urgent referral and prompt treatment with anti-VEGF therapy to prevent rapid central vision loss. Regular follow-up is essential to assess treatment response, detect new or recurrent neovascularisation and adjust therapy as needed. Patients should also be advised on self-monitoring (e.g. using an Amsler grid) to identify early changes in their vision and seek timely assessment.

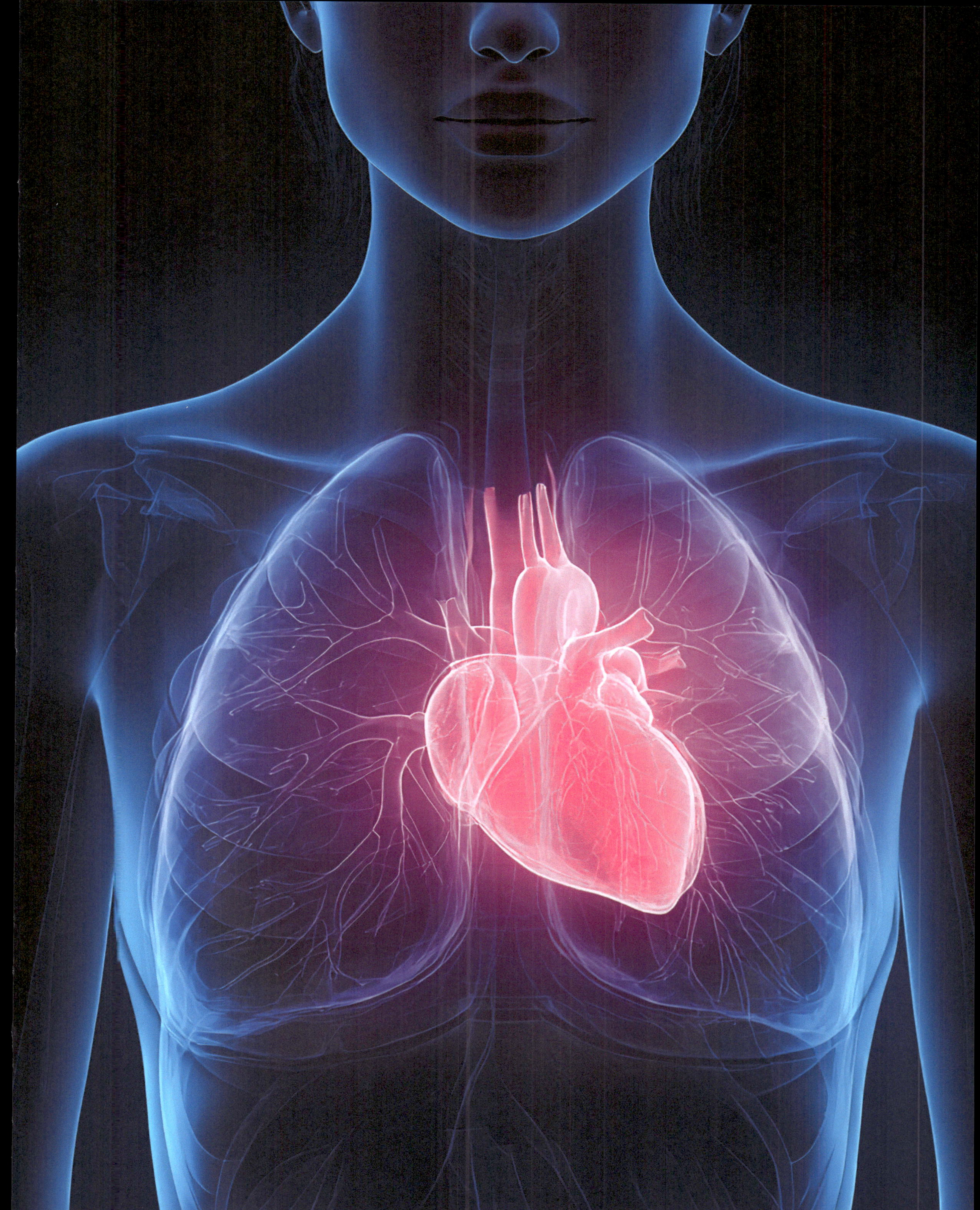

72 Conjunctivitis

Figure 72.1 The eye and associated structures (the conjunctiva).

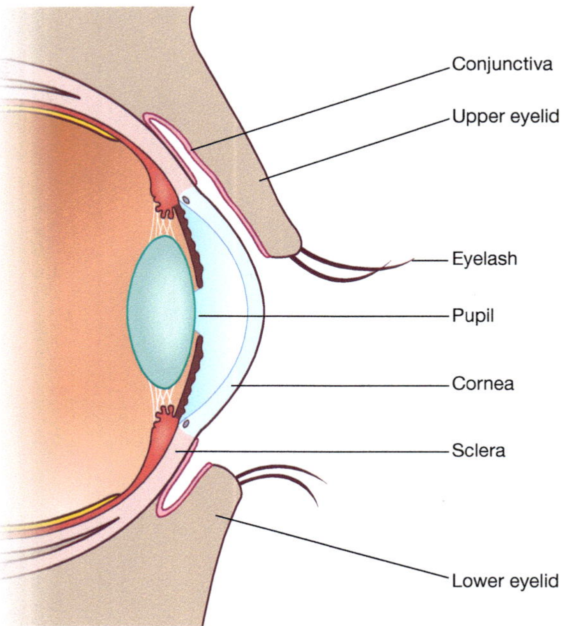

Figure 72.2 Conjunctivitis.

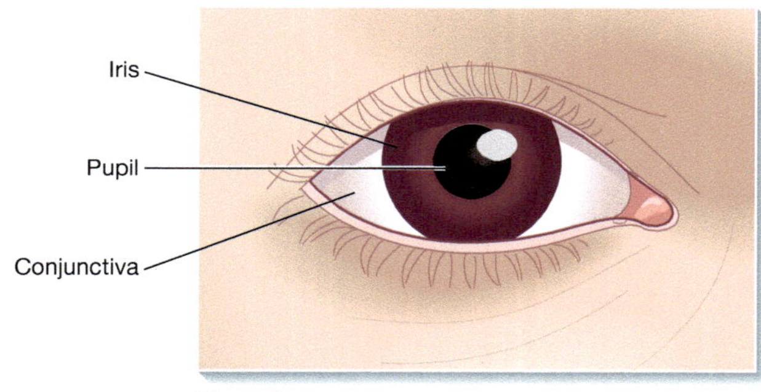

Normal eye

Conjunctivitis

Figure 72.3 Some causes of conjunctivitis.

- Viruses
- Bacteria
- Allergies
- A chemical splash in the eye
- A foreign object in the eye
- In newborns, a blocked tear duct

Overview

Allergies, viruses or bacteria can cause conjunctivitis. See Figure 72.1, the eye and associated structures. Common bacterial causes include *Staphylococcus* spp., *Streptococcus* spp., *Chlamydia trachomatis* and *Neisseria gonorrhoeae*. Mild conjunctivitis is generally self-limiting and non-threatening. Severe forms, such as gonococcal conjunctivitis, can lead to corneal damage and blindness and may indicate a serious underlying systemic infection.

Pathophysiology

Conjunctivitis is the inflammation of the conjunctiva, the transparent mucous membrane covering the sclera and inner eyelids. If the cornea is involved, the condition is termed keratoconjunctivitis; if the eyelids are involved, it is called blepharoconjunctivitis. Inflammation may be infective (bacterial, viral and chlamydial) or non-infective (allergic, chemical or mechanical) and can be acute or chronic.

The epithelial layer of the conjunctiva serves as the primary defence against infection. Disruption of this barrier due to trauma, foreign bodies or contact lens use allows microbial invasion. Normally, the conjunctiva is colonised by commensal organisms such as *Staphylococcus* and *Streptococcus* species. Infection occurs when the balance between host defence and microbial virulence is disturbed (e.g. by changes in local flora, contamination or spread from adjacent sites).

Once infection is established, immune responses are triggered, including:

- Recruitment of neutrophils, lymphocytes and macrophages
- Release of cytokines and chemokines
- Increased vascular permeability, leading to hyperaemia, oedema and exudate

These mechanisms produce the characteristic signs and symptoms of conjunctivitis: redness, discharge, irritation and tearing. Most cases are self-limiting, but severe infections, such as gonococcal conjunctivitis, can rapidly progress to corneal damage and vision loss. Box 72.1 highlights some of the causes of conjunctivitis.

Signs and symptoms

Conjunctivitis, commonly referred to as 'pink eye', typically presents with redness in one or both eyes, accompanied by itchiness, irritation or a gritty sensation. Patients may experience tearing and discharge, which often forms a crust overnight and can make it difficult to open the eyes in the morning. While the condition frequently affects both eyes, it may initially present unilaterally, particularly in bacterial infections.

Pain is usually mild and related to irritation; however, severe pain or photophobia may indicate corneal involvement or a more serious underlying ocular condition that requires urgent assessment. On examination, the conjunctiva may show dilated vessels (conjunctival injection) and oedema (chemosis) (see Figure 72.2). Small nodular structures known as follicles may be seen, especially in viral or chlamydial conjunctivitis, whereas papillae, elevated vascularised lesions, are more characteristic of allergic or bacterial forms. These signs, together with the patient's symptoms, help guide the clinical diagnosis and management.

Investigations

In most cases of conjunctivitis, a detailed history and careful examination of the eyes are sufficient to establish the diagnosis. The condition is usually identified rapidly without the need for laboratory tests. However, further investigations may be required in certain circumstances, and the patient should be referred to a specialist if necessary. Conjunctival scrapings and cultures are generally reserved for severe bacterial conjunctivitis, suspected gonococcal infections or cases that do not respond to standard antibacterial therapy. Additional referral is indicated if there are atypical features, significant pain, corneal involvement or visual impairment.

Management

Patients should be advised to discontinue contact lens wear until at least 24–48 hours after symptoms have fully resolved. They should also be counselled on measures to reduce the risk of transmission, including avoiding rubbing the eyes, not sharing towels or make-up and practising good hand hygiene. Patients should return for review if symptoms worsen within a week or persist for longer than 10 days.

Supportive care is often sufficient for mild cases. Artificial tears can provide comfort and relieve irritation. In cases of bacterial conjunctivitis, antibiotic eye drops may be prescribed and typically resolve the infection within several days. Drops are generally preferred over ointments because ointments can smear, blur vision and be impractical during the day. However, ointments maintain the medication in the eye for longer periods and may be easier to apply for individuals with poor dexterity, such as the elderly. An effective approach is to use drops during the day and ointment at night.

Bacterial conjunctivitis

Antibiotic eye ointments, such as chloramphenicol, are sometimes prescribed for bacterial conjunctivitis, particularly in more severe cases. Ointment application may blur vision for up to 20 minutes, and patients should be advised accordingly. Signs and symptoms generally begin to improve within a few days of starting treatment. It is important to complete the prescribed course to reduce the risk of recurrence.

There is ongoing debate regarding the routine use of antibiotics for infective conjunctivitis, as many cases are mild and self-limiting, particularly in adults. Current guidance recommends antibiotics primarily for severe, persistent or high-risk cases.

Viral conjunctivitis

Most cases of viral conjunctivitis are self-limiting and require no specific treatment. The infection usually begins in one eye and spreads to the other within a few days. Supportive care such as artificial tears for comfort is often sufficient.

In cases caused by the herpes simplex virus, antiviral treatment (topical or oral) may be prescribed under specialist supervision. Patients should be advised to adhere to strict hygiene measures, including frequent handwashing, avoiding sharing towels or personal items and refraining from swimming, to reduce the risk of transmission.

Allergic conjunctivitis

The management of allergic conjunctivitis focuses on preventing the release of allergy mediators, controlling the inflammatory cascade and protecting the ocular surface from secondary damage. Where possible, avoidance of the triggering allergen is recommended. Supportive measures, such as cold compresses and artificial tears, can help relieve mild symptoms by soothing irritation and diluting allergens. Contact lenses should not be worn during an active episode or while using topical therapy.

Topical antihistamines provide rapid symptom relief but are not recommended for prolonged use (generally no longer than 6 weeks). Mast cell stabilisers are useful for longer-term control and prevention of recurrent symptoms. Topical corticosteroids may be used in severe cases but require careful monitoring due to potential adverse effects, including cataracts, glaucoma and secondary ocular infections. Decongestant drops can temporarily reduce redness but should only be used for the short term to avoid rebound hyperaemia.

Systemic therapy may be indicated when ocular allergy is associated with allergic rhinitis. Oral antihistamines can relieve both ocular and nasal symptoms, while intranasal corticosteroids can reduce ocular manifestations in people with significant nasal allergies, though long-term use carries risks of ocular and systemic adverse effects.

Clinical considerations

Effective infection prevention and control are essential when managing conjunctivitis. Patients should be advised to practise strict hand hygiene, washing hands thoroughly before and after touching their eyes or administering eye drops. Avoid rubbing or touching your eyes, which can exacerbate irritation and facilitate the spread of infection. Sharing of personal items, including towels, face cloths, pillowcases or make-up, should be avoided. Contact lenses should not be worn until at least 24–48 hours after symptoms have fully resolved. Patients should also be encouraged to clean frequently touched surfaces, such as door handles and taps, and to avoid swimming pools during the active infection to reduce transmission.

Death and dying

Chapters

73 Principles of end-of-life care

Figure 73.1 Multidisciplinary team members.

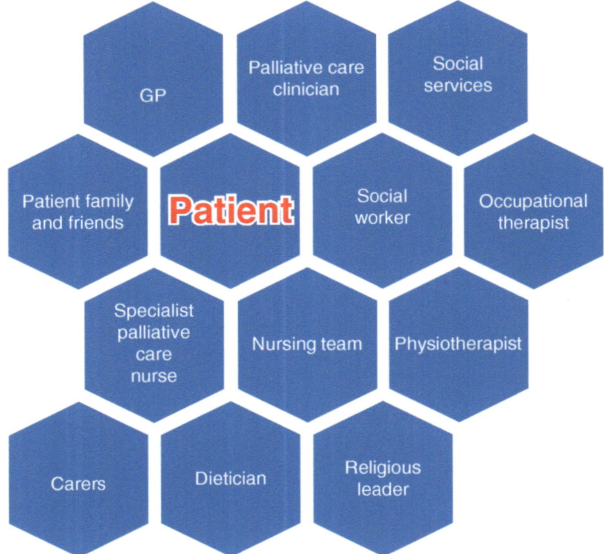

Source:
Peate 2021/with permission
of John Wiley & Sons

Table 73.1 The 6Cs and end-of-life care.

6Cs	Application in end-of-life care	Examples
Care	Providing holistic, person-centred care that meets physical, emotional, social and spiritual needs	Assisting with personal hygiene, ensuring comfort and providing support for emotional or spiritual concerns
Compassion	Showing empathy, kindness, and sensitivity to the patient's and family's experiences	Listening to a patient's fears, offering reassurance, sitting with a patient who is distressed
Competence	Having the necessary skills and knowledge to manage symptoms and provide safe, effective care	Administering pain relief correctly, recognising signs of deterioration and understanding palliative interventions
Communication	Using clear, honest and sensitive communication with patients, families and the healthcare team	Explaining what to expect in the final stages, answering questions such as 'Am I dying?' and involving family in care discussions
Courage	Being willing to face difficult situations, have sensitive conversations and advocate for the patient	Discussing end-of-life wishes, initiating conversations about DNAR orders and challenging care decisions that do not prioritise comfort
Commitment	Dedication to providing high-quality care and supporting the patient and family throughout the dying process	Regularly reviewing the patient's comfort, staying present during difficult moments, supporting family members emotionally

Overview

End-of-life care refers to the support and medical care that is offered to individuals (and their families) who are in the final stages of a life-limiting illness. The overall goal is to ensure comfort, dignity and quality of life, rather than focusing on curing the disease. Understanding the fundamental principles helps healthcare students provide compassionate and appropriate care to patients and their families.

End-of-life care

End-of-life care generally refers to the final weeks of a person's life, when their condition has significantly worsened and no further treatments are available to extend life. The National Institute for Health and Care Excellence has set standards that are related to end-of-life care for adults.

During the final weeks of a person's life, often the patient becomes increasingly tired; they may sleep for longer periods, eat very little and prefer to remain in bed. Many people recognise that they are becoming weaker and may wish to discuss what is happening to them, they will ask direct questions such as 'Am I dying?' It is important to respond to such questions with honesty and sensitivity, as this is often a signal to talk about their situation. Patients may feel anxious or frightened and will need reassurance.

As death approaches, the patient's condition will continue to decline, although the rate of deterioration varies widely between individuals. Therefore, when offering care and support to someone in the last weeks of life, it is essential to recognise when they are entering the terminal phase of their illness. Regular assessment is crucial to identify any changes or signs of deterioration. The frequency of review depends on the care setting: in hospitals, hospices or nursing homes, observations may be required several times per shift, whereas in community or home settings, reviews may be less frequent. Whilst it is still important to assess patients regularly as they approach death, the type, frequency and method of assessment should minimise disturbance, prioritising the person's comfort over routine monitoring.

If a patient appears to be becoming more unwell or showing signs that they are entering the final phase of life, this should be promptly reported to the appropriate healthcare professionals, such as the medical team, the patient's GP or the palliative care team, depending on the care setting. Providing psychological and emotional support for both the patient and their family is also an essential aspect of care during this time.

Person-centred care

Central to end-of-life care is a person-centred approach, which recognises the patient as a whole person rather than simply a set of symptoms or a disease. It involves respecting the patient's wishes, values and beliefs, and engaging them in decisions about their care whenever possible. Care should be tailored to meet the patient's physical, emotional, spiritual and social needs, and healthcare professionals should take time to listen to their concerns, answer questions honestly and provide reassurance as needed. By focusing on the individual, healthcare staff can ensure that care is meaningful, responsive and supportive during a vulnerable time.

Equally important is the principle of dignity and respect. Every patient deserves to be treated with kindness and compassion, even when they are very unwell or unable to communicate. Maintaining privacy and modesty during care, using respectful language and supporting the patient's right to make choices, such as where they wish to spend their final days, are all essential. Respecting cultural, spiritual and personal values helps preserve a patient's sense of control and self-worth, which can significantly influence their comfort and emotional well-being.

A core element of end-of-life care is comfort and symptom management. Patients may experience pain, breathlessness, nausea, anxiety and fatigue; those who are offering care and support have a responsibility to monitor these symptoms carefully, reporting any changes to senior staff. Interventions should prioritise comfort and peace rather than attempting to prolong life unnecessarily. Non-pharmacological approaches, such as adjusting the patient's position, providing gentle therapeutic touch or creating a calm environment, can complement medical management and help reduce distress.

In practice, these principles: person-centred care, dignity and respect, and comfort-focused symptom management, are closely interconnected. Together, they guide healthcare professionals in providing compassionate, responsive and effective care, ensuring that patients can spend their final days with as much comfort, control and dignity as possible. Table 73.1 outlines how the 6Cs are closely related to end-of-life care provision.

Effective end-of-life care

Effective end-of-life care relies heavily on clear, sensitive communication. Healthcare professionals should be honest yet compassionate when talking to patients and their families, providing information in simple, supportive language. Active listening is essential; patients and families often need to express fears, concerns or questions about the dying process. It is equally important to be aware of non-verbal cues, such as tone of voice, touch and body language.

End-of-life care also addresses emotional, social and spiritual needs as well as physical care. Patients and families may require emotional support, and healthcare professionals should be prepared to offer this directly or refer them to counsellors, chaplains or other specialists. Recognising and respecting religious or cultural practices is vital; encouraging families to spend time together and express their feelings, which can help foster connection and emotional well-being.

Families often need as much support as the patient; keeping them informed about changes in the patient's condition is essential. Encouraging families to participate in care, if they wish, and providing practical guidance about what to expect as death approaches can reduce anxiety and improve their experience of care.

End-of-life care is delivered by a multidisciplinary team, which may include doctors, nurses, healthcare assistants, social workers and chaplains. Each team member plays an important role, and good communication and coordination between team members ensures continuity and quality of care (see Figure 73.1).

Consideration must be given to ethical and legal issues. End-of-life care often involves sensitive decisions, and it is important to respect advance care plans or 'do not attempt resuscitation' (DNAR) orders. Always act in the patient's best interests and maintain confidentiality at all times, balancing honesty with sensitivity in discussions about prognosis and care choices.

Integrating effective communication, emotional support, family involvement, teamwork and ethical practice can help to provide compassionate, respectful and high-quality care at the end of life.

Clinical considerations

Providing end-of-life care can be emotionally and physically demanding. You should acknowledge your feelings, reflect on experiences and seek support from colleagues, mentors or counselling services. Maintaining professional boundaries while practising self-care, such as taking breaks, resting and managing stress, helps prevent burnout. Participating in debriefings and using reflective or mindfulness strategies can build resilience, enabling staff to continue offering compassionate and high-quality care.

74 Pain relief

Figure 74.1 The WHO analgesic ladder.

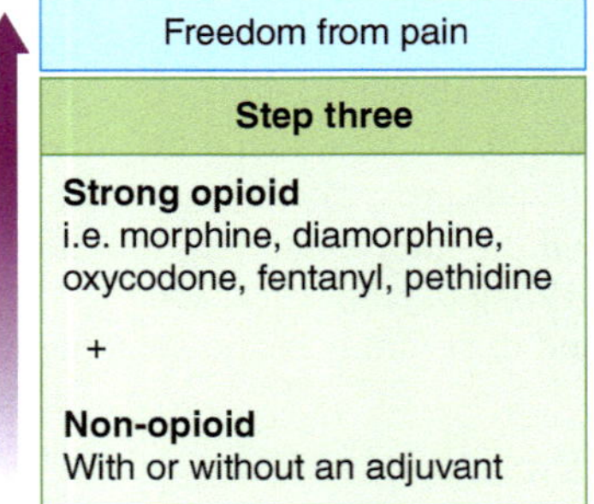

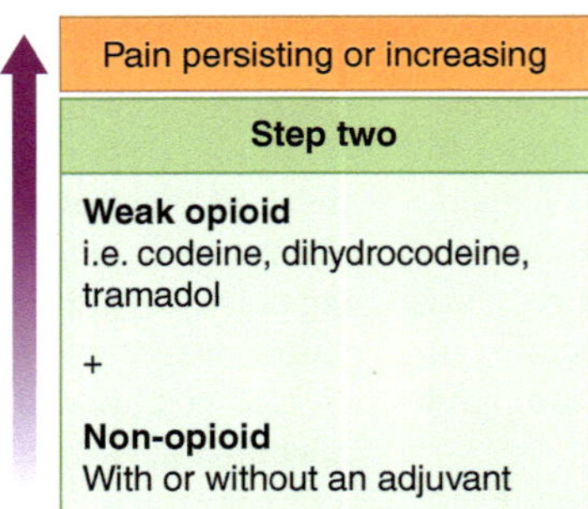

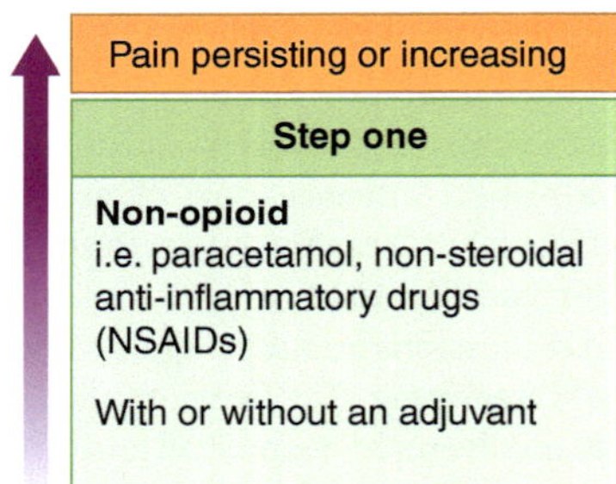

Source:
Peate & Mitchell 2022/with permission of John Wiley & Sons

Table 74.1 Principles of pain relief in end-of-life care.

Principle	Application	Examples
Assessment	Regular, holistic evaluation of pain using validated tools.	Using the Abbey Pain Scale for non-verbal patients; documenting pain scores at each review.
Individualisation	Tailoring analgesia to the patient's needs, preferences and comorbidities.	Adjusting opioid dose for renal impairment; respecting patient wishes about sedation.
Multimodal approach	Combining pharmacological and non-pharmacological strategies.	Opioids with adjuvant drugs; positioning, relaxation or heat packs.
Communication	Clear, compassionate dialogue with patients, families and the healthcare team.	Explaining opioid side effects; involving family in comfort measures.
Safety	Monitoring for adverse effects and balancing relief with quality of life.	Watching for constipation, nausea, delirium or respiratory depression.
Continuity	Ensuring seamless care across settings and providers.	Coordinating with GPs, hospices and community nurses.

Overview

Pain is one of the most common and distressing symptoms experienced by people approaching the end of life. Uncontrolled pain can undermine dignity, independence and emotional well-being; for families, it can be deeply upsetting to witness. The overall goal of pain relief in end-of-life care is not to cure the underlying disease but to ensure comfort, dignity and quality of life during the remaining time.

Understanding the principles of pain management helps healthcare professionals to provide safe, compassionate and appropriate care, recognising that pain is not only physical but also influenced by emotional, social and spiritual factors. Effective relief requires careful assessment, timely interventions and a willingness to adapt treatment as the patient's condition changes (see Table 74.1, and overview of pain relief in end-of-life care).

During the final weeks and days of life, patients may become weaker, less able to communicate or unable to swallow oral medication. Anticipating these changes and planning for alternative routes of administration, such as subcutaneous infusion, is essential. Honest and sensitive communication is important; there may be concerns about the use of strong painkillers, sedation or the possibility of hastening death.

Pain assessment

Accurate assessment is the foundation of effective pain relief. Patients who can communicate should be encouraged to describe their pain in their own words, including location, intensity, quality and impact. Tools such as the Numerical Rating Scale can support consistency between staff. For patients who cannot self-report, observational tools such as the Abbey Pain Scale are valuable, focusing on behaviours such as facial expression, body movements and vocalisation.

Assessment is continuous. Pain can change rapidly as illness progresses; regular reassessment ensures treatment remains appropriate. Documentation of baseline pain, triggers and response to interventions is essential; family members often provide useful insights, particularly for patients with dementia or delirium.

Pharmacological management

The WHO analgesic ladder remains a helpful framework, though in end-of-life care, many patients require strong opioids from the outset (see Figure 74.1). Non-opioids such as paracetamol may still provide benefit for mild or background pain; NSAIDs can be useful for bone or inflammatory pain if tolerated.

Morphine is a first-line strong opioid. Alternatives such as oxycodone, fentanyl or alfentanil may be used in these circumstances. Oral administration is preferred when possible, but as swallowing becomes difficult, subcutaneous routes via syringe driver provide reliable continuous delivery. Breakthrough doses should always be available for episodic pain, usually calculated as one-sixth of the total 24-hour dose.

Side effects must be anticipated and managed proactively. Chapter 75 of this book discusses symptom control.

Adjuvant drugs play an important role in specific pain syndromes. Neuropathic pain may respond to gabapentin, pregabalin or low-dose amitriptyline. Corticosteroids can relieve pain from liver capsule distension or raised intracranial pressure. Bone pain may be eased by radiotherapy, bisphosphonates or denosumab, though these are not always feasible in the final stages of life.

Non-pharmacological approaches

Medication is only one part of pain relief. Simple physical measures such as careful positioning, pressure-relieving equipment and supportive mattresses can reduce discomfort. Heat or cold packs and relaxation techniques may also help. A calm environment, familiar music and consistent routines can reduce anxiety and improve comfort. Families can be encouraged to participate in comfort measures, such as hand massage or creating a peaceful environment, which can strengthen bonds and provide reassurance.

Communication and person-centred care

Pain relief must be grounded in open, sensitive communication. Patients may worry about addiction, sedation or the possibility that opioids will hasten death. Healthcare professionals should address these concerns honestly, explaining that the aim is comfort and dignity, not shortening life. Preferences about alertness, sedation and timing of doses should be explored and respected.

Families also need clear explanations, particularly when syringe drivers are introduced. Understanding why continuous infusion is recommended, how it works and how effectiveness is monitored can reduce anxiety.

Ethical and legal considerations

Pain relief at the end of life must always be provided in line with professional guidance, legal requirements and the patient's best interests. The principle of double effect is relevant: medicines given with the intention of relieving pain may have foreseeable but unintended side effects, such as increased drowsiness.

Advance care planning, DNACPR decisions and treatment escalation plans should be integrated with pain management. Where patients lack capacity, decisions must be made in their best interests, taking into account prior wishes, values and the views of those close to them.

The multidisciplinary team

Effective pain relief depends on teamwork. Prescribing and pain assessment are shared responsibilities across the team: doctors, advanced nurse practitioners, specialist paramedics and prescribing pharmacists may all be involved in medication decisions. Pharmacists advise on drug interactions and formulations, and allied health professionals contribute physical and psychological strategies. Spiritual and emotional support is provided by a range of roles, including chaplains, faith leaders and pastoral carers. Effective communication and coordination between team members ensure continuity and can prevent gaps in care.

Pain relief is a central element of end-of-life care. Careful assessment, appropriate use of medicines, integration of non-pharmacological measures and sensitive communication can ensure that patients spend their final days with comfort and dignity. Developing confidence in pain management requires technical knowledge and the ability to listen, empathise and work collaboratively. Excellence in this area is measured not only by the absence of pain but also by the presence of dignity, peace and human connection at the end of life.

Clinical considerations

Providing pain relief at the end of life can be emotionally demanding. Staff may feel pressure to achieve perfect control or distress when symptoms remain difficult to manage. Reflective practice, supervision and debriefing help staff process these experiences and maintain resilience. Attending to personal well-being, taking breaks and seeking peer support are important in preventing burnout. Professional boundaries, combined with compassion and presence, enable staff to remain steady and supportive during difficult encounters.

75 Symptom control

Table 75.1 End-of-life symptoms.

Type of symptom	Description in end-of-life care
Remitting symptoms	Symptoms that temporarily improve or resolve but may recur. For example, episodes of breathlessness or nausea may come and go depending on disease progression or interventions. Regular monitoring allows timely reassessment and adjustment of symptom management strategies.
Chronic symptoms	Persistent or long-lasting symptoms that require ongoing management. Examples include fatigue, low mood or constipation in advanced illness. Continuous evaluation and tailored interventions help maintain patient comfort and dignity.
Relapsing symptoms	Symptoms that previously resolved but return intermittently. For instance, agitation, breathlessness or vomiting may reappear despite prior control. Early recognition and intervention are crucial to prevent distress and optimise quality of life.
Breakthrough symptoms	These are sudden, short-term increases in the intensity of a symptom that occur despite otherwise stable or well-controlled baseline management. They typically appear between scheduled doses of medication or as a result of new or worsening disease processes.

Table 75.2 Pharmacological and non-pharmacological approaches to symptom control.

Type of intervention	Examples	Notes/considerations
Pharmacological	• Antiemetics (for nausea) • Aperients (for constipation) • Oxygen or opioids (for breathlessness) • Anxiolytics (for agitation)	Doses may need adjustment based on effectiveness and patient tolerance.
Non-pharmacological	• Positioning to relieve breathlessness • Gentle massage • Relaxation techniques • Environmental adjustments (lighting, noise) • Cooling fans or humidified air	Focus on comfort and support; interventions tailored to individual patient needs.

Overview

Symptom relief and symptom control encompass a broad range of approaches, reflecting the complex and individual nature of experiences at the end of life. Effective management of symptoms is central to providing compassionate, patient-centred care, ensuring that individuals maintain the highest possible quality of life in their final days.

Effective symptom control is a key component of high-quality end-of-life care. As individuals approach the final stages of life, they may experience multiple distressing symptoms that can affect their physical comfort, emotional well-being and overall quality of life. Symptom control focuses on alleviating suffering, maintaining dignity and ensuring that patients can spend their remaining time as comfortably as possible.

Common symptoms

Patients at the end of life may experience a wide range of symptoms, which can vary in severity and pattern. Pain is one of the most feared and distressing symptoms at the end of life. It can result from the disease itself, such as tumour invasion into bones or nerves, or from other causes such as muscle wasting, immobility or pressure sores (see Chapter 74 of this book). Common physical symptoms include:

- Breathlessness (dyspnoea)
- Fatigue and weakness
- Nausea and vomiting
- Constipation or bowel changes
- Agitation, anxiety or confusion

Symptoms may present as remitting, chronic, relapsing or breakthrough, highlighting the need for continuous assessment and flexible management strategies (see Table 75.1).

Pathophysiology

As a person approaches the end of life, their body undergoes complex physiological and biochemical changes that affect all major organ systems. These changes arise from underlying disease, treatment effects and the body's natural process of shutting down.

The severity and pattern of symptoms may vary over time, influenced by the individual's diagnosis, treatment and overall decline.

Breathlessness (Dyspnoea)

Breathlessness, or dyspnoea, is the subjective sensation of difficult or uncomfortable breathing, often developing in people approaching the end of life due to a combination of mechanical, physiological and neurological changes. In some cases, mechanical factors play a major role. For example, tumour growth within the chest, the presence of pleural effusion (fluid around the lungs) or ascites (fluid in the abdomen) can physically restrict lung expansion, making breathing more difficult and shallow.

Gas exchange may be impaired by conditions such as pneumonia, pulmonary oedema, or diseases that reduce lung compliance, as these limit the diffusion of oxygen into the bloodstream and the elimination of carbon dioxide. This can lead to hypoxia (low oxygen levels) and hypercapnia (raised carbon dioxide levels), contributing to the distressing sensation of breathlessness. As death approaches, irregular and shallow breathing often develops with the accumulation of secretions in the throat.

Fatigue and weakness

These are among the most common and persistent symptoms near the end of life, arising from a combination of metabolic, inflammatory, nutritional factors and treatment-related factors. Anaemia and cachexia limit the transport of oxygen to muscles, reducing strength and endurance. Even when a person rests, their muscles may feel weak, and everyday activities can become exhausting. Medications commonly used in end-of-life care, including opioids and sedatives, may also contribute to increased drowsiness and lethargy.

Fatigue often becomes profound, leaving the person with minimal strength for daily activities. It is a hallmark of the body's decreasing ability to maintain normal physiological function.

Nausea and vomiting

Nausea and vomiting are common symptoms at the end of life and arise from multiple interacting mechanisms. One major pathway is chemical stimulation, where drugs, toxins or metabolic disturbances such as uraemia or hypercalcaemia activate the chemoreceptor trigger zone in the medulla of the brain, initiating the vomiting reflex.

Gastrointestinal irritation is another important contributor. Conditions such as constipation, bowel obstruction or delayed gastric emptying stimulate nerve endings in the gut, particularly the vagus nerve, which sends signals to the brain to trigger nausea and vomiting.

The vestibular system can also play a role. Changes in motion or increases in intracranial pressure affect the inner ear balance system, which in turn can activate vomiting pathways in the brain.

Higher brain centres can trigger nausea in response to emotional or psychological factors such as anxiety, fear or pain. These triggers illustrate how complex and multifactorial nausea and vomiting can be, and why a holistic approach to symptom management is essential in end-of-life care.

The severity of nausea and vomiting ranges from mild queasiness to persistent vomiting. Managing underlying causes, adjusting medication and using targeted antiemetics are essential.

Constipation and bowel changes

Constipation and bowel changes are common at the end of life and result from a combination of physiological, treatment-related and disease-related factors. Opioid medications are a major contributor, slowing intestinal motility, reducing secretions and increasing water absorption from the stool, making bowel movements more difficult.

Dehydration and reduced dietary intake further contribute to harder, drier stools that are difficult to pass. In some cases, tumour-related obstruction or nerve damage affecting the gut can restrict bowel movement even more, worsening constipation. If untreated, faecal impaction can develop, sometimes causing overflow diarrhoea.

Agitation, anxiety and confusion

These are common neuropsychiatric symptoms at the end of life, often caused by delirium. Delirium can arise from a variety of factors, including metabolic imbalances such as hypoxia, kidney or liver failure, infection or medication toxicity.

At a neurochemical level, changes in neurotransmitter balance, particularly increased dopamine and reduced acetylcholine, disrupt normal brain function, contributing to confusion and agitation.

In the final stages of life, cerebral hypoperfusion, reduced blood flow to the brain and decreased oxygen delivery further impair consciousness, leading to fluctuating awareness, restlessness and, eventually, a decline into drowsiness or coma.

Symptoms can fluctuate, with alternating periods of lucidity and confusion. In the final hours, reduced responsiveness and eventual coma typically precede death.

Management

Symptom management at the end of life involves pharmacological and non-pharmacological interventions (see Table 75.2). The combination of both approaches often provides the most effective symptom relief and supports holistic care.

End-of-life care extends beyond physical symptom control. It also involves addressing emotional, social and spiritual needs. Collaborative communication with patients and their families is essential; symptom control becomes part of a broader strategy to enhance quality of life, reduce suffering and preserve dignity.

> **Clinical considerations**
>
> At the end of life, symptoms are often multifactorial, progressive and interconnected. As organ systems fail, the body loses the ability to maintain equilibrium, and symptoms intensify. Recognising the physiological basis of these changes supports holistic and compassionate care, helping to relieve distress and uphold the patient's dignity and comfort.

76 Care after death

Figure 76.1 Diagnosing death.

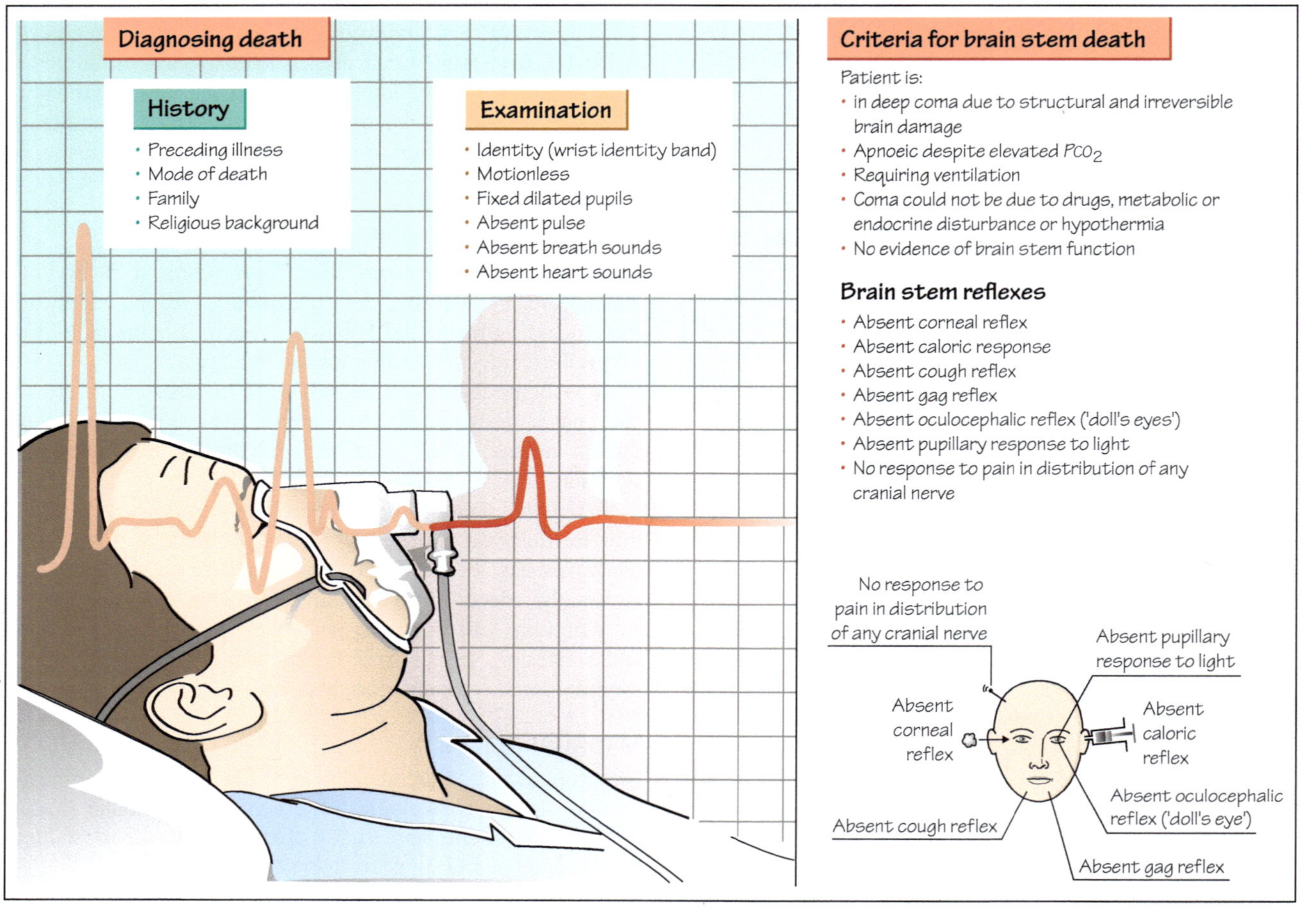

Source:
Gleadle, J. 2011/John Wiley & Sons

Table 76.1 Diagnosing death.

Step	Action	Details/considerations
1	Confirm authorised personnel	Only healthcare professionals legally permitted to diagnose death may perform the assessment. Follow local policy and institutional protocols.
2	Prepare the patient and environment	Ensure privacy, dignity and comfort. Gather all relevant clinical information, including vital signs, history and current interventions.
3	Initial clinical assessment	Assess for the absence of responsiveness, respiration and pulse. Check pupils for fixed and dilated reaction if relevant. Ensure no reversible causes (e.g. hypothermia, drug overdose) are present.
4	Neurological assessment (if applicable)	For brainstem death: assess brainstem reflexes (pupillary response, corneal reflex, oculocephalic reflex and gag/cough reflex) following approved protocols (see Figure 76.1).
5	Confirm cessation of circulation	For circulatory death: confirm absent heartbeat and pulse over the required observation period as per local guidelines. Use appropriate monitoring equipment.
6	Ancillary tests (if required)	Perform additional investigations only if mandated by local policy (e.g. EEG, cerebral blood flow studies) to confirm death in complex cases.
7	Document findings	Record the date, time, personnel involved, method of assessment and results. Include any special circumstances (e.g. organ donation consideration). Documentation must meet legal and institutional standards.
8	Communicate with family	Explain findings clearly and compassionately. Allow time for questions and emotional support. In organ donation cases, provide information sensitively and according to consent and legal requirements.
9	Follow institutional protocols for post-mortem care	Arrange for care of the deceased, preservation and transfer. Respect cultural, religious and family preferences, including consideration for organ donation procedures.

Overview

Supporting end-of-life planning, diagnosing death and caring for the deceased can be emotionally and professionally challenging. Supporting patients to plan for end-of-life care involves facilitating discussions about advance directives, palliative options and personal wishes, often in the context of complex emotional responses and cultural considerations. Accurately diagnosing death requires a thorough understanding of physiological signs, legal requirements and institutional protocols, while maintaining sensitivity and compassion for the patient and their family. Caring for the deceased demands respect, dignity and adherence to legal and organisational procedures, which can be distressing, particularly for healthcare professionals who have developed a therapeutic relationship with the patient. Providing structured support, debriefing opportunities and training in emotional resilience are essential to help staff manage the psychological impact of these experiences while ensuring high standards of compassionate care.

Supporting end-of-life planning

Supporting patients to plan for the end of life is a hallmark of patient-centred care. Advance care planning allows individuals to express preferences about medical interventions, place of care and comfort measures, and includes documentation such as advance directives or do not attempt cardiopulmonary resuscitation (DNACPR) orders. Effective facilitation requires clear, empathetic communication, active listening and respect for patient autonomy. Patients may experience a range of emotions, including fear, anxiety, denial or sadness, and healthcare professionals must provide reassurance and psychological support while guiding informed decision-making.

Cultural and spiritual considerations are critical during end-of-life planning. Patients' beliefs can shape preferences regarding treatment, dying rituals and organ donation. Those who offer people care and support must approach these discussions with cultural competence, asking open, respectful questions and avoiding assumptions. Multidisciplinary collaboration, including palliative care specialists, social workers and chaplains, ensures that physical, emotional, social and spiritual needs are addressed holistically. Importantly, discussions about end-of-life planning should include conversations about organ donation where appropriate. Healthcare professionals must sensitively confirm and document patients' donation preferences and provide families with clear information, ensuring that choices are respected and aligned with the patient's values.

Diagnosing death

The diagnosis of death is often obvious; the body is cool, motionless and pale. Accurately diagnosing death is a critical responsibility that combines clinical precision with ethical and legal awareness. Only those healthcare professionals who are legally authorised are permitted to confirm death, and local policy and institutional procedures must be followed at all times. Clinicians must recognise the irreversible cessation of vital functions, adhering to established guidelines that may include assessment of neurological and circulatory criteria. Thorough documentation is essential, both to meet legal requirements and to provide clarity for families and the healthcare team.

In the context of organ donation, precise diagnosis of death is particularly critical. For donation after brainstem death (DBD) or donation after circulatory death (DCD), strict protocols to confirm death before organ retrieval must be complied with. Adherence to legal, ethical and institutional standards ensures that the process is valid and transparent and maintains public trust in transplantation systems. Communication with families during this process must be compassionate, clear and sensitive to their emotional state, as they are navigating grief while making decisions about organ donation.

Following legal requirements and local policy not only protects patients and families but also safeguards healthcare professionals by ensuring that the diagnosis of death is conducted correctly and appropriately documented. This is especially important in complex situations, such as suspected organ donation or cases involving unclear clinical presentation, where adherence to protocols ensures both ethical integrity and professional accountability. Table 76.1 and Figure 76.1 provide an overview of the diagnosis of death.

Caring for the deceased

Caring for the deceased is a fundamental aspect of professional practice, emphasising dignity, respect and cultural sensitivity. Post-mortem care involves proper positioning of the body, maintaining privacy and adhering to infection prevention and control and organisational protocols. Healthcare teams must also accommodate religious or cultural rituals, demonstrating respect for the patient's identity and offering reassurance to families.

When organ donation is involved, additional considerations arise. The body must be managed in a way that allows for organ preservation while maintaining dignity and respecting cultural or religious practices. Staff must provide clear explanations to families about the procedures, including timing and physical interventions involved in organ retrieval, while offering emotional support. Caring for patients who have donated organs can be emotionally challenging, particularly when staff have established therapeutic relationships. Structured support, debriefing and reflective practice are essential to manage emotional strain and prevent compassion fatigue or moral distress.

Supporting end-of-life planning, diagnosing death, caring for the deceased and facilitating organ donation are integral components of compassionate, patient-centred healthcare. Each domain demands technical skill, ethical discernment and emotional sensitivity. By fostering open communication, respecting cultural and spiritual values and providing structured support for families and staff, healthcare professionals can deliver dignified care at the end of life. Ultimately, excellence in this domain is measured not only by clinical accuracy but also by the compassion, respect and holistic support provided to patients, families and colleagues during one of life's most profound transitions.

Appendix 1: Prefixes and suffixes

Prefix: A prefix is positioned at the beginning of a word to modify or change its meaning. 'Pre' means 'before'. Prefixes may also indicate a location, number or time.

Suffix: The ending part of a word that changes the meaning of the word.

Prefix or suffix	Meaning	Example(s)
a-, an-	not, without	analgesic, apathy
ab-	from, away from	abduction
abdomin(o)-	of or relating to the abdomen	abdomen
acous(io)-	of or relating to hearing	acoumeter, acoustician
acr(o)-	extremity, topmost	acrocrany, acromegaly, acroosteolysis, acroposthia
ad-	at, increase, on, toward	adduction
aden(o)- aden(i)-	of or relating to a gland	adenocarcinoma, adenology, adenotome, adenotyphus
adip(o)-	of or relating to fat or fatty tissue	adipocyte
adren(o)-	of or relating to adrenal glands	adrenal artery
-aemia	blood condition	anaemia
aer(o)-	air, gas	aerosinusitis
aesthes-	sensation	anaesthesia
alb-	denoting a white or pale colour	albino
alge(si)-	pain	analgesic
-algia, alg(i)o-	pain	myalgia
all(o-)	denoting something as different, or as an addition	alloantigen, allopathy
ambi-	denoting something as positioned on both sides, describing both of two	ambidextrous
amni-	pertaining to the membranous foetal sac (amnion)	amniocentesis
an-	not, without	analgesia
ana-	back, again, up	anaplasia
andr(o)-	pertaining to a man	android, andrology
angi(o)-	blood vessel	angiogram
ankyl(o)-, ancyl(o)-	denoting something as crooked or bent	ankylosis
ante-	describing something as positioned in front of another thing	antepartum
anti-	describing something as 'against' or 'opposed to' another	antibody, antipsychotic
arteri(o)-	of or pertaining to an artery	arteriole, artery
arthr(o)-	of or pertaining to the joints, limbs	arthritis
articul(o)-	joint	articulation
-ase	enzyme	lactase
-asthenia	weakness	myasthenia gravis
ather(o)-	fatty deposit, soft gruel-like deposit	atherosclerosis
atri(o)-	an atrium (esp. heart atrium)	atrioventricular
aur(i)-	of or pertaining to the ear	aural
aut(o)-	self	autoimmune
axill-	of or pertaining to the armpit (uncommon as a prefix)	axilla
bi-	twice, double	binary
bio-	life	biology
blephar(o)-	of or pertaining to the eyelid	blepharoplast
brachi(o)-	of or relating to the arm	brachium of inferior colliculus
brady-	'slow'	bradycardia
bronch(i)-	bronchus	bronchiolitis obliterans
bucc(o)-	of or pertaining to the cheek	buccolabial
burs(o)-	bursa (fluid sac between the bones)	bursitis
carcin(o)-	cancer	carcinoma
cardi(o)-	of or pertaining to the heart	cardiology
carp(o)-	of or pertaining to the wrist	carpopedal
-cele	pouching, hernia	hydrocele, varicocele
-centesis	surgical puncture for aspiration	amniocentesis

Prefix or suffix	Meaning	Example(s)
cephal(o)-	of or pertaining to the head (as a whole)	cephalalgia
cerebell(o)-	of or pertaining to the cerebellum	Cerebellum
cerebr(o)-	of or pertaining to the brain	Cerebrology
chem(o)-	chemistry, drug	chemotherapy
chol(e)-	of or pertaining to bile	cholecystitis
cholecyst(o)-	of or pertaining to the gall bladder	cholecystectomy
chondr(i)o-	cartilage, gristle, granule, granular	chondrocalcinosis
chrom(ato)-	colour	haemochromatosis
-cidal, -cide	killing, destroying	bactericidal
cili-	of or pertaining to the cilia, the eyelashes and eyelids	Ciliary
circum-	denoting something as 'around' another	circumcision
col-, colo-, colono-	Colon	colonoscopy
colp(o)-	of or pertaining to the vagina	colposcopy
contra	Against	contraindicate
coron(o)-	Crown	coronary
cost(o)-	of or pertaining to the ribs	costochondral
crani(o)-	belonging or relating to the cranium	craniology
-crine, crin(o)	to secrete	endocrine
cry(o)-	Cold	cryoablation
cutane-	Skin	subcutaneous
cyan(o)-	denotes a blue colour	cyanopsia
cycl-	circle, cycle	cyclodialysis
cyst(o)-, cyst(i)-	of or pertaining to the urinary bladder	cystotomy
cyt(o)-	Cell	cytokine
-cyte	Cell	leukocyte

Prefix or suffix	Meaning	Example(s)
-dactyl(o)-	of or pertaining to a finger, toe	dactylology, polydactyly
dent-	of or pertaining to teeth	dentist
dermat(o)- derm(o)-	of or pertaining to the skin	dermatology
-desis	Binding	arthrodesis
dextr(o)-	right, on the right side	dextrocardia
di-	Two	diplopia
dia-	through, during, across	dialysis
dif-	apart, separation	different
digit-	of or pertaining to the finger (rare as a root)	digit
-dipsia	suffix meaning (condition of) thirst	polydipsia, hydroadipsia, oligodipsia
dors(o)-, dors(i)-	of or pertaining to the back	dorsal, dorsocephalad
duodeno-	duodenum, twelve: the upper part of the small intestine (twelve inches long on average), connects to the stomach	duodenal atresia
dynam(o)-	force, energy, power	hand strength dynamometer
-dynia	Pain	vulvodynia
dys-	bad, difficult, defective, abnormal	dysphagia, dysphasia

Prefix or suffix	Meaning	Example(s)
ec-	out, away	ectopia, ectopic pregnancy
ect(o)-	outer, outside	ectoblast, ectoderm
-ectasia, -ectasis	expansion, dilation	bronchiectasis, telangiectasia
-ectomy	denotes a surgical operation or removal of a body part, resection, excision	mastectomy
-emesis	vomiting condition	haematemesis
-aemia	blood condition	anaemia
encephal(o)-	of or pertaining to the brain; also see cerebro	encephalogram
endo-	denotes something as 'inside' or 'within'	endocrinology, endospore
eosin (o)-	Red	eosinophil granulocyte
enter(o)-	of or pertaining to the intestine	gastroenterology
epi-	on, upon	epicardium, epidermis, epidural, episclera, epistaxis
erythr(o)-	denotes a red colour	erythrocyte
ex-	Out of, away from	excision, exophthalmos
exo-	denotes something as 'outside' another	exoskeleton
extra-	Outside	extradural haematoma

Prefix or suffix	Meaning	Example(s)
faci(o)-	of or pertaining to the face	facioplegic
fibr(o)-	Fibre	fibroblast
fore-	before or ahead	foreword

Prefix or suffix	Meaning	Example(s)
fossa-	a hollow or depressed area; trench or channel	fossa ovalis
front-	of or pertaining to the forehead	frontonasal
galact(o)-	Milk	galactorrhoea
gastr(o)-	of or pertaining to the stomach	gastric bypass
-genic	formative, pertaining to producing	cardiogenic shock
gingiv-	of or pertaining to the gums	gingivitis
glauc(o)-	denoting a grey or bluish-grey colour	glaucoma
gloss(o)-, glott(o)-	of or pertaining to the tongue	glossology
gluco-	Sweet	glucocorticoid
glyc(o)-	Sugar	glycolysis
-gnosis	knowledge	diagnosis, prognosis
gon(o)-	seed, semen, also reproductive	gonorrhoea
-gram, -gramme	record or picture	Angiogram
-graph	instrument used to record data or pictures	electrocardiograph
-graphy	process of recording	angiography
gyn(aec)o-	Woman	gynaecomastia
halluc-	to wander in mind	Hallucinosis
haemat-, haemato- (haem-)	of or pertaining to blood	haematology
haemangi-, haemangio-	blood vessels	haemangioma
hemi-	one-half	cerebral hemisphere
hepat- (hepatic-)	of or pertaining to the liver	Hepatology
heter(o)-	denotes something as 'the other' (of two), as an addition, or different	heterogeneous
hist(o)-, histio-	Tissue	Histology
home(o)-	Similar	homoeopathy
hom(o)-	denotes something as 'the same' as another or common	homosexuality
hydr(o)-	Water	hydrophobe
hyper-	denotes something as 'extreme' or 'beyond normal'	hypertension
hyp(o)-	denotes something as 'below normal'	hypovolaemia
hyster(o)-	of or pertaining to the womb, the uterus	hysterectomy, hysteria
iatr(o)-	of or pertaining to medicine, or a physician	Iatrogenic
-iatry	denotes a field in medicine of a certain body component	podiatry, psychiatry
-ics	organised knowledge, treatment	Obstetrics
ileo-	Ileum	ileocecal valve
infra-	Below	infrahyoid muscles
inter-	between, among	interarticular ligament
intra-	Within	Intramural
ipsi-	Same	ipsilateral hemiparesis
ischio-	of or pertaining to the ischium, the hip joint	ischioanal fossa
-ism	condition, disease	Dwarfism
-ismus	spasm, contraction	hemiballismus
iso-	denoting something as being 'equal'	isotonic
-ist	one who specialises in	pathologist
-itis	Inflammation	tonsillitis
-ium	structure, tissue	pericardium
juxta (iuxta)	near to, alongside or next to	juxtaglomerular apparatus
karyo-	Nucleus	eukaryote
kerat(o)-	cornea (eye or skin)	keratoscope
kin(e)-, kin(o), kinaesi(o)-	Movement	kinaesthesia
kyph(o)-	Humped	kyphoscoliosis
labi(o)-	of or pertaining to the lip	labiodental
lacrim(o)-	Tear	lacrimal canaliculi
lact(i)-, lact(o)	Milk	lactation
lapar(o)-	of or pertaining to the abdominal wall, flank	laparotomy

Prefix or suffix	Meaning	Example(s)
laryng(o)-	of or pertaining to the larynx, the lower throat cavity where the voice box is	laryngeal oedema
latero-	Lateral	lateral pectoral nerve
-lepsis, -lepsy	attack, seizure	epilepsy, narcolepsy
lept(o)-	light, slender	leptomeningeal
leuc(o)-, leuk(o)-	denoting a white colour	leukocyte
lingua(a)-, lingu(o)-	of or pertaining to the tongue	linguistics
lip(o)-	Fat	liposuction
lith(o)-	stone, calculus	lithotripsy
log(o)-	Speech	logogram
-logist	denotes someone who studies a certain field	oncologist, pathologist
-logy	denotes the academic study or practice of a certain field	haematology, urology
lymph(o)-	Lymph	lymphoedema
lys(o)-, -lytic	Dissolution	lysosome
-lysis	destruction, separation	paralysis
macr(o)-	large, long	macrophage
-malacia	Softening	osteomalacia
mamm(o)-	of or pertaining to the breast	mammogram
mammill(o)-	of or pertaining to the nipple	mammillaplasty, mammillitis
manu-	of or pertaining to the hand	manufacture
mast(o)-	of or pertaining to the breast	mastectomy
meg(a)-, megal(o)-, -megaly	enlargement, million	splenomegaly, megametre
melan(o)-	black colour	Melanin
mening(o)-	Membrane	Meningitis
meta-	after, behind	metacarpus
-meter	instrument used to measure or count	sphygmomanometer
-metry	process of measuring	Optometry
metr(o)-	pertaining to conditions or instruments of the uterus	metrorrhagia
micro-	denoting something as small, or relating to smallness, millionth	Microscope
milli-	Thousandth	Millilitre
mon(o)-	Single	infectious mononucleosis
morph(o)-	form, shape	morphology
muscul(o)-	Muscle	musculoskeletal system
my(o)-	of or relating to muscle	Myoblast
myc(o)-	Fungus	onychomycosis
myel(o)-	of or relating to bone marrow or spinal cord	Myeloblast
myri-	ten thousand	Myriad
myring(o)-	Eardrum	myringotomy
narc(o)-	numb, sleep	Narcolepsy
nas(o)-	of or pertaining to the nose	Nasal
necr(o)-	Death	necrosis, necrotising fasciitis
neo-	New	Neoplasm
nephr(o)-	of or pertaining to the kidney	Nephrology
neur(i)-, neur(o)-	of or pertaining to nerves and the nervous system	neurofibromatosis
normo-	Normal	Normocapnia
ocul(o)-	of or pertaining to the eye	Oculist
odont(o)-	of or pertaining to teeth	Orthodontist
odyn(o)-	Pain	Stomatodynia
-oesophageal, oesophago-	Gullet	Oesophagus
-oid	resemblance to	Sarcoidosis
-ole	small or little	Bronchiole
olig(o)-	denoting something as 'having little, having few'	Oliguria
-oma (singular) -omata (plural)	tumour, mass, collection	sarcoma, teratoma
onco-	tumour, bulk, volume	Oncology
onych(o)-	of or pertaining to the nail (of a finger or toe)	Onychophagy
oo-	of or pertaining to an egg, a woman's egg, the ovum	Oogenesis
oophor(o)-	of or pertaining to the woman's ovary	Oophorectomy
ophthalm(o)-	of or pertaining to the eye	Ophthalmology

Prefix or suffix	Meaning	Example(s)
optic(o)-	of or relating to chemical properties of the eye	opticochemical biopsy
orchi(o)-, orchid(o)-, orch(o)-	testis	orchiectomy, orchidectomy
-osis	a condition, disease or increase	harlequin-type ichthyosis, psychosis, osteoporosis
osseo-	bony	Osseous
ossi-	bone	peripheral ossifying fibroma
ost(e)-, oste(o)-	bone	Osteoporosis
ot(o)-	of or pertaining to the ear	Otology
ovo-, ovi-, ov-	of or pertaining to the eggs, the ovum	oogenesis
oxo-	addition of oxygen	Oxygenate

Prefix or suffix	Meaning	Example(s)
pachy-	Thick	Pachyderma
palpebr-	of or pertaining to the eyelid (uncommon as a root)	Palpebra
pan-, pant(o)-	denoting something as 'complete' or containing 'everything'	panophobia, panopticon
papill-	of or pertaining to the nipple (of the chest/breast)	Papillitis
papul(o)-	indicates papulosity, a small elevation or swelling in the skin, a pimple, swelling	Papulation
para-	alongside of, abnormal	Paracyesis
-paresis	slight paralysis	Hemiparesis
parvo-	small	Parvovirus
path(o)-	disease	Pathology
-pathy	denotes (with a negative sense) a disease or disorder	sociopathy, neuropathy
pector-	Breast	pectoralgia, pectoriloquy, pectorophony
ped-, -ped-, -pes	of or pertaining to the foot, -footed	Pedoscope
paed-, paedo-	of or pertaining to the child	paediatrics. paedophilia
pelv(i)- pelv(o)-	hip bone	Pelvis
-penia	deficiency	Osteopenia
-pepsia	denotes something relating to digestion, or the digestive tract	Dyspepsia
peri-	denoting something with a position 'surrounding' or 'around' another	Periodontal
-pexy	Fixation	Nephropexy
phaco-	lens-shaped	phacolysis, phacometer, phacoscotoma
-phage -phagia	forms terms denoting conditions relating to eating or ingestion	Sarcophagia
-phago-	eating, devouring	Phagocyte
phagist-	forms nouns that denote a person who 'feeds on' the first element or part of the word	Lotophagi
-phagy	forms nouns that denote 'feeding on' the first element or part of the word	Haematophagy
pharmaco-	drug, medication	Pharmacology
pharyng(o)-	of or pertaining to the pharynx, the upper throat cavity	pharyngitis, pharyngoscopy
phleb(o)-	of or pertaining to the (blood) veins, a vein	phlebography, phlebotomy
-phobia	exaggerated fear, sensitivity	arachnophobia
phon(o)-	Sound	phonograph, symphony
phos-	of or pertaining to light or its chemical properties, now historic and used rarely; see the common root phot(o)- below	phosphene
phot(o)-	of or pertaining to light	photopathy
phren(i)-, phren(o)-, phrenic	the mind	phrenic nerve, schizophrenia, diaphragm
-plasia	formation, development	achondroplasia
-plasty	surgical repair, reconstruction	rhinoplasty
-plegia	paralysis	paraplegia
pleio-	more, excessive, multiple	pleomorphism
pleur(o)-, pleur(a)	of or pertaining to the ribs	pleurogenous
-plexy	stroke or seizure	cataplexy
pneum(o)-	of or pertaining to the lungs	pneumonocyte, pneumonia
pneumat(o)-	air, lung	pneumatic
-poiesis	production	haematopoiesis
poly-	denotes a 'plurality' of something	polymyositis

Prefix or suffix	Meaning	Example(s)
post-	denotes something as 'after' or 'behind' another	postoperation, post-mortem
pre-	denotes something as 'before' another (in (physical) position or time)	premature birth
presby(o)-	old age	presbyopia
prim-	denotes something as 'first' or 'most important'	primary
proct(o)-	anus, rectum	proctology
prot(o)-	denotes something as 'first' or 'most important'	protoneuron
pseud(o)-	denotes something false or fake	pseudoephedrine
psych(e)-, psych(o)	of or pertaining to the mind	psychology, psychiatry
psor-	Itching	psoriasis
-ptosis	falling, drooping, downward placement, prolapse	apoptosis, nephroptosis
-ptysis	(a spitting), spitting, haemoptysis, the spitting of blood derived from the lungs or bronchial tubes	haemoptysis
pulmon-, pulmo-	of or relating to the lungs	pulmonary
pyel(o)-	Pelvis	pyelonephritis
py(o)-	Pus	pyometra
pyr(o)-	Fever	antipyretic
quadr(i)-	Four	quadriceps
radio-	Radiation	radio wave
ren(o)-	of or pertaining to the kidney	renal
retro-	backward, behind	retroversion, retroverted
rhin(o)-	of or pertaining to the nose	rhinoceros, rhinoplasty
rhod(o)-	denoting a rose-red colour	rhodophyte
-rrhage	burst forth	haemorrhage
-rrhagia	rapid flow of blood	menorrhagia
-rrhaphy	surgical suturing	aortorrhaphy
-rrhexis	Rupture	karyorrhexis
-rrhoea	flowing discharge	diarrhoea
-rupt	break or burst	erupt, interrupt
salping(o)-	of or pertaining to tubes, e.g. Fallopian tubes	salpingectomy, salpingopharyngeus muscle
sangui-, sanguine-	of or pertaining to blood	Sanguine
sarco-	muscular, flesh-like	Sarcoma
scler(o)-	Hard	scleroderma
-sclerosis	Hardening	atherosclerosis, multiple sclerosis
scoli(o)-	Twisted	Scoliosis
-scope	instrument for viewing	stethoscope
-scopy	use of an instrument for viewing	Endoscopy
semi-	one-half, partly	semiconscious
sial(o)-	saliva, salivary gland	Sialagogue
sigmoid(o)-	sigmoid, s-shaped curvature	sigmoid colon
sinistr(o)-	left, left side	sinistrotorsion
sinus-	of or pertaining to the sinus	sinusitis
somat(o)-, somatico-	body, bodily	somatic
-spadias	slit, fissure	hypospadias, epispadias
spasmo-	Spasm	spasmodic dysphonia
sperma-, spermo-, spermato-	semen, spermatozoa	spermatogenesis
splen(o)-	Spleen	splenectomy
spondyl(o)-	of or pertaining to the spine, the vertebra	spondylitis
squamos(o)-	denoting something as 'full of scales' or 'scaly'	squamous cell
-stalsis	contraction	peristalsis
-stasis	stopping, standing	cytostasis, homeostasis
-staxis	dripping, trickling	epistaxis
sten(o)-	denoting something as 'narrow in shape' or pertaining to narrowness	stenography
-stenosis	abnormal narrowing in a blood vessel or other tubular organ or structure	restenosis, stenosis
stomat(o)-	of or pertaining to the mouth	stomatogastric, stomatognathic system
-stomy	creation of an opening	colostomy
sub-	Beneath	subcutaneous tissue

Prefix or suffix	Meaning	Example(s)
super-	in excess, above, superior	superior vena cava
supra-	above, excessive	supraorbital vein
tachy-	denoting something as fast, irregularly fast	tachycardia
-tension, -tensive	Pressure	hypertension
tetan-	rigid, tense	tetanus
thec-	case, sheath	intrathecal
therap-	treatment	hydrotherapy, therapeutic
therm(o)-	Heat	thermometer
thorac(i)-, thorac(o)-, thoracico-	of or pertaining to the upper chest, the area above the breast and under the neck	thorax
thromb(o)-	of or relating to a blood clot, clotting of blood	thrombus, thrombocytopenia
thyr(o)-	Thyroid	thyroid
thym-	Emotions	dysthymia
-tome	cutting instrument	dermatome
-tomy	act of cutting; incising, incision	gastrotomy
tono-	tone, tension, pressure	tonometry
top(o)-	place, topical	topical anaesthetic
tort(i)-	twisted	Torticollis
tox(i)- tox(o)- toxic(o)-	toxin, poison	toxoplasmosis
trache(a)-	Trachea	tracheotomy
trachel(o)-	of or pertaining to the neck	tracheloplasty
trans-	denoting something as moving or situated 'across' or 'through'	Transfusion
tri-	Three	Triangle
trich(i)- trichia trich(o)-	of or pertaining to hair, hair-like structure	Trichocyst
-tripsy	Crushing	Lithotripsy
-trophy	nourishment, development	pseudohypertrophy
tympan(o)-	Eardrum	tympanocentesis
-ula, -ule	Small	Nodule
un(i)-	One	unilateral hearing loss
ur(o)-	of or pertaining to urine or the urinary system; (specifically) pertaining to the physiological chemistry of urine	Urology
uter(o)-	of or pertaining to the uterus or womb	Uterus
vagin-	of or pertaining to the vagina	Vagina
varic(o)-	swollen or twisted vein	Varicose
vas(o)-	duct, blood vessel	vasoconstriction
vasculo-	blood vessel	vasculopathy
ven-	of or pertaining to the (blood) veins, a vein (used in terms pertaining to the vascular system)	vein, venospasm
ventr(o)-	of or pertaining to the belly; the stomach cavities	ventrodorsal
ventricul(o)-	of or pertaining to the ventricles; any hollow region inside an organ	cardiac ventriculography
-version	turning	anteversion, retroversion
vesic(o)-	of or pertaining to the bladder	vesical arteries
viscer(o)-	of or pertaining to the internal organs, the viscera	viscera
xanth(o)-	denoting a yellow colour, an abnormally yellow colour	xanthopathy
xen(o)-	foreign, different	xenograft
xer(o)-	dry, desert-like	xerostomia
zo(o)-	animal, animal life	zoology
zym(o)-	fermentation	enzyme, lysozyme

Appendix 2: Glossary of Terms

Acquired: an acquired disorder is a medical condition that develops post-foetally.

Acute: of sudden onset

Aetiology: the study of the cause of a disease

Aggregate: the clumping together in the blood

Agonist: a substance that acts like another substance and therefore stimulates an action

Allergen: a substance that can produce hypersensitivity reactions in the body

Anaemia: a condition characterised by a deficiency of red blood cells or haemoglobin, leading to reduced oxygen-carrying capacity of the blood.

Anaphylaxis: a severe, systemic allergic response characterised by vasodilation and bronchoconstriction

Anoxia: total depletion of oxygen

Antigens: substances (often proteins) causing the formation of an antibody that reacts specifically with that antigen.

Aplastic anaemia: a disease in which the bone marrow and the blood stem cells that reside there are damaged, resulting in reduced blood cells.

Apoptosis: a process of programmed cell death

Arteries: blood vessels that transport blood away from the heart

Ascites: the build-up of fluid in the space between the lining of the abdomen and abdominal organs (the peritoneal cavity)

Atheromatous plaques: a deposit or degenerative accumulation of lipid-containing plaques on the innermost layer of the wall of an artery.

Atrophy: decrease in size

Autoimmune: an autoimmune disorder is a condition that occurs when the immune system mistakenly attacks and destroys healthy body tissue.

Azotaemia: see uraemia

Basophils: a type of white blood cell

Benign: a non-malignant neoplasm

Biologic (biological therapy): a therapeutic product derived from living organisms, such as proteins, monoclonal antibodies or vaccines, used to modify immune responses or target specific components of disease processes (e.g. tumour necrosis factor inhibitors in autoimmune disease).

Blebbing: protrusions of the cell membrane

Calculi: stones

Capillaries: small blood vessels where exchange between blood and the tissue cells takes place

Carcinogens: cancer-causing substances

Carcinoma: a malignancy originating in epithelial tissues

Cardiac: output volume of blood pumped out every minute by the ventricle

Chronic: a disease developing gradually and lasting longer than 3 months

Cilia: hair-like projections that sweep dust and other foreign particles out

Colonoscopy: an examination that views the inside of the colon (large intestine) and rectum, using a tool called a colonoscope

Congenital: a condition existing at birth and often before birth

Coronary revascularisation: the restoration of perfusion to the coronary arteries as a result of ischaemia

Cyanosis: blue discolouration, usually of the lips and fingers

Cytokines: small proteins released by cells that mediate and regulate immunity, inflammation and haematopoiesis.

Cytotoxic drugs: chemotherapy drugs

Defaecate: to pass stool (motion)

Demyelination: to destroy or remove the myelin sheath of (a nerve fibre), as through disease

Diagnosis: the process of identifying a disease or condition based on signs, symptoms and test results.

Diaphoresis: excessive sweating

Dysfunction: impaired or abnormal functioning of a tissue, organ or system.

Dyspnoea: difficulty in breathing

Embolism: obstruction of a blood vessel by a foreign substance (e.g. blood clot, air bubble and fat globule).

Engulfing: swallowing up

Enzymes: are biological catalysts – catalysts are substances that increase the rate of chemical reactions without being used up.

Enzymes: proteins that speed up chemical reactions in a cell

Eosinophils: a type of white blood cell

Epigastric: relating to the abdominal region lying between the hypochondriac regions and above the umbilical region

Erythropoietin: a hormone that stimulates the production of red blood cells in the bone marrow

Exacerbation: an increase in the severity of a disease or any of its signs or symptoms

Fatigue: extreme tiredness

Fibrinogen: a protein in the blood plasma that is essential for the coagulation of blood and is converted to fibrin by the action of thrombin in the presence of ionised calcium

Fibrosis: excessive formation of fibrous connective tissue during repair, often leading to scarring.

Fistula: an abnormal connection between an organ, vessel or intestine and another structure

Genetics: concerns the process of trait inheritance from parents to offspring

Genotoxic: pertaining to agents known to damage DNA, thereby causing mutations, which can result in cancer

Goblet cells: glandular epithelial cells found in the lining of the digestive and respiratory tracts that secrete mucus

Haemopoiesis: the formation of blood cells in the living body (especially in the bone marrow)

Haemostasis: the process of stopping bleeding through vascular constriction, platelet aggregation and coagulation.

Hemiparesis: weakness

Homeostasis: the maintenance of a stable internal environment within physiological limits.

Hydronephrosis: a condition where one or both kidneys become stretched and swollen as a result of a build-up of urine inside the kidney(s)

Hypercalcaemia: high levels of calcium in the blood

Hyperkalaemia: high levels of potassium in the blood

Hyperplasia: an increase in cell number

Hypersensitivity reaction: an altered immunological response to an antigen resulting in a pathological immune response upon re-exposure

Hypertrophy: an increase in size

Hypoalbuminaemia: a medical condition where levels of albumin in blood serum are abnormally low

Hypocellular: containing less than the normal number of cells

Hypoglycaemia: low blood glucose

Hypokalaemia: low levels of potassium in the blood

Hyponatraemia: low levels of sodium in the blood

Hypoperfusion: decreased blood flow through an organ, as in hypovolemic shock; if prolonged, it may result in permanent cellular dysfunction and death.

Hypoxaemia: a lower than normal oxygen content of the blood as measured in an arterial blood sample

Idiopathic: having no demonstrable cause

Immune response: a defence function of the body that produces antibodies to destroy invading antigens and malignancies

Immunoglobulins: antibodies

Immunosuppressants: powerful medicines that dampen down the activity of the body's immune system

Inflammation: swelling

Inflammatory response: tissue reaction to injury or to an antigen; can include pain, swelling, itching, redness, heat and loss of function.

Inotrope: a drug that alters the force or energy of muscular contractions

Integrin: a transmembrane receptor that mediates the attachment between a cell and its surroundings, such as other cells or the extracellular matrix

Ischaemia: insufficient perfusion of oxygenated blood to a body organ or part

Kernig's sign: inability to extend the knee while the hip is flexed at a 90° angle

Kinin: polypeptide hormones that are formed locally in the tissues and cause dilation of blood vessels and contraction of smooth muscle

Lethargy: lack of energy

Macrophages: a cell that ingests and destroys microbes and foreign matter

Malaise: a vague feeling of bodily discomfort, as at the beginning of an illness

Malignant: a cancerous neoplasm

Mast cells: a cell found in the connective tissue that releases histamine during inflammation

Mesothelial cells: a membrane that forms the lining of several body cavities, the pleura, peritoneum and pericardium

Mesothelial tissue: also surrounds the male internal reproductive organs and covers the internal reproductive organs of women

Metaplasia: reversible replacement of one mature cell type by another less mature type

Metastasise: spread of the tumour cells

Microemboli: tiny blood clots

Mucoprotein: any of a group of organic compounds, such as the mucins, that consist of a complex of proteins and glycosaminoglycans and are found in body tissues and fluids

Murphy's sign: elicited by firmly placing a hand at the costal margin in the right upper abdominal quadrant and asking the patient to breathe deeply; if the gallbladder is inflamed, the patient will experience pain and catch their breath as the gallbladder descends and contacts the palpating hand

Mutation: altered or changed

Necrosis: death of cells or tissues through injury or disease, especially in a localised area of the body

Negative feedback: mechanisms that usually result in a response that balances a change in the system

Neoplasia: growth of cells and tissue into new areas, resulting in a tumour; can be benign or malignant

Nucleation: is the process where droplets of liquid can condense from a vapour, or bubbles of gas can form in a boiling liquid.

Oedema: accumulation of excess fluid in the interstitial spaces of tissues.

Oesophagus: gullet

Oligodendrocytes: myelin-producing cells

Oncogene: a gene that, when mutated or overexpressed, can lead to uncontrolled cell growth and cancer development.

Orthopnoea: difficulty in breathing that occurs when lying flat, relieved by sitting or standing upright; commonly associated with left-sided heart failure and pulmonary congestion.

Orthostasis: maintenance of an upright standing posture

Pancytopenia: a medical condition in which there is a reduction in the number of red and white blood cells, as well as platelets

Pathogenesis: events leading to the development of a disease and the signs and symptoms occurring as the disease progresses

Pathology: the study of changes in cell/tissue structure related to disease or death

Pathophysiology: the study of the disturbance of normal mechanical, physical and biochemical functions, either caused by a disease or resulting from a disease or abnormal syndrome or condition that may not qualify to be called a disease

Petechiae: pinpoint-sized reddish-purple spots on the skin

Petechial: rashes, small spots

Phagocytes: white blood cells

Phagocytose: to envelop and destroy bacteria and other foreign material

Photophobia: aversion to light

Pluripotent: capable of differentiating into one of many cell types

Polyps: small growths on the inner lining of the colon

Proctitis: inflammation of the rectum

Prognosis: the predicted outcome or course of a disease.

Pyuria: pus in the urine

Reticulin: a scleroprotein from the connective fibres of reticular tissue

Sclera: the white of the eye

Selectins: a family of cell adhesion molecules

Sepsis: a life-threatening organ dysfunction caused by a dysregulated host response to infection.

Septicaemia: blood infection

Serosal: a serous membrane, especially one that lines the pericardial, pleural and peritoneal cavities, enclosing their contents

Shock: a condition of severely inadequate blood flow to the body's peripheral tissues, associated with life-threatening cellular dysfunction; also known as hypoperfusion

Sigmoidoscope: a procedure used to see inside the sigmoid colon and rectum

Sign: an objective finding observed by a clinician (e.g. fever, rash).

Sinusoids: small blood vessels, similar to capillaries

Stenosis: narrowing of any canal or opening (e.g. the intestine, a blood vessel or a heart valve)

Supersaturation: to cause (a chemical solution) to be more highly concentrated than is normally possible under given conditions of temperature and pressure

Symptom: a subjective experience reported by the patient (e.g., pain, fatigue).

Syndrome: a group of signs and symptoms that occur together and characterise a particular condition.

Systemic: a condition that affects the entire body

Tachycardia: rapid heart rate

Tachypnoea: rapid breathing

Thromboxane: a substance made by platelets that causes blood clotting and constriction of blood vessels

Tinnitus: the perception of a noise in one or both ears (e.g. a ringing in the ears)

Toxin: a poisonous substance produced by microorganisms, animals or plants that can cause harm to tissues.

Trigone: a smooth triangular area on the inner surface of the bladder limited by the apertures of the ureters and urethra

Tumour (Neoplasm): an abnormal mass of tissue resulting from uncontrolled cell proliferation; may be benign or malignant.

Uraemia: the accumulation of waste products, normally excreted in the urine, in the blood causes severe headaches, vomiting, etc.

Urethral sphincter: one of two muscles used to control the exit of urine in the urinary bladder through the urethra

Vasculitis: inflammation of the wall of a blood vessel

Vasoconstriction: narrowing of blood vessels, decreasing blood flow.

Vasodilation: widening of blood vessels, increasing blood flow.

Venules: small veins

Wheezing: a coarse whistling sound produced when airways are partially obstructed

Further Reading

Banasik, J.L. (2021). *Pathophysiology*, 7e. Elsevier, St. Louis.

Braun, C.A. & Anderson, C.M. (2011). *Pathophysiology: A Clinical Approach*, 2e. Wolters Kluwer/Lippincott, Baltimore.

Dlugasch, L. & Story, L. (2021). *Applied Pathophysiology*. Jones & Bartlett, Burlington.

Huether, S.E., McCance, K.L., Brashers, V.L. & Rote, N.S. (2019). *Pathophysiology: The Biologic Basis for Disease in Adults and Children*, 8e. Elsevier, St. Louis.

Finlay, I., Richards, M., Maskell, R. et al. (2025). *Palliative Care and End-of-Life Care: Opportunities for England (Volume 2)*, The Commission on Palliative and End-of-Life Care.

Peate, I., Clare, C. & Wheeldon, A. (2026). *Fundamentals of Applied Pathophysiology: An Essential Guide for Nursing and Healthcare Students*, 5e. Wiley, Oxford.

Peate, I. & Evans, S. (2026). *Anatomy and Physiology for Nurses at a Glance*, 4e. Wiley, Oxford.

Roiger, D. & Bullock, N. (2019). *Anatomy, Physiology and Disease: Foundations for the Health Professions*, 3e. McGraw Hill, New York.

VanMeter, K.C. & Hubert, R.J. (2022). *Study Guide for Pathophysiology for the Health Professions*, 7e. Elsevier, St. Louis.

Index

Note: Page numbers in *italics* and **bold** refers to figures and tables respectively.